Medical Terminology

get connected!

Suzanne S. **FRUCHT**

Associate Professor Emeritus
Northwest Missouri State University
Maryville, MO

Pearson

Boston   Columbus   Indianapolis   New York   San Francisco   Upper Saddle River
Amsterdam   Cape Town   Dubai   London   Madrid   Milan   Munich   Paris   Montreal   Toronto
Delhi   Mexico City   Sao Paulo   Sydney   Hong Kong   Seoul   Singapore   Taipei   Tokyo

Library of Congress Cataloging-in-Publication Data

Frucht, Suzanne S.
  Medical terminology : get connected! / Suzanne S. Frucht. — 1st ed.
    p. ; cm.
  Includes index.
  ISBN-13: 978-0-13-112112-6
  ISBN-10: 0-13-112112-X
  1. Medicine—Terminology. I. Title.
  [DNLM: 1. Medicine—Terminology—English. W 15]
  R123.F78 2012
  610.1'4—dc22

                                        2010046325

Notice: The author and the publisher of this volume have taken care that the information and technical recommendations contained herein are based on research and expert consultation, and are accurate and compatible with the standards generally accepted at the time of publication. Nevertheless, as new information becomes available, changes in clinical and technical practices become necessary. The reader is advised to carefully consult manufacturers' instructions and information material for all supplies and equipment before use, and to consult with a healthcare professional as necessary. This advice is especially important when using new supplies or equipment for clinical purposes. The author and publisher disclaim all responsibility for any liability, loss, injury, or damage incurred as a consequence, directly or indirectly, of the use and application of any of the contents of this volume.

Publisher: Julie Levin Alexander
Publisher's Assistant: Regina Bruno
Editor-in-Chief: Mark Cohen
Associate Editor: Melissa Kerian
Editorial Assistant: Rosalie Hawley
Development Editor: Danielle Doller
Director of Marketing: David Gesell
Executive Marketing Manager: Katrin Beacom
Marketing Specialist: Michael Sirinides
Managing Production Editor: Patrick Walsh
Production Liaison: Christina Zingone

Production Editor: Amy L. Saucier, Laserwords
Senior Media Editor: Amy Peltier
Media Project Managers: Lorena Cerisano
  and Julita Navarro
Manufacturing Manager: Alan Fischer
Art Director: Mary Siener
Cover/Interior Designer: Mary Siener
Composition: Laserwords
Printing and Binding: Quebecor World Color
Cover Printer: Lehigh-Phoenix Color/Hagerstown
Illustrator: Body Scientific International, LLC

Case Study Credits: chapter's 5, 6 & 11, Shutterstock, Monkey Business Images; chapter's 7 & 8, Shutterstock, Yuri Arcurs; chapter 9, Shutterstock, Chubykin Arkady; chapter 10, Shutterstock, FineCollection; chapter 12, Shutterstock, Leifstiller; chapter 13, Shutterstock, Terence Mendoza; chapter 14, Shutterstock, Brian Eichhorn; chapter 15, Ronald Sumners; chapter 16, Shutterstock, Varina and Jay Patel; chapter 17, Shutterstock, lofoto.

10 9 8 7 6 4 3 2 1

PEARSON

www.pearsonhighered.com

ISBN-13: 978-0-13-112112-6
ISBN-10: 0-13-112112-X

Brief Contents

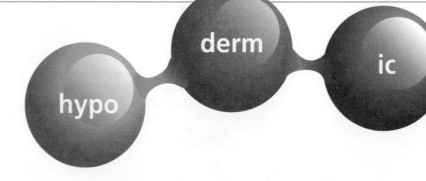

Make the Connection!

Welcome to your first leap into the study of medical language. You may be curious about the title of this book and why it is so important to "get connected." In this socially networked world, where we can organize the meaningful aspects of our lives and link them with others, it is clear that successful experiences involve making connections. Medical terminology is no different. Let us illustrate.

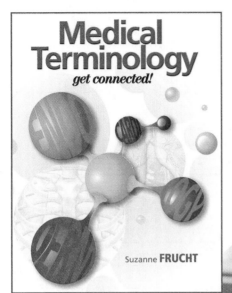

Medical Terminology
get connected!

Suzanne **FRUCHT**

Medical Terminology is about connecting...

*with peers and classmates **to help you study***

word parts **to form medical terms**

laryng

-itis

organs and structures **that comprise body systems**

*with colleagues and patients **for accurate medical communication***

This text will give you the ability to build and interpret medical terms with accuracy and confidence. It will demonstrate the interconnectedness of body structures and systems. It will provide you with activities and online resources that will foster peer-to-peer study opportunities. And finally, it will help you acquire the tools necessary to communicate effectively in a professional healthcare environment.

So let's get connected with the features of this book.

What Makes This Book Different

You will quickly notice that this book is not arranged like most other medical terminology texts. Others present medical terms within the framework of basic human anatomy and physiology, creating a mini-A&P course. Rather, this book organizes and presents terms by medical specialty. This gives you an immediate window into how the healthcare world is organized—around medical specialties, and not by organ systems.

This is a true introductory-level "essentials" text focusing solely on medical terminology, and on teaching how to construct and translate medical terms. Designed to be fun, accessible, and eye-catching, it guides readers step-by-step toward mastery of relevant word parts, understanding word roots, and assembling words. To help you learn meanings, correct spelling, pronunciation, and other components of each term, the book contains numerous exercises, tips, and colorful figures for learning and practice. It is flexible enough to be used either in support of lectures, or as a workbook to support independent study.

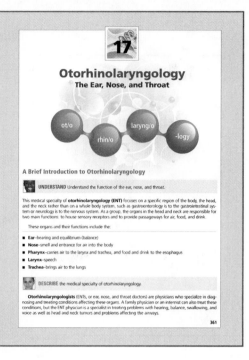

17

Otorhinolaryngology
The Ear, Nose, and Throat

ot/o   laryng/o
rhin/o   -logy

A Brief Introduction to Otorhinolaryngology

UNDERSTAND Understand the function of the ear, nose, and throat.

This medical specialty of **otorhinolaryngology (ENT)** focuses on a specific region of the body, the head, and the neck rather than on a whole body system, such as gastroenterology is to the gastrointestinal system or neurology is to the nervous system. As a group, the organs in the head and neck are responsible for two main functions: to house sensory receptors and to provide passageways for air, food, and drink.

These organs and their functions include the:

- **Ear**–hearing and equilibrium (balance)
- **Nose**–smell and entrance for air into the body
- **Pharynx**–carries air to the larynx and trachea, and food and drink to the esophagus
- **Larynx**–speech
- **Trachea**–brings air to the lungs

DESCRIBE the medical specialty of otorhinolaryngology.

Otorhinolaryngologists (ENTs, or ear, nose, and throat doctors) are physicians who specialize in diagnosing and treating conditions affecting these organs. A family physician or an internist can also treat these conditions, but the ENT physician is a specialist in treating problems with hearing, balance, swallowing, and voice as well as head and neck tumors and problems affecting the airways.

361

Here is a summary of the key objectives of the book.

DESCRIBE each of the medical specialties

Each chapter in Section Two begins with a brief description of its particular medical specialty, along with some examples of healthcare workers in this specialty and some conditions that they treat.

DEFINE relevant combining forms, suffixes, and prefixes

DEFINE otorhinolaryngology-related combining forms, prefixes, and suffixes.

Otorhinolaryngology Combining Forms

The following list presents new combining forms important for building and defining otorhinolaryngology terms.

adenoid/o	adenoids	nas/o	nose
audi/o	hearing	ot/o	ear
audit/o	hearing	pharyng/o	pharynx (throat)
aur/o	ear	rhin/o	nose
cochle/o	cochlea	sinus/o	sinus
epiglott/o	epiglottis	tonsill/o	tonsils
laryng/o	larynx (voice box)	trache/o	trachea (windpipe)
myring/o	tympanic membrane (eardrum)	tympan/o	tympanic membrane (eardrum)

The following list presents combining forms that are not specific to the ear, nose, or throat but are also used for building and defining otorhinolaryngology terms.

gastr/o	stomach	neur/o	nerve
myc/o	fungus	py/o	pus

Suffix Review

These suffixes and prefixes were introduced in Chapters 2 and 3. They are being reviewed in this chapter because they are especially important suffixes in otorhinolaryngology terms.

-al	pertaining to	-ory	pertaining to
-algia	pain	-osis	abnormal condition
-ar	pertaining to	-osmia	smell
-eal	pertaining to	-otomy	cutting into
-ectomy	surgical removal	-phonia	voice
-gram	record	-plasty	surgical repair
-ic	pertaining to	-plegia	paralysis
-itis	inflammation	-rrhea	discharge, flow

This section in each chapter introduces the word parts that build the terms most common to each medical specialty.

Each medical specialty chapter presents a quick visual summary of the appropriate organs. To reinforce the combining forms introduced in the preceding section, this art is labeled with both the names and combining forms of each organ.

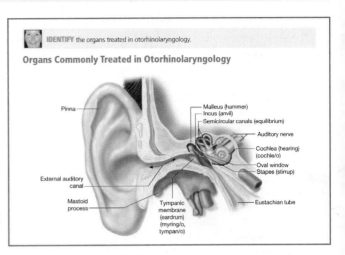

IDENTIFY the organs treated in otorhinolaryngology.

Organs Commonly Treated in Otorhinolaryngology

- Pinna
- Malleus (hammer)
- Incus (anvil)
- Semicircular canals (equilibrium)
- Auditory nerve
- Cochlea (hearing) (cochle/o)
- Oval window
- Stapes (stirrup)
- External auditory canal
- Mastoid process
- Tympanic membrane (eardrum) (myring/o, tympan/o)
- Eustachian tube

BUILD medical terms from word parts

BUILD otorhinolaryngology medical terms from word parts.

Building Otorhinolaryngology Terms

This section presents word parts most often used to build otorhinolaryngology terms. Following the explanation of the term, you have the opportunity to begin building your own vocabulary. Read the meaning for each term and then fill in the blanks to build a single medical term. Use the slashes to divide prefixes, word roots, combining vowels, and suffixes. To help you out you will find a key to the word parts underneath the blanks: / for word roots, // for prefix, cv for combining vowel, and s for suffix. Remember that not every term will contain all these word parts, it's up to you to decide which to use. As you gain experience, this process becomes easier. Answers can be found at the back of the book.

1. adenoid/o–combining form meaning **adenoids**
   The adenoids are one of three pairs of **tonsils** located in pharynx; also called **pharyngeal tonsils;** tonsils house large number of white blood cells that protect body by removing foreign invaders from air, food, and drink passing through pharynx
   a. surgical removal of adenoids _____/_____
   b. adenoid inflammation _____/_____

2. audi/o–combining form meaning **hearing**
   a. study of hearing _____/____/____
   b. one who studies hearing _____/____/____
   c. process of measuring hearing _____/____/____

Perhaps the heart of each chapter, this is where you will apply your knowledge. Each word part is explained and then followed by a list of phrases followed by a color-coded blank line divided by slash marks. These marks indicate how many word parts are necessary to build the term. You will complete this section by filling in the blanks as you work through this section.

EXPLAIN vocabulary terms

You will quickly learn that not all medical terms are built completely from word parts. This section defines this type of term. Note that some of these terms, such as *contusion* or *fibrillation,* have no word parts in them at all. While other terms, such as *coronary artery bypass graft* or *malignant melanoma,* contain some word parts, but the whole term is not built using word parts.

EXPLAIN otorhinolaryngology medical terms.

Otorhinolaryngology Vocabulary

The otorhinolaryngology terms presented in this section include eponyms, modern English words, and those that contain Latin or Greek word parts but are not constructed solely from these word parts. When you recognize word parts within a term they will give you a hint about the word's meaning. In these instances, look for the word parts to follow the term.

Term	Explanation
acoustic neuroma neur/o = nerve -oma = tumor	Benign tumor of auditory nerve sheath; symptoms include tinnitus, headache, vertigo, and progressive hearing loss
cochlear implant cochle/o = cochlea -ar = pertaining to	Hearing device surgically placed under skin behind ear; converts sound signals into magnetic impulses to stimulate auditory nerve 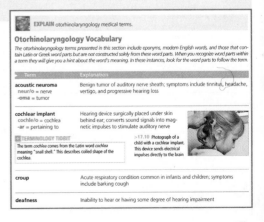
⊕ **TERMINOLOGY TIDBIT** The term *cochlea* comes from the Latin word *cochlea* meaning "snail shell." This describes coiled shape of the cochlea.	➤17.10 Photograph of a child with a cochlear implant. This device sends electrical impulses directly to the brain
croup	Acute respiratory condition common in infants and children; symptoms include barking cough
deafness	Inability to hear or having some degree of hearing impairment

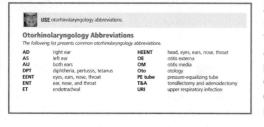

USE otorhinolaryngology abbreviations.

Otorhinolaryngology Abbreviations

The following list presents common otorhinolaryngology abbreviations.

AD	right ear	HEENT	head, eyes, ears, nose, throat
AS	left ear	OE	otitis externa
AU	both ears	OM	otitis media
DPT	diphtheria, pertussis, tetanus	Oto	otology
EENT	eyes, ears, nose, throat	PE tube	pressure-equalizing tube
ENT	ear, nose, and throat	T&A	tonsillectomy and adenoidectomy
ET	endotracheal	URI	upper respiratory infection

Abbreviations are an essential part of the medical language because they save time. However, only approved abbreviations may be used in order to prevent misunderstandings. This section of each chapter presents the most commonly used abbreviations for that medical specialty.

PRACTICE using medical terms

As with any newly learned skill, practice is essential. Each chapter closes with a large variety of exercises. These include real-life application exercises (Case Study and Transcription Practice), pronunciation practice (Sound It Out), as well as more typical types of recall exercises (labeling, fill-in-the-blank, matching, crossword puzzle). In addition, this section also includes exercises requiring higher levels of critical thinking (Med Term Analysis and Photomatch Challenge).

Build Medical Terms

Use each of the following word parts to build the indicated medical terms.

The combining form ot/o means ear.

1. study of ear _____
2. ear fungus abnormal condition _____
3. surgical repair of ear _____
4. ear inflammation _____
5. process of viewing ear _____

The combining form pharyng/o means pharynx.

6. involuntary muscle contraction of pharynx _____
7. pertaining to the pharynx _____

The suffix -phonia means voice.

8. without voice _____
9. difficult voice _____

The combining form trache/o means trachea.

10. trachea narrowing _____
11. trachea cutting into _____
12. enlarged trachea _____

The combining form tympan/o means tympanic membrane (eardrum).

13. eardrum surgical repair _____
14. instrument to measure the eardrum _____
15. eardrum rupture _____

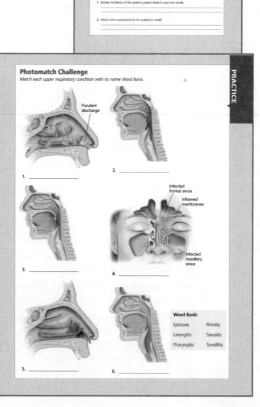

Photomatch Challenge

Match each upper respiratory condition with its name Word Bank.

Word Bank:

Epistaxis	Rhinitis
Laryngitis	Sinusitis
Pharyngitis	Tonsillitis

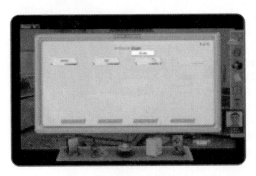

Get Connected to *MyMedicalTerminologyLab*

The ultimate personalized learning tool is available at **www. mymedicalterminologylab.com**. This online course correlates with the textbook and is available for purchase separately or for a discount when packaged with the book. MyMedicalTerminologyLab is an immersive study experience that takes place within Pearson General Hospital—a virtual world of fun quizzes, word games, videos, and other self-study challenges. The system allows learners to track their own progress through the course and use a personalized study plan to achieve success.

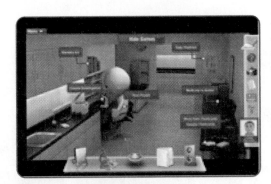

MyMedicalTerminologyLab saves instructors time by providing quality feedback, ongoing individualized assessments for students, and instructor resources all in one place. It offers instructors the flexibility to make technology an integral part of their course, or a supplementary resource for students.

Visit **www.mymedicalterminologylab.com** to log in to the course or purchase access. Instructors seeking more information about discount bundle options or for a demonstration, please contact your Pearson sales representative.

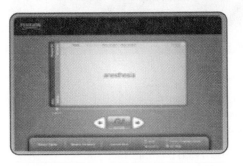

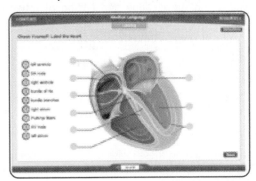

Comprehensive Instructional Package

Perhaps the most gratifying part of an educator's work is the "aha" learning moment when the light bulb goes off and a student truly understands a concept — when a connection is made. Along these lines, Pearson is pleased to help instructors foster more of these educational connections by providing a complete battery of resources to support teaching and learning. Qualified adopters are eligible to receive a wealth of materials designed to help instructors prepare, present, and assess. For more information, please contact your Pearson sales representative or visit **www.pearsonhighered.com/educator**.

About the Author

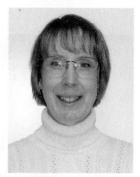

Suzanne S. Frucht was an Associate Professor of Physiology at Northwest Missouri State University (NWMSU). She holds baccalaureate degrees in biological sciences and physical therapy from Indiana University, an MS in biological sciences at NWMSU, and a PhD in molecular biology and biochemistry from the University of Missouri-Kansas City. For 14 years she worked full-time as a physical therapist in various health care settings, including acute care hospitals, extended care facilities, and home health. Based on her educational and clinical experience she was invited to teach medical terminology part-time in 1988 and became a full-time faculty member three years later as she discovered her love for the challenge of teaching. Before retiring in 2008, she taught a variety of courses including medical terminology, human anatomy, human physiology, and animal anatomy and physiology. She received the Governor's Award for Excellence in Teaching in 2003.

About the Illustrators

Marcelo Oliver is president and founder of Body Scientific International, LLC. He holds a masters degree in Medical and Biological Illustration from the University of Michigan. For the past 15 years, his passion has been to condense complex anatomical information into visual education tools for students, patients and medical professionals. Body Scientific's contributing medical artists in this publication were **Carol Gudanowski, Liana Bauman,** and **Dawn Scheuerman**. Their contribution in the publication was key in the creation and editing of artwork throughout. Body Scientific invites you to visit their website at **www.bodyscientific.com**.

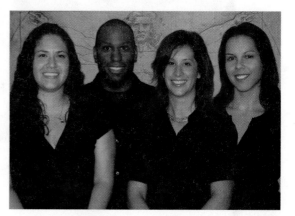

Acknowledgments

It is axiomatic that no textbook can ever reach the hands of students without the extraordinary contributions of many talented and dedicated professionals. *Medical Terminology: Get Connected* is certainly no exception and I would like to take this opportunity to acknowledge their contributions.

Foremost among those I wish to thank is editor-in-chief Mark Cohen, who promoted and supported the concept of a different type of medical terminology text. No author could ever have a more thoughtful champion in her corner than I have had in Mark. Danielle Doller, developmental editor, not only kept me on track but also knew every detail (and then some) necessary to bring a book to light. And when I needed to talk through ideas, no one could be a better sounding board for the good thoughts and a gentle critic of the others. It would be easy to see ancillaries as an afterthought, but I do not make that mistake! Melissa Kerian, developmental managing editor, made sure they were of the highest caliber. Marcello Oliver and his team of illustrators at Body Scientific International, LLC provided the outstanding art that enhances the text. Their skills are clear everywhere in the volume. Mary Siener produced a design that exceeded even my high expectations. And last, but certainly not least, words can never express my appreciation to the myriad reviewers whose comments and suggestions at each turn made this a better book.

Without the hard work and dedication of each of these individuals, there might be a book, but certainly not this one. I thank you all from the bottom of my heart.

—Suzanne Frucht

x

Editorial Development Team

The content and format of *Medical Terminology: Get Connected* are the result of an incredible collaboration of expert educators from all around. This book represents the collective insights, experience, and thousands of hours of work performed by members of this development team. Their influence will continue to have an impact for decades to come. Let us introduce the members of our team.

Reviewers

Steven G. Bassett, Ph.D.
Seton Hill University
Greensburg, Pennsylvania

Karen Boriack, RN, BSN, MA Ed.
Porterville College
Porterville, California

Ranelle Brew, Ed.D
Grand Valley State University
Grand Rapids, Michigan

Amanda J. Davis
Meridian Community College
Meridian, Mississippi

Dianne Davis, MS
West Virginia University at Parkersburg
Parkersburg, West Virginia

Duane A. Dreyer, Ph.D.
Miller-Motte College
Cary, North Carolina

Marie A. Fenske, Ed.D., RRT
GateWay Community College
Phoenix, Arizona

Melissa Mapp Francisco, BA, MAOM
Suwanee Hamilton Technical Center
Live Oak, Florida

Elaine Garcia, RHIT
Spokane Community College
Spokane, Washington

Krista L. Hoekstra, R.N., M.A.
Hennepin Technical College
Brooklyn Park, Minnesota

Traci Hotard, RHFA
Louisiana Technical College
Morgan City, Louisiana

Donna M. Kubesh, BS, MA, Ph.D
Luther College
Decorah, Iowa

Anita Lane, M.Ed., OTR
Navarro College
Corsicana, Texas

Molly Lee, Ph.D.
Harrisburg Area Community College
Harrisburg, Pennsylvania

Tricia Leggett, MSEd, R.T.(R)(QM)
Zane State College
Zanesville, Ohio

Sue Moe, RN
Northwest Technical College
East Grand Forks, Minnesota

Cynthia K. Moore, Ph.D., R.D.
University of Arkansas — Fayetteville
Fayetteville, Arkansas

Paulette Nitkiewicz, BSN, RN, CMA
Westmoreland County Community College
Youngwood, Pennsylvania

Tonya Oakley, B.S., R.T.(R)
Forsyth Technical Community College
Winston-Salem, North Carolina

Michelle Parolise, MBA, OTR/L
Santa Ana College
Santa Ana, California

Karen Plawecki, PhD, RD, LDN
University of Illinois
Urbana, Illinois

Martha L. Rew, MS, RD, LD
Texas Woman's University
Denton, Texas

Michael Sells, RN, Certified Surgical Tech
Kirkwood Community College
Cedar Rapids, Iowa

Don Steinert, MA, RRT, MT, CLS
University of the District of Columbia
Washington, D.C.

Halcyon Watkins, BS, DVM
Prairie View A&M University
Prairie View, Texas

Amy Way, Ph.D
Lock Haven University
Clearfield, Pennsylvania

Sherry B. Wilson, RN, MSN
Durham Technical Community College
Durham, North Carolina

Focus Group Members

Edward W. Kolk, DPM
Suffolk Community College
Brentwood, New York

Glenn Ross
The College of Westchester
White Plains, New York

Denise Vill'neuve, MA, RT(R)(CT)(M)
County College of Morris
Randolph, New Jersey

Photograph Contributors

Special thanks to the students of Keiser University who graciously provided profile photos for our use in the design of the objectives in each chapter. We are grateful to Alice Macomber, Regional Medical Assisting Program Director, for organizing this effort.

A Commitment to Accuracy

As a learner embarking on a career in health care you probably already know how critically important it is to be precise in your work. Patients and co-workers will be counting on you to avoid errors on a daily basis. Likewise, we owe it to you—the reader—to ensure accuracy in this book. We have gone to great lengths to verify that the information provided in *Medical Terminology: Get Connected!* is complete and correct. To this end, here are the steps we have taken:

1. **Editorial review**—We have assembled a large team of developmental consultants to critique every word and every image in this book. No fewer than 12 content experts have read each chapter for accuracy. In addition, some members of our developmental team were specifically assigned to focus on the precision of each illustration that appears in the book.

2. **Medical Illustrations**—A team of medically trained illustrators was hired to prepare each piece of art that graces the pages of this book. These illustrators have a higher level of scientific education than the artists for most textbooks, and they worked directly with the author and members of our development team to make sure that their work was clear, correct, and consistent with what is described in the text.

3. **Accurate Ancillaries**—The teaching and learning ancillaries are often as important to instruction as the textbook itself. Therefore we took steps to ensure accuracy and consistency of these components by reviewing every ancillary component.

While our intent and actions have been directed at creating an error-free text, we have established a process for correcting any mistakes that may have slipped past our editors. Pearson takes this issue seriously and therefore welcomes any and all feedback that you can provide along the lines of helping us enhance the accuracy of this text. If you identify any errors that need to be corrected in a subsequent printing, please send them to:

Pearson Health Science Editorial
Medical Terminology Corrections
One Lake Street
Upper Saddle River, NJ 07458

Thank you for helping Pearson reach its goal of providing the most accurate medical terminology textbooks available.

Section I – Basic Word Building

Section II – Medical Specialties

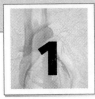

Introduction to Medical Terminology

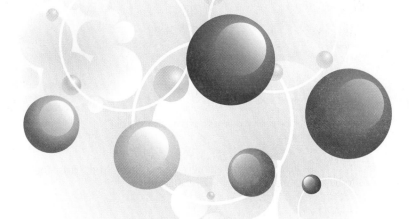

 IDENTIFY the three types of medical terms.

A Brief Introduction to Medical Terminology

In our daily lives, each of us is surrounded by medical terminology. Of course, health care professionals use it to communicate with each other (Figure 1.1>), but every person is exposed to these terms whether in the doctor's office, talking with friends, reading the newspaper, or watching television. Using medical terminology is an efficient method of conveying very specific and important information. Because each term has a precise meaning, detailed information can be quickly shared using only a few words. Therefore, everyone has something to gain from learning how to understand and use medical terminology whether in your professional or personal life.

There are three common types of medical terms:

1. Words built from **Latin** and **Greek** word parts; examples are *cardiology* and *tonsillectomy*.

2. Words based on a person's name, called **eponyms**; examples are Alzheimer disease and Parkinson disease. The current trend in writing eponyms is away from using the possessive form of the person's name, this text will follow that practice.

3. Words utilizing **modern English** words; examples are *magnetic resonance imaging* and *irritable bowel syndrome*.

1

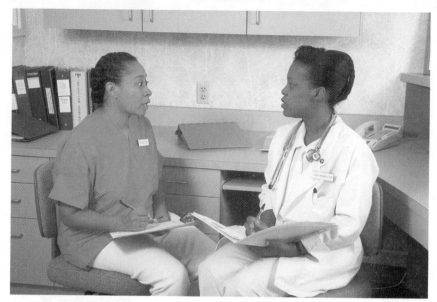

>1.1 A nurse and medical assistant review a patient's chart and plan daily care
Source: Shutterstock, Michaeljung

Without doubt, the majority of medical terms are based on Latin and Greek word parts. The remainder of this chapter teaches you how to build and analyze this type of medical term.

EXPLAIN the differences between prefixes, suffixes, word roots, and combining vowels.

Elements of Latin- and Greek-Based Medical Terms

Learning medical terminology is similar to learning a foreign language because the basis for the majority of medical terms is Latin or Greek. In mastering this "language of medicine" you will:

- Begin by memorizing individual word parts
- Learn to analyze and build terms from word parts
- Gain skill and confidence through repetitious use of terms
- Make these terms a permanent part of your professional vocabulary.

Latin- and Greek-based medical terms are constructed using word parts from four different categories: **word root, suffix, prefix,** and **combining vowel.**

Word Root

The word root is the foundation of most medical terms and gives the essential meaning of the term. It frequently but not always refers to a body structure, organ, or system. See examples in Table 1.1>.

TABLE 1.1   **EXAMPLES OF WORD ROOTS**

Word Root	Meaning
cardi	heart
gastr	stomach
hepat	liver
rhin	nose
cephal	head
arthr	joint
my	muscle
oste	bone
electr	electricity
carcin	cancer

Suffix

A suffix is found at the end of a medical term. The type of information it provides includes conditions, diseases, surgical procedures, and diagnostic procedures involving the word root. All medical terms *must* contain a suffix. See examples in Table 1.2>. *Note that when a suffix is written by itself, a hyphen is placed at the front.*

TABLE 1.2   **EXAMPLES OF SUFFIXES**

Suffix	Meaning	Used in Medical Term	Meaning of Medical Term
-ectomy	surgical removal	gastrectomy	surgical removal of stomach
-itis	inflammation	arthritis	joint inflammation
-megaly	enlarged	hepatomegaly	enlarged liver
-logy	study of	cardiology	study of the heart
-gram	record or picture	electrocardiogram	record of heart's electricity
-pathy	disease	myopathy	muscle disease

Prefix

A prefix is found at the beginning of a medical term. It often indicates information such as abnormal conditions, numbers, positions, or times. See examples in Table 1.3>. Many medical terms do not have a prefix. *Note that when a prefix is written by itself, a hyphen is placed at the end.*

TABLE 1.3   EXAMPLES OF PREFIXES

Prefix	Meaning	Used in Medical Term	Meaning of Medical Term
inter-	between	intervertebral	between vertebrae
a-	without	apnea	without breathing
dys-	abnormal, difficult, painful	dysuria	painful urination
sub-	below, underneath	subcutaneous	underneath the skin
bi-	two	bilateral	two sides
post-	after	postsurgical	after surgery

Combining Vowel

Combining vowels are used for two reasons: to connect word parts and to make medical terms easier to spell and pronounce. Combining vowels are placed either between a word root and suffix or between two word roots. They are not used between a prefix and word root. See Table 1.4> for examples. *Note that the slashes (/) are used to divide the term into its word parts.*

TABLE 1.4   EXAMPLES OF THE USE OF COMBINING VOWELS

Word with Combining Vowels	Meaning
rhin/o/plasty	surgical repair of the nose
hepat/o/megaly	enlarged liver
electr/o/cardi/o/gram	record of heart's electricity
oste/o/arthr/itis	bone and joint inflammation

However, combining vowels are *not* always necessary.

- To decide whether one is needed between a word root and suffix, you must look at the first letter of the suffix. Do *not* use a combining vowel between a word root and suffix if the suffix begins in a vowel. For example, the correct way to combine the word root *arthr* and suffix *-itis* is *arthr/itis,* not *arthr/o/itis.*
- Place a combining vowel between two word roots, even if the second word root begins with a vowel. The term, *gastr/o/enter/o/logy* is correct, while *gastr/enter/o/logy* is incorrect.

Combining Form

Combining forms consist of a word root and its combining vowel. Throughout this book, combining forms will be written with a slash (/) between the two word parts. For example, *electr/o is* the combining form meaning electricity. See Figure 1.2> for more examples of combining forms in the body.

A combining form is not another category of word part because it consists of two other word parts. However, word roots are normally presented as combining forms; these are easier to pronounce and therefore, to remember. Word roots will be given as combining forms throughout this text.

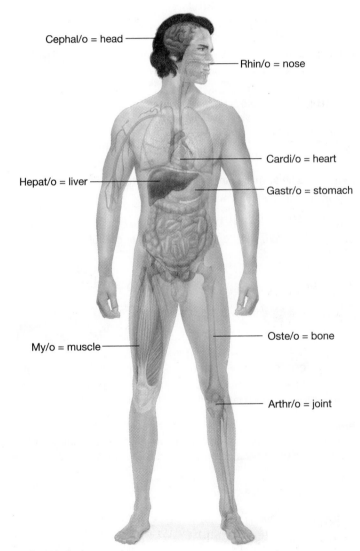

Cephal/o = head

Rhin/o = nose

Cardi/o = heart

Hepat/o = liver

Gastr/o = stomach

Oste/o = bone

My/o = muscle

Arthr/o = joint

>1.2 Common combining forms for body organs

Strategies for Analyzing Medical Terms

Using medical terms is a two-way street; you will need to learn both how to define medical terms used by other people and how to build medical terms for yourself. There are some specific strategies that will help you learn both.

> **+ TERMINOLOGY TIDBIT**
>
> Do not try to memorize every medical term. Instead, figure out how the word is formed from its components. In a short time, you will be able to do this automatically when seeing a new term.

Defining Medical Terms

When you first encounter an unfamiliar medical term, don't panic! Remember that the meaning of the individual word parts will give you the information needed to understand at least the basic meaning of the word.

Follow these simple steps:

1. Divide the term into its word parts.

2. Define each word part.

3. Put the meaning of the word parts together in order to see what the term is describing.

For example, follow the steps to define the term, *dysmenorrhea*.

1. Divide term into word parts: dys / men / o / rrhea

2. Define each word part

   - **dys-** → prefix meaning abnormal, painful
   - **men/o** → combining form meaning menstruation
   - **-rrhea** → suffix meaning flow

3. Put the meaning of individual word parts together: abnormal or painful menstrual flow. See Figure 1.3> for an overview of this process.

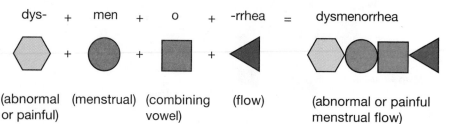

dys-　+　men　+　o　+　-rrhea　=　dysmenorrhea

(abnormal or painful)　(menstrual)　(combining vowel)　(flow)　(abnormal or painful menstrual flow)

>1.3 You can figure out the meaning of a medical term by dividing it into its word parts and then define each part

Building Medical Terms

Building medical terms is almost the reverse of defining them. Begin by selecting word parts that convey the meaning needed. Then place the word parts in the correct order to build a complete term.

For example, build a term for the phrase: fibrous skin tumor. First, choose word parts that represent each portion of the phrase.

- combining form, *fibr/o,* means *fibrous*
- combining form, *dermat/o,* means *skin*
- suffix, *-oma,* means *tumor*

Then place these word parts in the correct order to complete the whole term: *dermatofibroma*.

It is important to realize that not all possible combinations of word parts will build actual medical terms used by medical professionals. At the beginning of building medical terms, this is very frustrating, but do not give up! After working with medical terms for only a short period of time, you will find making correct choices easier and easier.

 DESCRIBE how to pluralize medical terms.

Rules for Building Plurals

Latin and Greek style medical terms do not follow the same pluralization rules used in English. Refer to the rules presented in Table 1.5> when deciding how to pluralize medical terms.

TABLE 1.5 RULES FOR PLURALIZING MEDICAL TERMS

➤ If the Word Ends In	Singular	Plural
–a, keep –a and add –e	vertebra	vertebrae
–ax, drop –x and add –ces	thorax	thoraces
–ex, drop –ex and add –ices	apex	apices
–ix, drop –x and add –ces	appendix	appendices
–ma, keep –ma and add –ta	sarcoma	sarcomata
–is, drop –is and add –es	metastasis	metastases
–on, drop –on and add –a	spermatozoon	spermatozoa
–us, drop –us and add –i	alveolus	alveoli
–um, drop –um and add –a	ovum	ova
–y, drop –y and add –ies	biopsy	biopsies
–x, drop –x and add –ges	phalanx	phalanges

Pronouncing Medical Terms

Often medical terms are difficult to pronounce because the word parts are unfamiliar to us, or they contain letter combinations that do not occur in English words. Refer to Table 1.6> for hints to pronounce these letter combinations. Refer to the audio glossary at www.mymedicalterminologylab.com for a phonetical pronunciation of each term presented in this book. Any syllable that should be stressed is written in upper case.

TABLE 1.6   HINTS FOR PRONOUNCING MEDICAL TERMS

Hint	Examples
-ae or -oe, pronounce only second letter	bursae (BER-see) coelom (SEE-loam)
c and g have soft sound if followed by e, i, or y	cerebrum (ser-REE-brum) gingivitis (jin-jih-VIGH-tis)
c and g have hard sound if followed by other letters	cardiac (CAR-dee-ak) gastric (GAS-trik)
-e or -es at end of word pronounced as separate syllable	syncope (SIN-koh-pee) nares (NAIR-eez)
ch- at beginning of word has hard k sound	cholesterol (koh-LES-ter-all) chemical (KIM-ih-call)
-i at end of word pronounced "eye"	bronchi (BRONG-keye) nuclei (NEW-clee-eye)
pn- at beginning of word, pronounce only n	pneumonia (new-MOH-nee-ah) pneumogram (NOO-moe-gram)
pn in middle of word, pronounce hard p and hard n	tachypnea (tak-ip-NEE-ah) hypopnea (high-POP-nee-ah)
ps- at beginning of word, pronounce only s	psychiatry (sigh-KIGH-ah-tree) psychology (sigh-KOL-oh-jee)

Recognizing Types of Medical Terms

Indicate whether each of the medical terms below is a Latin/Greek term, eponym, or modern English term.

1. hepatitis _latin / Greek_

2. ball and socket _modern English_

3. Bell palsy _eponym_

4. arthrogram _Latin / Greek_

5. cardiomegaly _Latin / Greek_

6. Addison disease _eponym_

7. activities of daily living _modern English_

8. Hodgkin disease _eponym_

9. pacemaker _modern English_

10. gastritis _Latin / Greek_

Forming Plurals

Fill in the following blanks with the missing singular or plural form of the term.

Singular	Plural
1. bursa	_bursae_
2. diverticulum	_diverticula_
3. _adenoma_	adenomata
4. ganglion	_ganglia_
5. index	_indices_
6. _diagnosis_	diagnoses
7. _alveolus_	alveoli

Practice Defining Medical Terms

These medical terms have already been subdivided into their word parts. Each word part has been defined for you. First, label each word part as a prefix, word root, suffix, or combining vowel. Then put together the meanings of all the word parts to define the term.

1. encephal/o/malacia
   - encephal is a __root word__ meaning brain
   - o is a __combining vowel__
   - -malacia is a __suffix__ meaning softening
   - *encephalomalacia* means __softening of the brain__

2. sub/cutane/ous
   - sub- is a __prefix__ meaning underneath
   - cutane is a __root word__ meaning skin
   - -ous is a __suffix__ meaning pertaining to
   - *subcutaneous* means __pertaining to under the skin__

3. hyster/o/pexy
   - hyster is a __root word__ meaning uterus
   - o is a __combining vowel__
   - -pexy is a __suffix__ meaning surgical fixation
   - *hysteropexy* means __surgical fixation of the uterus__

4. pan/sinus/itis
   - pan- is a __prefix__ meaning all
   - sinus is a __root word__ meaning sinuses
   - -itis is a __suffix__ meaning inflammation
   - *pansinusitis* means __inflammation of the sinuses__
      cul

5. angi/o/rrhaphy
   - angi is a __root word__ meaning vessel
   - o is a __combining vowel__
   - -rrhaphy is a __suffix__ meaning to suture
   - *angiorrhaphy* means __suture a vessel__

6. inter/ventricul/ar
   - inter- is a __prefix__ meaning between
   - ventricul is a __root word__ meaning ventricles
   - -ar is a __suffix__ meaning pertaining to
   - *interventricular* means __pertaining to between the ventricles__

Practice Building Medical Terms

Use the following list of word parts to build a medical term for each definition. The blanks following each definition provide an outline of the term showing the placement of prefixes, word roots, combining vowels, and suffixes.

Term	Category	Meaning
-ar	suffix	pertaining to
arthr	word root	joint
intra-	prefix	within
-logy	suffix	study of
laryng	word root	voice box
muscul	word root	muscle
neur	word root	nerve
o	combining form	
-oma	suffix	tumor
ophthalm	word root	eye
-plasty	suffix	surgical repair
scapul	word root	shoulder blade
-scope	suffix	instrument for viewing
sub-	prefix	below

1. surgical repair of the voice box — laryng / o / plasty
2. instrument for viewing a joint — arthr / o / scope
3. pertaining to below the shoulder blade — sub / scapul / ar
4. study of the eye — ophthalm / o / logy
5. nerve tumor — neur / oma
6. pertaining to within a muscle — intra / muscul / ar

mymedicalterminologylab

MyMedicalTerminologyLab is a premium online homework management system that includes a host of features to help you study. Registered users will find:

- Fun games and activities built within a virtual hospital
- Powerful tools that track and analyze your results—allowing you to create a personalized learning experience
- Videos, flashcards, and audio pronunciations to help enrich your progress
- Streaming lesson presentations and self-paced learning modules
- A space where you and your instructors can view and manage your assignments

2

Suffixes

EXPLAIN the role of suffixes in building medical terms.

A Brief Introduction to Suffixes

A suffix on the end of a medical term adds specific meaning to the term. All medical terms built from word parts must have a suffix. This can be illustrated with the combining form for heart, *cardi/o.* Using different suffixes changes the meaning of terms using **cardi/o.**

- **cardi/o + -logy** = *cardiology meaning study of heart*
- **cardi/o + -dynia** = *cardiodynia meaning heart pain*
- **cardi/o + -megaly** = *cardiomegaly meaning enlarged heart*

Most suffixes are not associated with only one medical specialty or body system. Therefore, you will use many of the same suffixes with each new set of combining forms introduced in each chapter. Suffixes can be placed into one of several categories. The following organizes the list and makes learning them easier by subdividing them into smaller groups:

- Suffixes indicating diseases or abnormal conditions
- Suffixes indicating a surgical procedure
- Suffixes indicating a diagnostic procedure
- General suffixes
- Suffixes indicating medical specialties or personnel
- Suffixes that convert word roots into adjectives

USE suffixes to indicate diseases or abnormal conditions.

Suffixes Indicating Diseases or Abnormal Conditions

Added to a word root, the following suffixes are used to indicate a diseased state or body abnormality.

Suffix	Meaning	Example (Definition)
-algia	pain	gastralgia (stomach pain)
-asthenia	weakness	myasthenia (muscle weakness)

> **TERMINOLOGY TIDBIT**
>
> The suffix *-asthenia* comes from combining the prefix *a-* meaning "without" and the Greek word *sthenos* meaning "strength."

Suffix	Meaning	Example (Definition)
-cele	hernia, protrusion	cystocele (protrusion of bladder)
-dynia	pain	cardiodynia (heart pain)
-cytosis	abnormal cell condition (too many)	erythrocytosis (too many red cells)
-ectasis	dilated, stretched out	bronchiectasis (dilated bronchi)
-edema	swelling	lymphedema (lymphatic swelling)
-emesis	vomiting	hematemesis (vomiting blood)
-emia	condition of the blood	oxemia (oxygen in blood)
-ia	state, condition	pneumonia (lung condition)
-iasis	abnormal condition	lithiasis (abnormal condition of stones)
-ism	state of, condition	hypothyroidism (state of low thyroid)
-itis	inflammation	dermatitis (skin inflammation)
-lith	stone	cystolith (bladder stone)
-lysis	destruction	osteolysis (bone destruction)
-lytic	destruction	thrombolytic (clot destruction)
-malacia	abnormal softening	chondromalacia (abnormal cartilage softening)

Suffix	Meaning	Example (Definition)
-megaly	enlargement, large	cardiomegaly (enlarged heart)
-oma	tumor, mass	carcinoma (cancerous tumor)
-osis	abnormal condition	cyanosis (abnormal condition of blue)
-pathy	disease	myopathy (muscle disease)
-penia	too few	cytopenia (too few cells)

+ TERMINOLOGY TIDBIT

The suffix -penia comes from the Greek word penia meaning "poverty."

Suffix	Meaning	Example (Definition)
-phobia	fear	photophobia (abnormal fear of light)
-plegia	paralysis	paraplegia (paralysis of both lower extremities)
-ptosis	drooping	proctoptosis (drooping rectum)
-rrhage	bursting forth	hemorrhage (bursting forth with blood)
-rrhagia	bursting forth	menorrhagia (bursting forth with menstrual flow)
-rrhea	discharge, flow	rhinorrhea (discharge from nose)

+ TERMINOLOGY TIDBIT

The suffixes -rrhea and -rrhagia are very similar but come from different Greek words. -rrhea comes from rhoia meaning "to flow"; -rrhagia comes from rhegnymi meaning "to burst forth" and now means excessive flow.

Suffix	Meaning	Example (Definition)
-rrhexis	rupture	hysterorrhexis (ruptured uterus)
-sclerosis	hardened condition	arteriosclerosis (hardening of artery)
-spasm	involuntary muscle contraction	bronchospasm (involuntary contraction of bronchi muscles)
-stasis	stopping	hemostasis (stopping blood flow)
-stenosis	narrowing	angiostenosis (narrowing of a vessel)
-toxic	poison	cytotoxic (poisonous to cells)
-uria	condition of the urine	hematuria (blood in urine)

USE suffixes to indicate surgical procedures.

Suffixes Indicating Surgical Procedures

The following are suffixes used to indicate surgical procedures. The word root paired with the surgical suffix indicates what area of the body is being operated on.

Suffix	Meaning	Example (Definition)
-clasia	surgical breaking	osteoclasia (surgical breaking of bone)
-desis	surgical fixation	arthrodesis (surgical fixation of joint)
-ectomy	surgical removal, excision	gastrectomy (surgically remove stomach)
-ostomy	surgically create an opening	colostomy (surgically create opening for colon [through abdominal wall])
-otomy	cutting into, incision	thoracotomy (cutting into chest)

> **+ TERMINOLOGY TIDBIT**
>
> The suffixes *-ectomy* and *-otomy* have very specific meanings that relate back to the original Greek words. *-ectomy* comes from *ektome* meaning "to cut out" while *-otomy* comes from *tomia* meaning "to cut into."

Suffix	Meaning	Example (Definition)
-pexy	surgical fixation	nephropexy (surgical fixation of kidney)
-plasty	surgical repair	dermatoplasty (surgical repair of skin)
-rrhaphy	suture	myorrhaphy (suture together muscle)
-tome	instrument to cut	dermatome (instrument to cut skin)
-tripsy	crushing	lithotripsy (crushing stone)

 USE suffixes to indicate diagnostic procedures.

Suffixes Indicating Diagnostic Procedures

The following are suffixes indicating common diagnostic procedures.

Suffix	Meaning	Example (Definition)
-centesis	puncture to withdraw fluid	arthrocentesis (puncture to withdraw fluid from joint)

> **+ TERMINOLOGY TIDBIT**
>
> The suffix *-centesis* comes from the Greek word *kentesis* meaning "to prick or pierce."

Suffix	Meaning	Example (Definition)
-gram	record or picture	electrocardiogram (record of heart's electricity)

Suffix	Meaning	Example (Definition)
-graph	instrument for recording	myograph (instrument for recording muscle)
-graphy	process of recording	electrocardiography (process of recording heart electricity)
-manometer	instrument for measuring pressure	sphygmomanometer (instrument for measuring pulse pressure)
-meter	instrument for measuring	audiometer (instrument to measure hearing)
-metry	process of measuring	audiometry (process of measuring hearing)
-scope	instrument for viewing	gastroscope (instrument to view stomach)
-scopy	process of visually examining	gastroscopy (process of visually examining stomach)

 USE general suffixes to create diminutive forms of medical terms.

General Suffixes

These suffixes belong to a group not specifically referring to a medical condition or procedure. However, they give general information about the condition of the word part.

Suffix	Meaning	Example (Definition)
-cle	small	vesicle (small bladder [blister])
-cyesis	pregnancy	salpingocyesis (fallopian tube pregnancy)
-cyte	cell	leukocyte (white cell)
-derma	skin condition	leukoderma (white skin condition)
-dipsia	thirst	polydipsia (frequent thirst)
-esthesia	feeling, sensation	anesthesia (without sensation)
-gen	that which produces	mutagen (that which produces mutations)
-genesis	produces, generates	osteogenesis (produces bone)
-genic	producing	carcinogenic (producing cancer)

+ TERMINOLOGY TIDBIT

The suffixes -genesis, -genic, and -gen all come from the Greek word gignesthai meaning "to be born."

Suffix	Meaning	Example (Definition)
-globin	protein	hemoglobin (blood protein)
-globulin	protein	immunoglobulin (protective protein)
-gravida	pregnancy	multigravida (many pregnancies)
-kinesia	movement	bradykinesia (slow movement)
-oid	resembling	lipoid (resembling fat)
-ole	small	arteriole (small artery)
-opia	vision	diplopia (double vision)
-opsy	view of	biopsy (view of life)
-osmia	sense of smell	anosmia (no sense of smell)
-oxia	oxygen	anoxia (without oxygen)
-para	to bear (offspring)	nullipara (to bear no children)
-partum	birth, labor	postpartum (after birth)
-pepsia	digestion	bradypepsia (slow digestion)
-phagia	eating, swallowing	dysphagia (difficulty swallowing)
-phasia	speech	aphasia (lack of speech)
-phil	attracted to	eosinophil (attracted to rosy [dye])
-phonia	voice	aphonia (without voice)
-plasm	formation, development	neoplasm (new formation)
-pnea	breathing	apnea (lack of breathing)
-poiesis	formation	hematopoiesis (blood formation)

Suffix	Meaning	Example (Definition)
-porosis	porous	osteoporosis (porous bone)
-ptysis	spitting up, coughing up	hemoptysis (spitting or coughing up blood)
-therapy	treatment	chemotherapy (treatment with chemicals)
-thorax	chest	hemothorax (blood in the chest)
-trophic	development	amyotrophic (without muscle development)
-trophy	nourishment, development	hypertrophy (excessive development)
-ule	small	venule (small vein)

 USE suffixes to indicate medical specialties or personnel.

Suffixes Indicating Medical Specialties or Personnel

The word root placed with these suffixes indicates the area of medicine in which the specialist works.

Suffix	Meaning	Example (Definition)
-er	one who	radiographer (one who takes x-rays)
-iatric	medical specialty	psychiatric (medical specialty of the mind)
-iatrist	physician	psychiatrist (physician specializing in the mind)
-iatry	treatment, medicine	podiatry (treatment of the foot)
-ician	specialist	pediatrician (specialist for children)
-ist	specialist	pharmacist (drug specialist)
-logist	one who studies	cardiologist (one who studies the heart)
-logy	study of	cardiology (study of the heart)

USE suffixes to convert word roots into nouns or adjectives.

USE suffixes to build additional medical terms.

Suffixes Used to Convert Word Roots into Adjectives

The following are suffixes used to convert word roots into adjectives. Often a term such as *ulcer* will need to be paired with a second term to indicate location. For example, *-ic* is combined with *gastr/o* to form the term *gastric* to give the adjective form for stomach. *Gastric* is then paired with *ulcer* to indicate that the ulcer is located in the stomach. The accepted meaning for these adjective suffixes is *pertaining to* or *relating to*.

Suffix	Meaning	Example (Definition)
-ac	pertaining to	cardiac (pertaining to heart)
-al	pertaining to	duodenal (pertaining to duodenum)
-an	pertaining to	ovarian (pertaining to ovary)
-ar	pertaining to	ventricular (pertaining to ventricle)
-ary	pertaining to	pulmonary (pertaining to lungs)
-atic	pertaining to	lymphatic (pertaining to lymph)
-eal	pertaining to	esophageal (pertaining to esophagus)
-ic	pertaining to	gastric (pertaining to stomach)
-ine	pertaining to	uterine (pertaining to uterus)
-ior	pertaining to	superior (pertaining to above)
-nic	pertaining to	embryonic (pertaining to embryo)
-ory	pertaining to	auditory (pertaining to hearing)
-ose	pertaining to	adipose (pertaining to fat)
-ous	pertaining to	venous (pertaining to vein)
-tic	pertaining to	hepatic (pertaining to liver)

Recognizing Categories of Suffixes

On each of the following blanks, indicate the category to which each suffix belongs and its translation. The suffix categories included in this exercise are disease/abnormal condition, surgical, diagnostic, and general.

Suffix	Meaning	Category
1. -plegia	paralysis	disease/ab. cond.
2. -metry	process of measuring	diagnostic
3. -cyte	cell	general
4. -otomy	cutting into	surgical
5. -lith	stone	disease/ab. cond.
6. -scope	insturment for viewing	diagnostic
7. -thorax	chest	general
8. -graphy	process of recording	diagnostic
9. -emesis	vomit	disease/ab. cond.
10. -clasia	surgical breaking	surgical
11. -lysis	destruction	disease/ab. cond.
12. -ectomy	surgical removing	surgical

Matching

Match each suffix to its definition.

E	1. -pepsia	A.	cell
L	2. -pnea	B.	formation, development
F	3. -phasia	C.	movement
H	4. -cyesis	D.	producing
C	5. -kinesia	E.	digestion
D	6. -genic	F.	speech
I	7. -dipsia	G.	therapy
A	8. -cyte	H.	pregnancy
K	9. -porosis	I.	thirst
G	10. -therapy	J.	vision
B	11. -plasm	K.	porous
J	12. -opia	L.	breathing

Choosing the Correct Adjective Form

One of the most difficult things to master in learning medical terminology is to use correct adjective forms. There are several ways to technically construct a word, but only one of them is an actual medical term. The rest simply aren't used. Unfortunately, there is no rule to help; you can learn this only by becoming familiar with which adjective form is correct. After a short while, a term will just "sound" correct and you won't forget it again.

The following exercise is a start to this process. Read the definition, sound out each choice, and circle the one that "sounds" correct to you.

1. **pertaining to the heart**
    (cardiac)   cardial   cardior   carditic

2. **pertaining to the ovary**
    ovarous   ovariac   (ovarian)   ovarial

3. **pertaining to the duodenum**
    duodenar   (duodenal)   duodeniac   duodentic

4. **pertaining to a ventricle**
    ventricultic   ventriculous   (ventricular)   ventriculac

5. **pertaining to the lungs**
    pulmonal   pulmontic   pulmonous   (pulmonary)

6. **pertaining to the esophagus**
    (esophageal)   esophagic   esophagous   esophagar

7. **pertaining to the stomach**
    gastran   (gastric)   gastral   gastreal

8. **pertaining to uterus**
    uterior   uterary   uterotic   (uterine)

9. **pertaining to a vein**
    (venous)   ventic   venary   veniac

10. **pertaining to the liver**
    hepatar   hepatary   (hepatic)   hepatac

Build Medical Terms

Now you are ready to start building actual medical terms. The following format will be used for this exercise and word building throughout the rest of this text:

- Translation phrase for the medical term
- Blank subdivided into prefix (if needed), word root, combining vowel (if needed), and suffix

Examples

- Instrument to view the stomach   gastr / o / scope
- Enlarged liver   hepat / o / megaly
- Pertaining to the kidney   ren / al
- Inflammation of skin   dermat / itis

Remember that whether or not to use a combining vowel depends on the first letter of the suffix. If it begins in a consonant, use a combining vowel (first two examples). If the suffix begins with a vowel, a combining vowel is not necessary (last two examples). Refer back to Chapter 1 if you need more help with this rule. Finally, you will need a short list of combining forms to use with the suffixes you learned in this chapter. The following list contains several common combining forms for use in these exercises.

Combining Form	Meaning		
angi/o	vessel	hepat/o	liver
arteri/o	artery	my/o	muscle
arthr/o	joint	nephr/o	kidney
bronch/o	bronchus	neur/o	nerve
col/o	colon	rhin/o	nose
cyst/o	bladder	thorac/o	chest
dermat/o	skin	trache/o	trachea
gastr/o	stomach		

1. Surgical removal of stomach   _gastr_ / _ectomy_
2. Instrument to view inside the stomach   _gastr_ / _o_ / _scope_
3. Process of visually examining the stomach   _gastr_ / _o_ / _scopy_
4. Stomach pain   _gastr_ / _algia_ or _gastr_ / _o_ / _dynia_
5. Bladder stone   _cyst_ / _o_ / _lith_
6. Instrument to view inside the bladder   _cyst_ / _o_ / _scope_
7. Process of visually examining the bladder   _cyst_ / _o_ / _scopy_
8. Surgically create an opening in the bladder   _cyst_ / _ostomy_
9. Pertaining to the bladder   _cyst_ / _ic_

10. Surgical repair of a vessel   angi / o / plasty

11. Vessel tumor   angi / oma

12. Process of recording a vessel   angi / o / graphy

13. Picture of a vessel   angi / o / gram

14. Narrowing vessel   angi / o / stenosis

15. Hardening of an artery   arteri / o / sclerosis

16. Involuntary muscle contraction in an artery   arteri / o / spasm

17. Ruptured artery   arteri / o / rrhexis

18. Small artery   arteri / ole

19. Inflamed joint   arthr / itis

20. Instrument to view inside a joint   arthr / o / scope

21. Process of visually examining a joint   arthr / o / scopy

22. Surgical repair of a joint   arthr / o / plasty

23. Puncture to withdraw fluid from a joint   arthr / o / centesis

24. Study of the skin   dermat / o / logy

25. One who studies the skin   dermat / o / logist

26. Inflamed skin   dermat / itis

27. Suture the skin   dermat / o / rrhaphy

28. Abnormal condition of the skin   dermat / osis

29. Inflamed liver   hepat / itis

30. Liver tumor   hepat / oma

31. Enlarged liver   hepat / o / megaly

32. Liver cell   hepat / o / cyte

33. Pertaining to the liver   hepat / ic

34. Discharge from the nose — rhin / o / rrhea

35. Surgical repair of the nose — rhin / o / plasty

36. Bursting forth from the nose — rhin / o / rrhagia

37. Inflamed bronchus — bronch / itis

38. Instrument to view inside the bronchus — bronch / o / scope

39. Process of visually examining the bronchus — bronch / o / scopy

40. Surgically create an opening into the trachea — trache / o / stomy

41. Cut into the trachea — trache / o / tomy

42. Protrusion of the trachea — trache / o / cele

43. Softening of the trachea — trache / o / malacia

44. Pertaining to the trachea — trache / al

45. Surgically create an opening into the colon — col o s / o / stomy

46. Surgical removal of the colon — col / ectomy

47. Surgical fixation of the colon — col / o / pexy

48. Study of the kidney — nephr / o / logy

49. One who studies the kidney — nephr / o / logist

50. Softening of the kidney — nephr / o / malacia

51. Abnormal condition of the kidney — nephr / o / sis

52. Kidney disease — nephr / o / pathy

53. Surgical fixation of the kidney — nephr / o / pexy

54. Cut into the chest — thorac / o / tomy

55. Puncture to withdraw fluid from the chest — thorac / o / centesis

56. Chest pain — thorac / o / dynia or thorac / algia

57. Study of the nerves — neur / o / logy

58. One who studies the nerves   neur / o / logist

59. Surgical repair of a nerve   neur / o / plasty

60. Crushing a nerve   neur / o / tripsy

61. Nerve pain   neur / algia or neur / o / dynia

62. Suture a muscle   my / o / rrhaphy

63. Muscle disease   my / o / pathy

64. Muscle pain   my / algia or my / o / dynia

65. Instrument to cut muscle   my / o / tome

66. Instrument for recording a muscle   my / o / graph

67. Record of a muscle   my / o / gram

68. Process of recording a muscle   my / o / graphy

Crossword Puzzle

Use the definitions given to complete the crossword puzzle. All answers are suffixes, but do not include the hyphen in your answers.

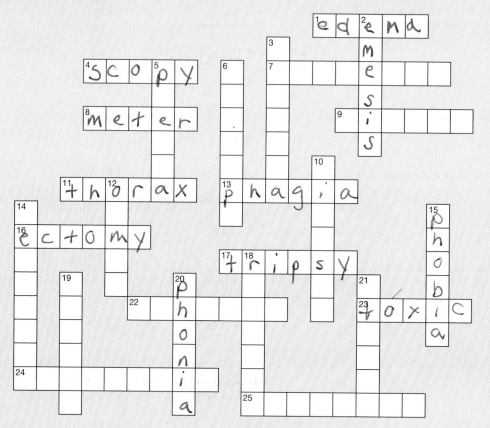

ACROSS

1 Swelling
4 Process of visually examining
7 Weakness
8 Instrument for measuring
9 Thirst
11 Chest
13 Eating, swallowing
16 Surgical removal
17 Crushing
22 Suture
23 Poison
24 Hardened
25 Narrowing

DOWN

2 Vomiting
3 Abnormal softening
5 Paralysis
6 Treatment
10 Movement
12 Sense of smell
14 Puncture to withdraw fluid
15 Fear
18 Rupture
19 Enlargement
20 Voice
21 Drooping

Prefixes

EXPLAIN the role of prefixes in building medical terms.

A Brief Introduction to Prefixes

A prefix at the beginning of a medical term adds specific information to the term. A good example uses the suffix meaning development, *-trophy*. Using different prefixes changes the meaning of each medical term.

- *hyper-* + *-trophy* = hypertrophy meaning *excessive development*
- *dys-* + *-trophy* = dystrophy meaning *abnormal development*
- *a-* + *-trophy* = atrophy meaning *lack of development*

Few prefixes are associated with only one medical specialty or body system. Therefore, you will use many of the same prefixes with each new set of combining forms introduced in each chapter. Prefixes can be placed into one of several categories. This organizes the list and makes learning them easier by subdividing them into smaller groups. These categories are:

- Prefixes indicating diseases or abnormal conditions
- Prefixes indicating directions or body positions
- Prefixes indicating numbers or quantity measurements
- Prefixes indicating time
- General prefixes

A few prefixes have multiple translations. Therefore, they appear in more than one category. For example, the prefix *hypo-* can be translated as *below,* placing it in the direction or body position category, or as *insufficient,* placing it in the number or quantity measurement category.

Prefixes Indicating Diseases or Abnormal Conditions

Used with word roots or suffixes, the following prefixes indicate a diseased state or body abnormality.

Prefix	Meaning	Example (Definition)
a-	without	aphasia (without speech)
an-	without	anoxia (without oxygen)
anti-	against	antibiotic (against life)
brady-	slow	bradycardia (slow heart beat)
de-	without	dehydration (without water)
dys-	painful, difficult	dyspnea (painful breathing)

> **+ TERMINOLOGY TIDBIT**
>
> The prefix *dys-* comes from the Greek word *dus*, which has a general negative meaning. It can be translated several ways such as "bad, difficult, abnormal, incorrect," and "painful."

Prefix	Meaning	Example (Definition)
pachy-	thick	pachyderma (thick skin)
tachy-	fast	tachycardia (fast heart beat)

Prefixes Indicating Directions or Body Positions

Used with word roots or suffixes, the following prefixes indicate directions or body positions.

Prefix	Meaning	Example (Definition)
ante-	in front of	anteorbital (in front of eye socket)
endo-	within, inner	endoscope (instrument for viewing within)
epi-	above, upon	epigastric (above stomach)

Prefix	Meaning	Example (Definition)
ex-	outward	exophthalmos (eyes [bulging] outward)
extra-	outside of	extraocular (outside of eye)
hypo-	below	hypogastric (below stomach)
infra-	below, under	infraorbital (below eye socket)
inter-	between	intervertebral (between vertebrae)
intra-	inside, within	intravenous (inside vein)

> **+ TERMINOLOGY TIDBIT**
>
> The prefixes *inter-* and *intra-* are commonly confused. Both come from Latin words, *intra* meaning "within" and *inter* meaning "between."

Prefix	Meaning	Example (Definition)
para-	alongside, near	paranasal (alongside nose)
peri-	around, near	periodontal (around tooth)
retro-	backward, behind	retroperitoneal (behind the peritoneum)
sub-	beneath, under	subcutaneous (under skin)
supra-	above	suprapubic (above pubic bone)
trans-	across, through	transurethral (across urethra)

USE prefixes to indicate numbers or quantity measurements.

Prefixes Indicating Numbers or Quantity Measurements

Used with word roots or suffixes, the following prefixes indicate the number of items or quantity measurement.

Prefix	Meaning	Example (Definition)
bi-	two	bilateral (two sides)
di-	two	diplegic (paralysis of two extremities)

Prefix	Meaning	Example (Definition)
hemi-	half	hemiplegia (paralysis of one side [half] of body)
hyper-	excessive, more than normal	hyperemesis (excessive vomiting)
hypo-	insufficient, less than normal	hypocalcemia (insufficient calcium in blood)

➕ **TERMINOLOGY TIDBIT**

The prefix *hypo-* is used several different ways. It comes from the Greek word *hupo* meaning "under" and is used to indicate a smaller than normal amount. It is also used to indicate a position underneath another structure.

Prefix	Meaning	Example (Definition)
micro-	small	microscope (instrument for viewing small things)
mono-	one	monoplegia (paralysis of one extremity)
multi-	many	multigravida (more than one pregnancy)
nulli-	none	nulligravida (no pregnancies)
pan-	all	pansinusitis (inflammation of all sinuses)
poly-	many, much	polyarteritis (many inflamed arteries)
primi-	first	primigravida (first pregnancy)
quadri-	four	quadriplegia (paralysis of all four extremities)
tri-	three	triplegia (paralysis of three extremities)
ultra-	excess	ultrasound (excess [high] sound wave frequency)
uni-	one	unilateral (one side)

USE prefixes to indicate time.

Prefixes Indicating Time

Used with word roots or suffixes, the following prefixes indicate time periods.

Prefix	Meaning	Example (Definition)
ante-	before	antepartum (before birth)
neo-	new	neonate (newborn)
post-	after	postpartum (after birth)
pre-	before	premenstrual (before menstruation)

 USE prefixes to build additional medical terms.

General Prefixes

These prefixes belong to a group not specifically referring to a disease, abnormal condition, direction, body position, number, or time. However, they give general information about the term to which they are added.

Prefix	Meaning	Example (Definition)
auto-	self	autograft (graft from one's own body)
eu-	normal, good	eupnea (normal breathing)
hetero-	different	heterograft (graft from a different species)
homo-	same	homograft (graft from same species)
per-	through	percutaneous (through skin)

➕ TERMINOLOGY TIDBIT

The prefix *eu-* comes from the Greek word *eu* and has a general positive meaning. It can be translated as "good, normal," or "well." It is the opposite of *dys-*.

Recognizing Categories of Prefixes

On each of the following blanks, indicate the category to which each prefix belongs and its translation. The categories included in this exercise are disease/abnormality prefixes, direction/body position prefixes, number prefixes, and time prefixes.

Prefix	Translation	Category
1. dys-	painful, difficult	disease/ab. cond.
2. hypo-	low	direction/b.p
3. nulli-	none	number
4. brady-	slow	time
5. an-	without	disease/ab. cond.
6. neo-	new	time
7. inter-	between	direction/b.p
8. post-	after	time
9. macro-		
10. peri-	around, near	direction/b.p.
11. epi-	above, upon	direction/b.p.
12. anti-	against	disease/ab. cond.

Matching

Match each prefix to its definition.

G	1. auto-	A.	same
D	2. poly-	B.	four
L	3. per-	C.	fast, rapid
A	4. homo-	D.	many
J	5. eu-	E.	first
K	6. pan-	F.	inside, within
E	7. primi-	G.	self
B	8. quadri-	H.	different
F	9. intra-	I.	excessive, above normal
H	10. hetero-	J.	normal, good
I	11. hyper-	K.	all
C	12. tachy-	L.	through

Build Medical Terms

Now you are ready to practice using prefixes to build medical terms. The following format will be used for this exercise:

■ *Translation phrase for the medical term*

■ *Blank subdivided into prefix and word root/suffix*

You will need additional word parts for this practice exercise. The following list contains word roots that have already been joined with a suffix making them ready to combine with a prefix.

Word Root + Suffix	Meaning
-cardia	heart
-carditis	heart inflammation
-cellular	pertaining to cells
-dermal	pertaining to skin
-graft	skin graft
-lateral	pertaining to the side
-operative	operation
-para	woman who has given birth
-pepsia	digestion
-phagia	eating
-plegia	paralysis
-pnea	breathing
-scapular	pertaining to the scapula
-trophy	development
-uria	condition of the urine

1. Fast heart   _____/_____

2. Slow heart   _____/_____

3. Inflammation inside the heart   _____/_____

4. Inflammation around the heart   _____/_____

5. Inflammation of the entire heart   _____/_____

6. Pertaining to inside the cell   _____/_____

7. Pertaining to outside the cell   _____/_____

8. Pertaining to several cells   _____/_____

9. Pertaining to one cell   _____/_____

10. Pertaining to within the skin   _____/_____

11. Pertaining to beneath the skin   _____/_____

12. Pertaining to above the skin

_____/_____

13. Graft from same source

_____/_____

14. Graft from other source

_____/_____

15. Graft from self

_____/_____

16. Pertaining to two sides

_____/_____

17. Pertaining to one side

_____/_____

18. Before an operation

_____/_____

19. After an operation

_____/_____

20. Within an operation

_____/_____

21. First birth

_____/_____

22. No births

_____/_____

23. Many births

_____/_____

24. No eating

_____/_____

25. Abnormal eating

_____/_____

26. Eating too much

_____/_____

27. Without digestion

_____/_____

28. Abnormal digestion

_____/_____

29. Slow digestion

_____/_____

30. Without development

_____/_____

31. Abnormal development

_____/_____

32. Half paralysis

_____/_____

33. Four paralysis

_____/_____

34. One paralysis

_____/_____

35. No breathing

_____/_____

36. Normal breathing _____/_____

37. Fast breathing _____/_____

38. Slow breathing _____/_____

39. Excessive breathing _____/_____

40. Deficient breathing _____/_____

41. Pertaining to below the scapula _____/_____

42. Pertaining to above the scapula _____/_____

43. Pertaining to beneath the scapula _____/_____

44. Condition of no urine _____/_____

45. Condition of much urine _____/_____

46. Condition of abnormal urine _____/_____

PEARSON mymedicalterminologylab

MyMedicalTerminologyLab is a premium online homework management system that includes a host of features to help you study. Registered users will find:

- Fun games and activities built within a virtual hospital
- Powerful tools that track and analyze your results—allowing you to create a personalized learning experience
- Videos, flashcards, and audio pronunciations to help enrich your progress
- Streaming lesson presentations and self-paced learning modules
- A space where you and your instructors can view and manage your assignments

Crossword Puzzle

Use the definitions given to complete the crossword puzzle. All answers are prefixes, but do not include the hyphen in your answers.

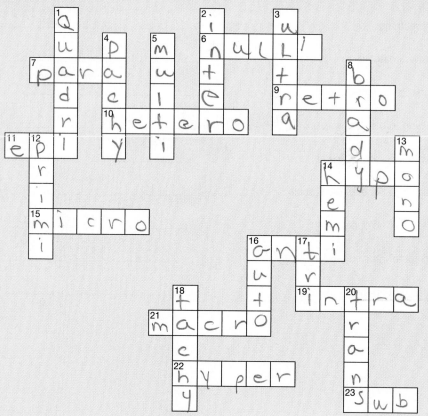

ACROSS

6 None
7 Alongside, near
9 Backward, behind
10 Different
11 Above, upon
14 Deficient, below normal
15 Small
16 Against
19 Inside, within
21 Large
22 Excessive, above normal
23 Beneath, under

DOWN

1 Four
2 Between
3 Excess
4 Thick
5 Many
8 Slow
12 First
13 One
14 Half
16 Self
17 Three
18 Fast
20 Across, through

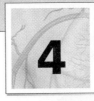

4

Anatomical Terminology

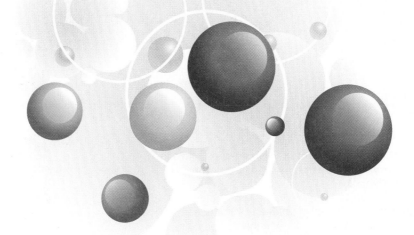

Anatomical Combining Forms

abdomin/o	abdomen		later/o	side
anter/o	front (side of body)		lumb/o	low back
brachi/o	arm		medi/o	middle
caud/o	tail		nas/o	nose
cephal/o	head		orbit/o	eye socket
cervic/o	neck		or/o	mouth
chondr/o	cartilage		ot/o	ear
crani/o	skull		patell/o	patella, kneecap
cubit/o	elbow		proxim/o	nearest (to beginning of structure)
dist/o	farthest (away from beginning of structure)		pelv/o	pelvis
			poster/o	back (side of body)
dors/o	back (side of body)		thorac/o	chest
femor/o	femur, thigh bone		scapul/o	scapula, shoulder blade
gastr/o	stomach		spin/o	spine
genit/o	genitals		stern/o	sternum, breast bone
glute/o	buttocks		super/o	above, upper
infer/o	below, lower		ventr/o	belly (side of body)
inguin/o	groin		vertebr/o	vertebra, back bone

Suffix Review

These suffixes and prefixes were introduced in Chapters 2 and 3. They are being reviewed in this chapter because they are especially important for building anatomical terms.

-al	pertaining to		**-ic**	pertaining to
-ar	pertaining to		**-ior**	pertaining to
-iac	pertaining to			

Prefix Review

ante-	in front of		**hypo-**	below
epi-	above		**retro-**	behind

 VISUALIZE patients in the anatomical position.

Anatomical Position

When describing body positions or using direction terms, health professionals visualize the patient in the **anatomical position** (see Figure 4.1>).

Therefore, it is not necessary to describe the patient's actual position. It does not matter whether the patient is lying down or sitting up or whether the health professional is on the patient's right or left side. Unless stated otherwise, it is assumed that the patient is:

+ TERMINOLOGY TIDBIT

The term *anatomy* comes from combining two Greek words: *ana* meaning "apart" and *tome* meaning "to cut." It was necessary to cut apart the body in order to study its internal structure.

- Standing upright
- Legs together
- Feet pointing forward
- Arms down to side
- Palms facing forward
- Eyes looking straight ahead

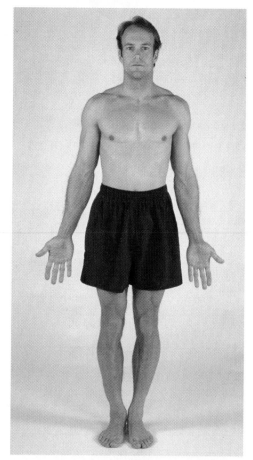

>4.1 The anatomical position: Standing upright, gazing straight ahead, arms down at sides, palms facing forward, fingers extended, legs together, and toes point forward.

Planes and Sections

The human body is three dimensional. Therefore, it can be divided into sections along three different planes: frontal (coronal), sagittal, and transverse (see Figure 4.2>). A two-dimensional image of the body, for example an x-ray, taken along one of the planes is called a *section*. Each plane yields a different section.

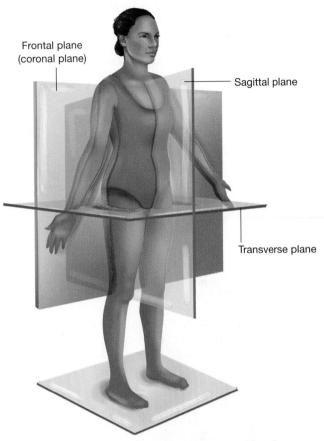

>4.2 The planes of the body. The sagittal plane is vertical from front to back, the frontal plane is vertical from left to right, and the transverse plane is horizontal.

1. **Frontal (or coronal) plane:** A vertical plane that runs from side to side; it slices body into anterior and posterior portions; a cut along frontal plane produces a **frontal** or **coronal section** (see Figure 4.3A>).

2. **Sagittal plane:** Also a vertical plane but runs from front to back; it slices body into left and right portions; a cut along the sagittal plane produces a **sagittal section** (see Figure 4.3B>).

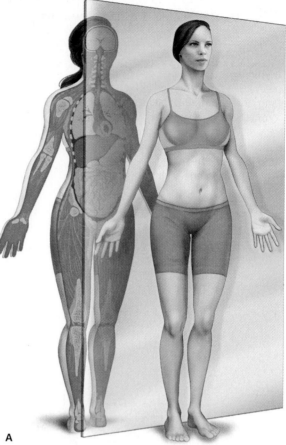

A

>4.3   Figures illustrating how the different body sections are formed. (A) Frontal or coronal section, (B) sagittal section, (C) transverse section.

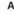

B

3. **Transverse plane:** Only horizontal plane; slices body into upper and lower portions; a cut along transverse plane produces a **transverse section** (see Figure 4.3C➤).

The terms **longitudinal section** and **cross-section** are often used to describe internal views of the body. A lengthwise slice along the long axis of a structure produces a longitudinal section. A cut down the length of the arm is an example of a longitudinal section. A cross-section is produced by a slice perpendicular to the long axis of a structure. A cut across the upper arm yields a cross-section view.

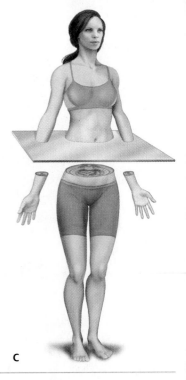

C

USE correct directional terms.

Directional Terminology

Directional terms indicate the position of a structure *in relation* to another structure. For example, the heart is above the stomach. The position of these two organs relative to each other can be expressed as either the heart is superior to the stomach or the stomach is infe-

➕ **TERMINOLOGY TIDBIT**

Remember when using direction terms that you assume that the patient is in the anatomical position unless otherwise noted.

rior to the heart. This example also demonstrates another characteristic of direction terms: They come in opposite pairs; for each directional term there is a second term than means the opposite (see Figure 4.4➤).

Building Direction Terms
Most directional terms are Latin-style terms and therefore can be built from word parts. They consist of a word root and an adjective suffix, usually *–ic, –ior,* or *–al.*

For each word root and suffix that follows, build the corresponding directional term. Terms not built from word parts are simply defined and presented with their definition.

1. **anter/o + -ior**

   a. pertaining to front (side of body) _____/_____

2. **caud/o + -al**

   a. pertaining to the tail _____/_____

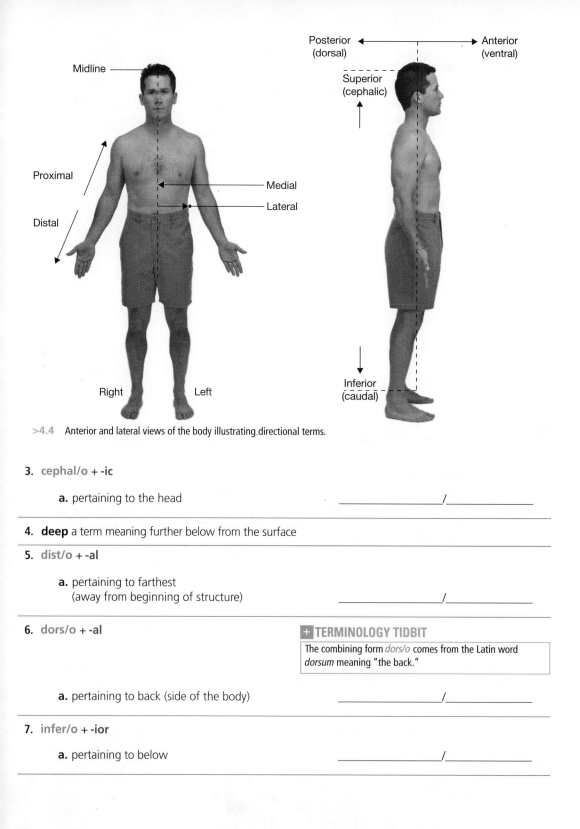

>4.4 Anterior and lateral views of the body illustrating directional terms.

3. **cephal/o + -ic**

    a. pertaining to the head   _____/_____

4. **deep** a term meaning further below from the surface

5. **dist/o + -al**

    a. pertaining to farthest
    (away from beginning of structure)   _____/_____

6. **dors/o + -al**

    a. pertaining to back (side of the body)   _____/_____

7. **infer/o + -ior**

    a. pertaining to below   _____/_____

➕ TERMINOLOGY TIDBIT

The combining form *dors/o* comes from the Latin word *dorsum* meaning "the back."

8. **later/o + -al**

    a. pertaining to the side   _____/_____

9. **medi/o + -al**

    a. pertaining to the middle   _____/_____

10. **poster/o + -ior**

    a. pertaining to back (side of body)   _____/_____

11. **prone** a term meaning to lie face down (see Figure 4.5A>)

+ TERMINOLOGY TIDBIT

The term *prone* comes from the Latin word *pronus* meaning "leaning forward."

>4.5A   The ~~supine~~ position.   *prone*

12. **proxim/o + -al**

    a. pertaining to nearest (to beginning of structure)   _____/_____

13. **superficial** a term meaning nearer the surface

14. **super/o + -ior**

    a. pertaining to above   _____/_____

15. **supine** a term meaning to lie face up (see Figure 4.5B>)

+ TERMINOLOGY TIDBIT

The term *supine* comes from the Latin word *supinus* meaning "bent backwards."

>4.5B   The ~~prone~~ position.   *supine*

16. **ventr/o + -al**

+ TERMINOLOGY TIDBIT

The combining form *ventr/o* comes from the Latin word *venter* meaning "the belly."

    a. pertaining to belly (side of body)   _____/_____

Body Surface Terminology

The different regions of the body are named so they can be easily and accurately referred to. Many are named for a body structure underlying the region. For example: the sternal region overlies the sternum and the abdominal region overlies the abdominal cavity (see Figure 4.6>).

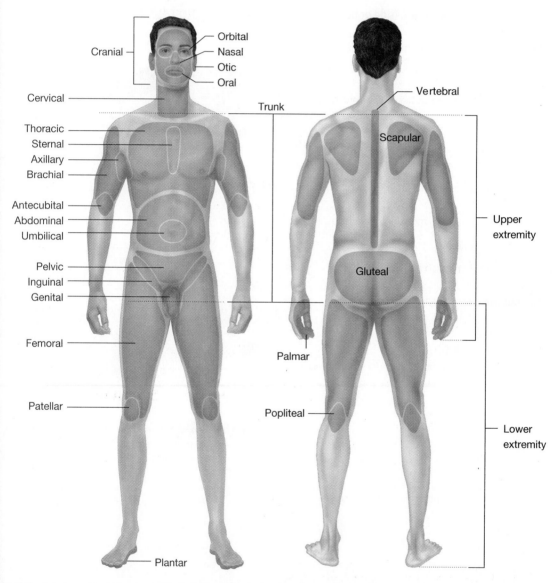

>4.6   Anterior and posterior views of the body illustrating the location of various body regions.

Building Body Surface Terms

Like directional terms, many body surface terms are Latin-style words consisting of a word root and suffix.

For each of the following word roots and suffixes, build the corresponding term for that body surface region. Terms not built from word parts are simply defined. One cautionary note: Some of the following terms may appear to be built from word parts but are not.

1. **abdomin/o + -al**

  a. pertaining to the abdomen   _____/_____

2. **ante- + cubit/o + -al**

  a. pertaining to in front of the elbow   _____/_____/_____

3. **axillary** a term meaning underarm area

4. **brachi/o + -al**

  a. pertaining to the arm   _____/_____

5. **cervic/o + -al**

  a. pertaining to the neck   _____/_____

6. **crani/o + -al**

  a. pertaining to the skull   _____/_____

7. **femor/o + -al**

  a. pertaining to the femur/thigh   _____/_____

8. **genit/o + -al**

  a. pertaining to the genitals   _____/_____

9. **glute/o + -al**

  a. pertaining to the buttocks   _____/_____

10. **inguin/o + -al**

  a. pertaining to groin   _____/_____

11. **lower extremity** a phrase used to refer to the entire leg

12. **nas/o + -al**

  a. pertaining to the nose   _____/_____

13. orbit/o + -al

    a. pertaining to the eye socket   _____/_____

14. or/o + -al

    a. pertaining to the mouth   _____/_____

15. ot/o + -ic

    a. pertaining to the ear   _____/_____

16. palmar a term meaning the palm of the hand

17. patell/o + -ar

    a. pertaining to the kneecap   _____/_____

18. pelv/o + -ic

    a. pertaining to the pelvis   _____/_____

19. plantar a term meaning the sole of the foot

20. popliteal a term meaning the creased area behind the knee

21. thorac/o + -ic

    a. pertaining to the chest   _____/_____

22. scapul/o + -ar

    a. pertaining to the shoulder blade   _____/_____

23. stern/o + -al

    a. pertaining to breast bone   _____/_____

24. trunk a term meaning the torso, excluding the head and extremities

25. umbilical a term meaning the region around the navel

26. upper extremity a phrase used to refer to the entire arm

27. vertebr/o + -al

    a. pertaining to vertebra/back bone   _____/_____

 PLACE internal organs into the correct body cavity.

Body Cavities

The majority of the body's internal organs, or **viscera,** are found within one of four body cavities (see Figure 4.7▶). Two of these cavities, the **cranial cavity** and **spinal cavity,** are on the dorsal side of the body. The other two, the **thoracic cavity** and **abdominopelvic cavity,** are ventral. The organs within the cavities are usually found within protective membrane sacs.

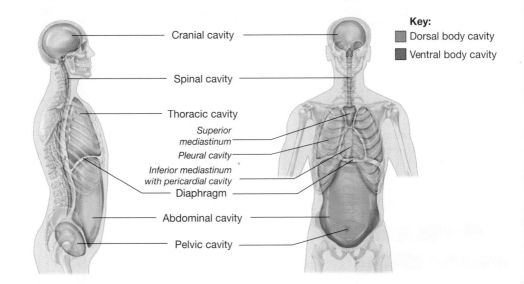

Cranial cavity	**Key:**
Spinal cavity	▨ Dorsal body cavity
Thoracic cavity	▧ Ventral body cavity
Superior mediastinum	
Pleural cavity	
Inferior mediastinum with pericardial cavity	
Diaphragm	
Abdominal cavity	
Pelvic cavity	

Lateral view   **Anterior view**

>4.7   The dorsal (in red) and ventral (in blue) body cavities.

Cavity	Description
Cranial **crani/o** = skull **-al** = pertaining to	Dorsal cavity; lies inside skull and contains the brain; brain is protected by membrane sac called the **meninges**.
Spinal **spin/o** = spine **-al** = pertaining to	Dorsal cavity; formed by canal through vertebrae; contains the spinal cord; spinal cord is also protected by the meninges.
Thoracic **thorac/o** = chest **-ic** = pertaining to	Superior of two ventral cavities; found enclosed by ribs and separated from abdominopelvic cavity by **diaphragm** muscle; contains organs such as the lungs, heart, esophagus, trachea, aorta, and thymus gland; it can be subdivided into one central and two side regions. ■ **Mediastinum:** central region; contains the heart, trachea, esophagus, aorta, and thymus gland; heart is encased in the pericardial sac. ■ **Pleural cavities:** side regions; each contains a lung; sac protecting lungs is called the **pleura**.
Abdominopelvic **abdomin/o** = abdomen **pelv/o** = pelvis **-ic** = pertaining to	Inferior of two ventral cavities; large cavity generally subdivided into abdominal and pelvic cavities; however, no clear structure indicating where one cavity stops and the other begins; organs of abdominopelvic cavity are protected by membrane covering called the **peritoneum**. ■ **Abdominal cavity:** houses the stomach, liver, gallbladder, spleen, pancreas, and portions of colon and intestine. ■ **Pelvic cavity:** contains the urinary bladder, ureters, urethra, and portions of colon and intestine in both genders; in females also contains the uterus, ovaries, fallopian tubes, and vagina; in males also contains the prostate gland, seminal vesicles, bulbourethral gland, and portion of vas deferens.

Know what is in each cavity

The only major abdominopelvic organs that lie outside of the peritoneum are the kidneys. These organs lie along either side of the vertebral column just under the lower ribs. Because they lie behind the peritoneum, their position is called *retroperitoneal* (retro- = behind).

 USE either anatomical divisions or clinical divisions to describe the abdominopelvic cavity.

Divisions of the Abdominopelvic Cavity

Because it is so large, the abdominopelvic cavity is commonly divided into regions. Health personnel can use two methods to do this: **clinical divisions** and **anatomical divisions.**

When using the clinical divisions, the abdominopelvic cavity is divided into four equal quadrants that cross at the navel (see Figure 4.8>). Each quadrant is named by its position as follows:

- **Right upper quadrant** (RUQ): contains right lobe of liver (bulk of liver), right kidney, upper portion of right ureter, pancreas (small section), gallbladder, and portions of colon and intestine
- **Right lower quadrant** (RLQ): contains lower portion of right ureter, portions of colon and intestine, appendix, right ovary and fallopian tube (in females), and right vas deferens and seminal vesicle (in males)
- **Left upper quadrant** (LUQ): contains stomach, spleen, left lobe of liver (smaller), pancreas (most of organ), left kidney, upper portion of left ureter, portions of colon and intestines
- **Left lower quadrant** (LLQ): contains lower portion of left ureter, portions of colon and intestine, sigmoid colon, left ovary and fallopian tube (in females), and left vas deferens and seminal vesicle (in males)

The urinary bladder, rectum, uterus (in females), and prostate gland (in males) are midline structures and therefore do not actually fall into any one quadrant.

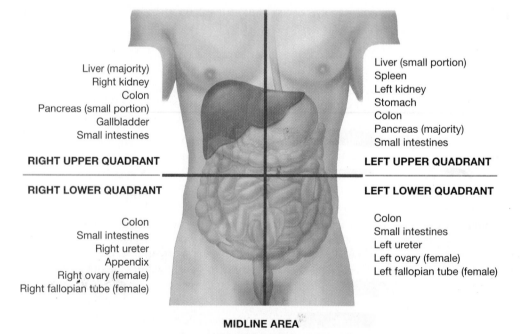

Liver (majority)
Right kidney
Colon
Pancreas (small portion)
Gallbladder
Small intestines

RIGHT UPPER QUADRANT

RIGHT LOWER QUADRANT

Colon
Small intestines
Right ureter
Appendix
Right ovary (female)
Right fallopian tube (female)

Liver (small portion)
Spleen
Left kidney
Stomach
Colon
Pancreas (majority)
Small intestines

LEFT UPPER QUADRANT

LEFT LOWER QUADRANT

Colon
Small intestines
Left ureter
Left ovary (female)
Left fallopian tube (female)

MIDLINE AREA

Bladder - Uterus (female) - Prostate (male)

>4.8 The clinical divisions of the abdomen. The abdominopelvic cavity is divided into four quadrants.

Anatomical divisions are smaller. This system divides the abdominopelvic cavity into nine sections like a tic-tac-toe board (see Figure 4.9>). The nine regions are as follows:

- **Right hypochondriac** (hypo- = below; chondr/o = cartilage; -iac = pertaining to): right lateral side of upper row under lower ribs that are connected to the sternum by cartilage
- **Epigastric** (epi- = above; gastr/o = stomach; -ic = pertaining to): middle area of upper row overlying stomach
- **Left hypochondriac:** left lateral side of upper row
- **Right lumbar** (lumb/o = low back; -ar = pertaining to): right lateral side of middle row near waist
- **Umbilical:** middle area of middle row containing navel (also called *umbilicus*)
- **Left lumbar:** left lateral side of middle row
- **Right inguinal** (inguin/o = groin; -al = pertaining to): right lateral side of lower row near groin
- **Hypogastric** (hypo- = below; gastr/o = stomach; -ic = pertaining to): middle area of lower row
- **Left inguinal:** left lateral side of lower row

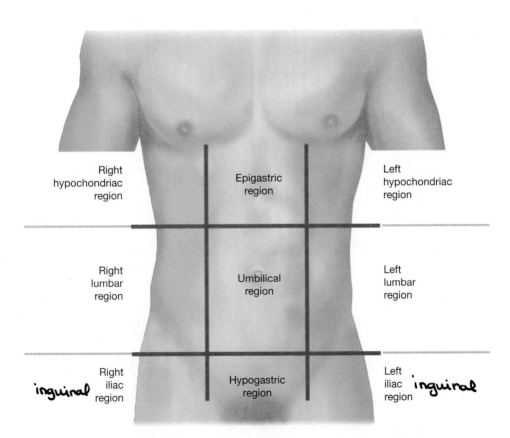

>4.9   The anatomical divisions of the abdomen. The abdominopelvic cavity is divided into nine regions.

Directional Terms

For each of the following directional terms, write a directional term that could be used to indicate the opposite direction.

1. anterior _____

2. caudal _____

3. cephalic _____

4. deep _____

5. distal _____

6. dorsal _____

7. inferior _____

8. lateral _____

9. medial _____

10. posterior _____

11. proximal _____

12. superficial _____

13. superior _____

14. ventral _____

15. supine _____

Fill in the Blank

Fill in the blank to complete each of the following sentences.

1. The _____ cavity contains the spinal cord.

2. The sac protecting the lungs is called the _____.

3. The cranial and spinal cavities are found on the _____ side of the body.

4. The _____ is the only major abdominopelvic internal organ found outside the peritoneum.

5. The heart, lungs, esophagus, aorta, and thymus gland are found in the _____ cavity.

6. The _____ protects the organs of the abdominopelvic cavity.

7. The cranial cavity contains the _____.

8. The pericardium covers the _____.

9. The urinary bladder is found in the _____ cavity.

10. The brain and spinal cord are protected by a sac called the _____.

11. The liver is found in the _____ cavity.

12. The central region of the thoracic cavity is called the _____.

Labeling Exercise—External Surface Anatomy

Write the name of each area on the numbered line. Also use this space to write the combining form where appropriate.

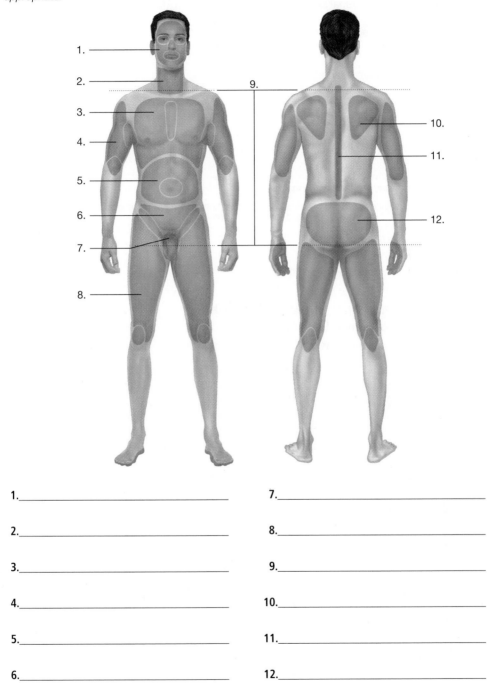

1._____

2._____

3._____

4._____

5._____

6._____

7._____

8._____

9._____

10._____

11._____

12._____

Matching—Planes and Sections

Match each body plane and section to its definition. Answers may be used more than once.

_____ **1.** Also called the *coronal plane*

_____ **2.** Section produced by cut at right angle to long axis of structure

_____ **3.** Plane that divides the body into left and right portions

_____ **4.** The two vertical planes

_____ **5.** Plane that divides body into anterior and posterior portions

_____ **6.** Section produced by the coronal plane

_____ **7.** Divides the body into upper and lower portions

_____ **8.** The only horizontal plane

_____ **9.** Section cut along long axis of the structure

A. Frontal plane

B. Sagittal plane

C. Transverse plane

D. Longitudinal section

E. Frontal section

F. Cross-section

Matching—Organs and Clinical Divisions of the Abdominopelvic Cavity

Match each organ to the quadrant in which you would expect to find the majority of that organ.

_____ **1.** Liver

_____ **2.** Left ureter

_____ **3.** Spleen

_____ **4.** Stomach

_____ **5.** Colon

_____ **6.** Gallbladder

_____ **7.** Right ovary

_____ **8.** Sigmoid colon

_____ **9.** Left kidney

_____ **10.** Uterus

_____ **11.** Pancreas

_____ **12.** Small intestine

_____ **13.** Appendix

A. RUQ

B. RLQ

C. LUQ

D. LLQ

E. In all quadrants

F. Midline

Labeling Exercise—Anatomical Divisions of the Abdominopelvic Cavity

Write the name for each anatomical division of the abdominopelvic cavity on the line provided.

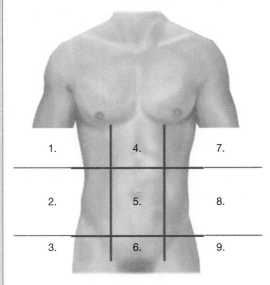

1. _____

2. _____

3. _____

4. _____

5. _____

6. _____

7. _____

8. _____

9. _____

Crossword Puzzle

Use the definitions given to complete the crossword puzzle.

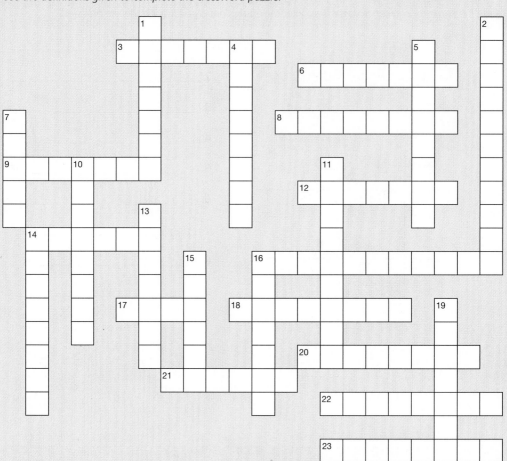

ACROSS

3 Term for thigh body region
6 Direction term referring to the side
8 Term for chest body region
9 Term for eye socket body region
12 Another name for frontal plane
14 Direction term referring to the tail
16 Direction term meaning nearer the surface
17 Direction term meaning away from the surface
18 Term for neck body region
20 Term for arm body region
21 Direction term referring to the middle
22 Direction term for front of body
23 Term for kneecap body region

DOWN

1 Direction term referring to the belly side of the body
2 Term for front of the elbow body region
4 Term for underarm body region
5 Plane divides body into left and right portions
7 Direction term meaning to lie face down
10 Term for groin body region
11 Direction term that means the same thing as dorsal
13 Term for buttocks body region
14 Direction term referring to the head
15 Direction term meaning to lie face up
16 Term for breast bone body region
19 Term for skull body region

Dermatology
Integumentary System

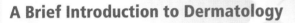

dermat/o

-logy

A Brief Introduction to Dermatology

 UNDERSTAND the functions of the skin.

The **skin,** or **integument**, is the largest organ in the body, weighing an average of 20 pounds. It serves several important functions.

- **Protection** – Skin is a continuous two-way barrier that prevents pathogens such as bacteria from invading the body and vital substances such as water from leaking out of the body.
- **Temperature regulation** – If the body is too hot, evaporation of sweat from sweat glands and dilation of blood vessels in skin helps to cool the body; if it needs to conserve heat, blood vessels constrict; additionally, the innermost layer of skin, the fatty subcutaneous layer, serves as insulation.
- **Sensation** – Skin contains many different sensory receptors that send information to the brain regarding the senses of touch, pressure, temperature, and pain.
- **Waste disposal** – A small amount of waste products, such as excess salt, is excreted from the body in sweat.

 DESCRIBE the medical specialty of dermatology.

    Dermatology is the branch of medicine concerned with the diagnosis and treatment of conditions involving the skin and its accessory structures, **hair** and **nails.** A **dermatologist** specializes in treating skin tumors, damaged skin from trauma and burns, skin infections, inflammatory skin conditions, and cosmetic disorders including hair loss, scars, and skin changes associated with aging.

    Plastic surgery is another branch of medicine that treats conditions involving the integumentary system as well as conditions of the musculoskeletal system, head and face, hands, breasts, and external genitalia. **Plastic surgeons** repair, reconstruct, or improve damaged or missing body structures.

55

Dermatology Combining Forms

The following list presents new combining forms important for building and defining dermatology terms.

aden/o	gland		lip/o	fat
adip/o	fat		melan/o	melanin, black
cutane/o	skin		onych/o	nail
cyan/o	blue		py/o	pus
dermat/o	skin		seb/o	sebum, oil
derm/o	skin		trich/o	hair
hidr/o	sweat		ungu/o	nail
kerat/o	keratin, hard, hornlike			

The following list presents combining forms that are not specific to the skin but are used for building and defining dermatology terms.

bi/o	life		myc/o	fungus
carcin/o	cancer		necr/o	death
chem/o	chemical		scler/o	hard
cry/o	cold		vesic/o	bladder, sac
erythr/o	red		xanth/o	yellow
ichthy/o	scaly		xer/o	dry
leuk/o	white			

Suffix Review

These suffixes introduced in Chapter 2 are being reviewed in this chapter because they are especially important for building dermatology terms.

-al	pertaining to		-oid	resembling
-cle	small		-oma	tumor, mass
-cyte	cell		-opsy	view of
-derma	skin condition		-ose	pertaining to
-ectomy	surgical removal		-osis	abnormal condition
-genic	producing		-ous	pertaining to
-ia	state, condition		-pathy	disease
-ic	pertaining to		-phagia	eating or swallowing
-itis	inflammation		-plasty	surgical repair
-logist	one who studies		-rrhea	flow, discharge
-logy	study of		-sclerosis	hardened condition
-malacia	abnormal softening		-tic	pertaining to
-megaly	enlargement, large		-tome	instrument used to cut

Prefix Review

These prefixes introduced in Chapter 3 are being reviewed in this chapter because they are especially important for building dermatology terms.

an-	without	pachy-	thick
epi-	above, upon	per-	through
hyper-	excessive, above	sub-	beneath, under
hypo-	below	trans-	across
intra-	inside, within		

 IDENTIFY the organs treated in dermatology.

Organs Commonly Treated in Dermatology

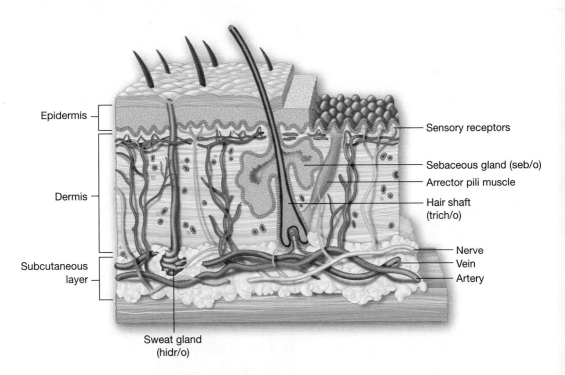

>5.1 Structures of the skin

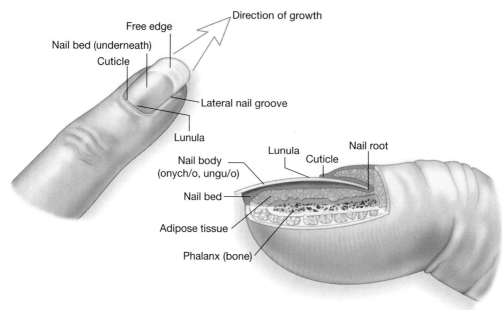

>5.2 Nail structure

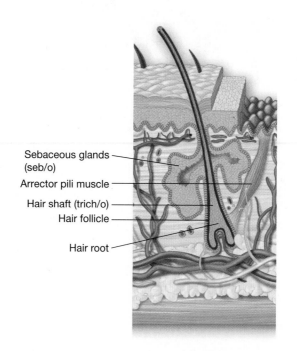

Sebaceous glands (seb/o)
Arrector pili muscle
Hair shaft (trich/o)
Hair follicle
Hair root

>5.3 Hair structure

Building Dermatology Terms

This section presents word parts most often used to build dermatology terms. Following the explanation of the term, you have the opportunity to begin building your own vocabulary. Read the meaning of each term and then fill in the blanks to build a single medical term. Use the slashes to divide prefixes, word roots, combining vowels, and suffixes. To help you out you will find a key to the word parts underneath the blanks: r for word root, p for prefix, cv for combining vowel, and s for suffix. Remember that not every term will contain all of these word parts; it is up to you to decide which to use. As you gain experience, this process will become easier. Answers can be found at the back of the book.

1. aden/o–combining form meaning **gland**

   A gland is an organ that secretes a substance; skin has two types: **sweat glands** and **sebaceous (oil) glands**

   a. surgical removal of a gland   _____ / _____
                                                            r   s

   b. inflammation of a gland   _____ / _____
                                                            r   s

   c. tumor in a gland   _____ / _____
                                                            r   s

   d. disease of a gland   _____ / ____ / _____
                                                            r   cv   s

   e. enlarged gland   _____ / ____ / _____
                                                            r   cv   s

2. adip/o–combining form meaning **fat**

   Fat tissue makes up the subcutaneous layer of the skin; forms continuous layer over the body; serves as insulation, energy storage, and protective padding layer

   a. pertaining to fat   _____ / _____
                                                            r   s

   b. fat cell   _____ / ____ / _____
                                                            r   cv   s

   c. tumor made of fat   _____ / _____
                                                            r   s

3. cutane/o–combining form meaning **skin**

   Skin is also called the **integument;** protective outer layer of the body; composed of three layers:

   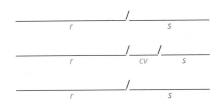

   - **Epidermis:** outer layer; composed primarily of dead keratinized cells that form protective barrier to keep out bacteria and other pathogens
   - **Dermis:** middle layer; strong, flexible connective tissue for strength; houses hair follicles, sweat glands, sebaceous glands, nerve endings, and blood vessels
   - **Subcutaneous layer:** inner layer; primarily fat that insulates the body and provides protective padding and energy storage

   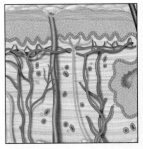

   >5.4 Skin

   a. pertaining to the skin   _____ / _____
                                                            r   s

b. pertaining to below the skin

_____/_____/_____
$\quad p \qquad\qquad r \qquad\qquad s$

c. pertaining to through the skin

_____/_____/_____
$\quad p \qquad\qquad r \qquad\qquad s$

4. **cyan/o**–combining form meaning **blue**

   Skin appears to be a blue color when its blood supply becomes deoxygenated

   a. abnormal condition of being blue

   _____/_____
   $\qquad\qquad r \qquad\qquad s$

   b. pertaining to being blue

   _____/____/_____
   $\qquad r \qquad cv \quad s$

5. **-derma**–suffix meaning **skin condition**

   This suffix is used with combining forms or prefixes to describe how skin looks or feels

   a. scaly skin condition

   _____/____/_____
   $\qquad r \qquad cv \quad s$

   b. hard skin condition

   _____/____/_____
   $\qquad r \qquad cv \quad s$

   c. yellow skin condition

   _____/____/_____
   $\qquad r \qquad cv \quad s$

   d. dry skin condition

   _____/____/_____
   $\qquad r \qquad cv \quad s$

   e. thick skin condition

   _____/_____
   $\qquad r \qquad s$

   f. red skin condition

   _____/____/_____
   $\qquad r \qquad cv \quad s$

   g. pus skin condition

   _____/____/_____
   $\qquad r \qquad cv \quad s$

   h. white skin condition

   _____/____/_____
   $\qquad r \qquad cv \quad s$

6. **dermat/o**–combining form meaning **skin**

   a. skin inflammation

   _____/_____
   $\qquad r \qquad s$

   b. study of the skin

   _____/____/_____
   $\qquad r \qquad cv \quad s$

   c. one who studies the skin

   _____/____/_____
   $\qquad r \qquad cv \quad s$

   d. abnormal condition of the skin

   _____/_____
   $\qquad r \qquad s$

   e. surgical repair of the skin

   _____/____/_____
   $\qquad r \qquad cv \quad s$

   f. abnormal skin fungus condition

   _____/__/_____/__
   $\quad r \quad cv \qquad r \qquad s$

g. disease of the skin

_____/_____/_____
　　　　　　　　r　　　CV　　S

h. hardened skin condition

_____/_____/_____
　　　　　　　　r　　　CV　　S

7. **derm/o**–combining form meaning **skin**

a. pertaining to the skin

_____/_____
　　　　　　　　r　　　　　　S

b. pertaining to over the skin

_____/_____/_____
　　p　　　　　　　r　　　　S

c. pertaining to within the skin

_____/_____/_____
　　p　　　　　　　r　　　　S

d. pertaining to under the skin

_____/_____/_____
　　p　　　　　　　r　　　　S

e. pertaining to across the skin

_____/_____/_____
　　p　　　　　　　r　　　　S

8. **hidr/o**–combining form meaning **sweat**

Sweat is secreted by sweat glands; the primary function is to cool the skin by evaporation; also contains a small amount of waste products such as sodium chloride, urea, and ammonia

a. abnormal condition of sweating

_____/_____
　　　　　　　　r　　　　　　S

b. abnormal condition with lack of sweating

_____/_____/_____
　　p　　　　　　　r　　　　S

c. sweat gland inflammation

_____/_____/_____
　　　　　　　r　　　　　r　　S

d. abnormal condition of excessive sweating

_____/_____/_____
　　p　　　　　　　r　　　　S

9. **kerat/o**–combining form meaning **keratin, hard, hornlike**

This hard protein is found in **hair, nails**, and cells of the epidermis; may become overgrown resulting in thick, hornlike layer of skin

a. hornlike skin condition

_____/_____/_____
　　　　　　　　r　　　CV　　S

b. hornlike abnormal condition

_____/_____
　　　　　　　　r　　　　　　S

c. producing keratin

_____/_____/_____
　　　　　　　　r　　　CV　　S

10. **lip/o**–combining form meaning **fat**

a. surgical removal of fat

_____/_____
　　　　　　　　r　　　　　　S

b. resembling fat

_____/_____
　　　　　　　　r　　　　　　S

c. fat tumor

_____/_____
r   s

d. fat cell

_____/____/_____
r   CV   s

---

11. **melan/o**–combining form meaning **melanin, black**

Melanin is the black pigment found in **melanocytes** that gives skin and hair its dark color; the more melanin present, the darker the hair or skin; provides protection against damage from sun exposure

a. black tumor

_____/_____
r   s

b. black cell

_____/____/_____
r   CV   s

c. pertaining to being black

_____/____/_____
r   CV   s

---

12. **onych/o**–combining form meaning **nail**

Nails are flat plates of keratin that cover ends of fingers and toes

>5.5 Nail

a. surgical removal of a nail

_____/_____
r   s

b. inflammation of a nail

_____/_____
r   s

c. softening of a nail

_____/____/_____
r   CV   s

d. abnormal nail fungus condition

_____/____/_____/__
r   CV   r   s

e. nail eating (biting)

_____/____/_____
r   CV   s

f. state of excessive nail (growth)

_____/_____/_____
p   r   s

---

13. **py/o**–combining form meaning **pus**

Pus is a semisolid fluid associated with certain bacterial infections; consists of tissue fluid, dead bacteria, debris from damaged cells, and dead white blood cells

a. producing pus

_____/____/_____
r   CV   s

b. discharge of pus

_____/____/_____
r   CV   s

---

14. seb/o–combining form meaning **oil**

Sebum is the oily secretion of **sebaceous glands**; lubricates the skin to keep it soft and from cracking

    a. flow of oil

    _____/___/_____
                     r   *cv*   *s*

---

15. trich/o–combining form meaning **hair**

A hair is a shaft of keratinized cells growing from the hair root (in dermis layer) up through the hair follicle and out above the surface of the skin

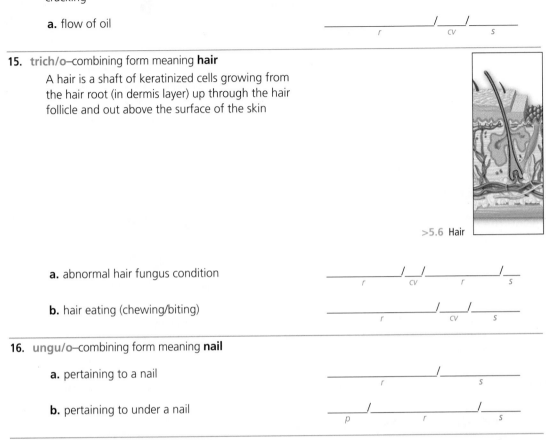

>5.6 **Hair**

    a. abnormal hair fungus condition

    _____/___/_____/__
                  r   *cv*   *r*   *s*

    b. hair eating (chewing/biting)

    _____/___/_____
                     r   *cv*   *s*

---

16. ungu/o–combining form meaning **nail**

    a. pertaining to a nail

    _____/_____
                     r   *s*

    b. pertaining to under a nail

    ____/_____/_____
      p   *r*   *s*

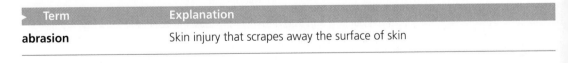

EXPLAIN dermatology medical terms.

Dermatology Vocabulary

The dermatology terms presented in this section include eponyms, modern English words, and those that contain Latin or Greek word parts but are not constructed solely from these word parts. When you recognize word parts within a term they will give you a hint about the word's meaning. In these instances, look for the word parts to follow the term.

► Term	Explanation
abrasion	Skin injury that scrapes away the surface of skin

Term	Explanation

abscess

Infection by pyogenic bacteria resulting in localized collection of pus

>5.7 Abscess with visible pus
Source: Courtesy of Jason L. Smith, MD

alopecia

Baldness

> ⊞ **TERMINOLOGY TIDBIT**
>
> The term *alopecia* comes from the Greek word *alopekia* meaning "fox mange," a condition that causes hair to fall out.

basal cell carcinoma (BCC)
  carcin/o = cancer
  -oma = tumor

Skin cancer in basal cell layer of the epidermis; very common cancer caused by sun exposure but rarely metastasizes or spreads

>5.8 Basal cell carcinoma
Source: Courtesy of Jason L. Smith, MD

biopsy (BX, bx)
  bi/o = life
  -opsy = to view

Surgical procedure to remove a piece of tissue by needle, knife, punch, or brush to examine under a microscope in order to make a diagnosis

boil

Bacterial infection of a hair follicle; also called a *furuncle*

burn, 1st degree

Mild burn that damages epidermis only; results in erythema but no blisters; generally, there is no scarring

>5.9 Illustration comparing the depth of the three types of burn

burn, 2nd degree

Burn damage that extends through the epidermis and into the dermis, causing blisters to form; scarring may occur

burn, 3rd degree

Burn damage to the full thickness of skin and into underlying tissues; infection and fluid loss are major concerns; usually requires skin grafts to cover burned areas; scarring will occur

cauterization

Intentional destruction of tissue by a caustic chemical, electric current, laser, or freezing

cellulitis

Inflammation of connective tissue cells of skin

chemabrasion
  chem/o = chemical

Removal of superficial layers of skin using chemicals; also called a *chemical peel*

contusion

Blunt trauma to skin that results in bruising

+ TERMINOLOGY TIDBIT

The term *contusion* comes from the Latin word *contusion* meaning "to bruise or crush."

cryosurgery
  cry/o = cold

Using extreme cold to freeze and destroy tissue

culture and sensitivity (C&S)

Laboratory test that grows a colony of bacteria removed from infected area in order to identify the specific type of bacteria and then determine its sensitivity to a variety of antibiotics

cyst

Fluid-filled sac under the skin

debridement

Removal of foreign material and dead or damaged tissue from a wound

decubitus ulcer (decub)

Open sore caused by pressure over bony prominences obstructing blood flow; can appear in bedridden patients who lie in one position too long and can be difficult to heal; commonly called a *bedsore* or a *pressure sore*

+ TERMINOLOGY TIDBIT

The term *decubitus* comes from the Latin word *decumbo*, meaning "lying down," which leads to the use of the term for a bedsore or pressure sore.

dermabrasion
  derm/o = skin

Scraping skin with rotating wire brushes or sandpaper; used to remove acne scars

dermatome
  derm/o = skin
  -tome = instrument to cut

Instrument that cuts out a small section of skin or a thin slice of skin to be used for a graft

ecchymosis

"Black and blue" skin bruise caused by blood collecting under skin after trauma

>5.10 Man lying supine on the ground with a large ecchymosis on his left lateral rib cage

erythema
  erythr/o = red

Redness of skin

fissure

Cracklike break in skin

gangrene

Tissue necrosis caused by loss of blood supply

+ **TERMINOLOGY TIDBIT**

The term *gangrene* comes from the Greek word *gangraina* meaning "an eating sore," which describes how this condition progresses by growing deeper and wider."

herpes simplex

Infection by herpes simplex virus (HSV) causing painful blisters around lips and nose; commonly called *fever blisters*

>5.11 Herpes simplex infection, commonly called "fever blisters"
Source: Courtesy of Jason L. Smith, MD

herpes zoster

Viral infection of a nerve root that causes the appearance of very painful blisters along the path of a nerve; commonly called *shingles*

impetigo

Inflammatory skin disease with pustules that rupture and become crusted

>5.12 Impetigo
Source: Courtesy of Jason L. Smith, MD

laceration

Jagged-edged skin wound caused by tearing of the skin; does not mean a skin cut

laser surgery

Removal of skin lesions and birthmarks using laser beam

lesion

General term than indicates the presence of some type of tissue abnormality

+ **TERMINOLOGY TIDBIT**

The term *lesion* comes from the Latin word *laedere* meaning "to injure."

macule

Flat, discolored spot on the skin surface; example is a freckle or birthmark

malignant melanoma (MM)
  melan/o = black
  -oma = tumor

Aggressive form of skin cancer that originates in a melanocyte; prone to metastasize or spread

>5.13 Malignant melanoma
Source: Courtesy of Jason L. Smith, MD

Term	Explanation
necrosis **necr/o** = death **-oma** = abnormal condition	Area of tissue death >5.14 Necrosis Source: Courtesy of Jason L. Smith, MD
nevus	Pigmented skin blemish, birthmark, or mole
nodule	Solid, raised clump of skin cells
onychia **onych/o** = nail	Inflamed nail bed
papule	Small, solid, raised lesion on surface of the skin
petechiae	Flat, pinpoint, purplish spots from bleeding under the skin
pruritus	Severe itching
psoriasis	Chronic inflammatory condition consisting of crusty papules forming patches with circular borders >5.15 Psoriasis Source: Courtesy of Jason L. Smith, MD
purpura	Purplish-red bruises usually occurring in people with thin, easily damaged skin >5.16 Purpura Source: Courtesy of Jason L. Smith, MD

Term	Explanation
pustule	Raised spot on the skin containing pus
skin graft (SG)	Transfer of the skin from a normal area to cover another site; used to treat burn victims and after some surgical procedure

squamous cell carcinoma (SCC)
  carcin/o = cancer
  -oma = tumor
	Skin cancer that begins in the epidermis but may grow into deeper tissue but does not generally metastasize to other areas of the body >5.17 Squamous cell carcinoma Source: Courtesy of Jason L. Smith, MD

tinea	Fungal skin disease resulting in itching, scaling lesions >5.18 Characteristic circular rash of tinea Source: Courtesy of Jason L. Smith, MD
ulcer	Open sore or lesion in the skin or mucous membrane
urticaria	Skin eruption of pale reddish wheals with severe itching; usually associated with food allergy, stress, or drug reactions ➕ **TERMINOLOGY TIDBIT** The term *urticaria* comes from the Latin word *urtica* meaning "nettle."
varicella	Viral infection with skin rash; commonly called *chicken pox* >5.19 Characteristic blistered rash of varicella (chicken pox) Source: Centers for Disease Control & Prevention

vesicle
  vesic/o = bladder, sac
  -cle = small
	Small, fluid-filled raised spot on the skin

wheal	Small, round, raised area on the skin that may be accompanied by itching; usually seen in allergic reactions

Dermatology Abbreviations

The following list presents common dermatology abbreviations.

BCC	basal cell carcinoma	**MM**	malignant melanoma
BX, bx	biopsy	**SG**	skin graft
C&S	culture and sensitivity	**SCC**	squamous cell carcinoma
decub	decubitus ulcer	**STSG**	split-thickness skin graft
Derm	dermatology	**Subcu, Subq**	subcutaneous
HSV	herpes simplex virus	**SQ**	subcutaneous
I&D	incision and drainage	**ung**	ointment
ID	intradermal		

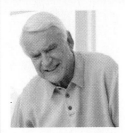

History of Present Illness

A 71-year-old male was referred to a dermatologist for evaluation of right foot ulcers that had not healed for 3 years. The ulcers first began as a tender, reddened, pustule on the lateral aspect of the right foot. The first ulcer appeared 3 months later and was quickly followed by the development of two additional ulcers. The lesions have not improved with treatment with oral antibiotics, topical anti-inflammatory cream, or whirlpool regimen.

Past Medical History

Patient was diagnosed with thromboangiitis obliterans 8 years ago. He had a vascular bypass for the right lower leg 5 years ago and for the left lower leg 2 years ago. He tests negative for diabetes mellitus.

Family and Social History

Patient is a retired night watchman. He is active and engages in extensive landscaping of his yard for a hobby. He smoked 2 packs of cigarettes per week beginning in his teenage years but stopped smoking at the time thromboangiitis obliterans was diagnosed. He denies alcohol or illicit drug use. He has been married for 49 years and has 3 married children. His mother died at age 75 following complications of type II diabetes mellitus necessitating bilateral below-the-knee amputations. His father is still alive at 93 years and in reasonable health for his age. He has no siblings.

Physical Examination

There are three ulcers on the lateral aspect of the right foot and ankle. Each measures approximately 3 by 4 cms. The ulcers are covered by necrotic tissue, and there are copious amounts of pus drainage from each. Erythema is noted in the skin around the edge of each ulcer.

Diagnostic Tests

C&S of drainage from each ulcer revealed staphylococcus bacterial infections that were found to be resistant to penicillin and sensitive to vancomycin, which is available only in IV form. Fungal scrapings were negative.

Diagnosis

Gangrene ulcers right lower leg.

Plan of Treatment

1. Admit to the hospital for IV antibiotic therapy, whirlpool, and surgical debridement of the ulcers
2. Schedule the patient for skin graft in the future when infection has cleared up and if lower leg circulation is sufficient to support healing of the grafts

Critical Thinking Questions

Answer the following questions regarding this case study. Do not just copy words out of the case study but translate all medical terms. In order to answer some of these questions, you may need to look up information in another chapter of this text, in a medical dictionary, or online. Answers are found at the back of the book.

1. Describe how the ulcers first appeared before they were actual ulcers.

2. Describe the treatments that have not healed the ulcers.

3. What medical condition does this patient not have that his mother did have?

4. Which of the following regarding the ulcers is NOT true?
   a. edges of ulcers are blue in color
   b. no fungi are present
   c. is covered in dead tissue
   d. a lot of pus is present

5. Explain what a C&S is. What does it mean that the bacteria are resistant to penicillin and sensitive to vancomycin?

6. The ulcers are infected by staphylococcus bacteria. Go to www.mayoclinic.com; type "staph infections" in the search box; and write a brief description about where this bacterium is found and how it causes serious infections.

7. This patient has ulcers that are caused by gangrene. What is the root cause of gangrene?

8. Explain each of the treatments planned when he is admitted to the hospital.

Sound It Out

The following are some of the key terms from this chapter written as their phonetic spelling. Sound out each term and write it in the blank. Pronunciations for all terms are included in the audio glossary at www.mymedicalterminologylab.com.

1. on-ih-koh-my-KOH-sis _____

2. cry-oh-SER-jer-ee _____

3. ah-BRAY-zhun _____

4. add-eh-POH-ma _____

5. kon-TWO-shun _____

6. SIST _____

7. al-oh-PEE-she-ah _____

8. an-hi-DROH-sis _____

9. BYE-op-see _____

10. kaw-ter-ih-ZAY-shun _____

11. sell-you-LYE-tis _____

12. kee-mah-BRAY-zhun _____

13. VAIR-ih-chell-a _____

14. ULL-ser _____

15. ek-ih-MOH-sis _____

16. de-BREED-mint _____

17. AB-sess _____

18. DER-mah-tohm _____

19. ep-ih-DER-mal _____

20. er-ih-THEE-mah _____

21. FISH-er _____

22. sigh-ah-NOH-sis _____

23. GANG-green _____

24. high-poh-DER-mik _____

25. im-peh-TYE-goh _____

26. PUS-tyool _____

27. VESS-ikl _____

28. add-eh-NOP-ah-the _____

29. KAIR-ah-tin _____

30. lip-OH-mah _____

31. NOD-yool _____

32. MACK-yool _____

33. LEE-shun _____

34. er-tih-KAY-ree-ah _____

35. mel-AN-oh-sight _____

36. sklair-ah-DER-mah _____

37. neh-KROH-sis _____

38. PAP-yool _____

39. zee-roh-DER-mah _____

40. soh-RYE-ah-sis _____

41. hi-drad-eh-NYE-tis _____

42. per-kyu-TAY-nee-us _____

43. der-mah-TALL-oh-jee _____

44. pye-oh-JEN-ik _____

45. on-ih-koh-FAY-jee-ah _____

46. seb-or-EE-ah _____

47. sub-kyoo-TAY-nee-us _____

48. TIN-ee-ah _____

49. UNG-gwal _____

50. loo-koh-DER-mah _____

Transcription Practice

Each of the following sentences is written in common English. Underline any words or phrases that can be replaced by a medical term. Then rewrite the entire sentence using medical terms. Answers are found at the end of book.

1. The specialist in treating skin conditions removed a sample of skin with a knife and examined it under a microscope to determine that the patient has a pigmented congenital skin blemish rather than aggressive skin cancer beginning in a melanocyte.

   _____

   _____

2. A laboratory test that grows a colony of bacteria to identify the type was performed to determine how best to treat the infected open sore.

   _____

   _____

3. The patient had a very large hair follicle with a bacterial infection surrounded by a large area of inflamed connective tissue skin cells around it.

   _____

   _____

4. Ms. Marks was lucky; when she tripped off the curb, she received only skin trauma that scraped away a layer of skin and blunt trauma to the skin resulting in bruises.

   _____

   _____

5. Mr. Brown's chronic exposure to toxins at work had left him with dry skin, scaly skin, and thick skin.

   _____

   _____

6. After years of nail biting, the patient developed a soft nail condition and an abnormal fungus nail condition that required surgical removal of the nail.

   _____

   _____

7. To repair the areas of full thickness burns, a transfer of skin from a normal area to cover another site was necessary.

   _____

   _____

8. Mr. Strong was concerned that the lump he could feel under his skin was a gland tumor, but it turned out to be only a fat tumor and was removed with a surgical removal of the fat.

   _____

   _____

9. The surgeon who uses surgery to improve the appearance of damaged skin helped Mr. Marsh decide whether to have abrasion using chemicals or abrasion using a rotating wire brush for his face lift.

_____

_____

10. New medical students often have difficulty telling the difference between a flat discolored spot, a raised solid lesion, and a fluid-filled sac under the skin.

_____

_____

Labeling Exercise

Write the name of each structure on the numbered line. Also use this space to write the combining form where appropriate.

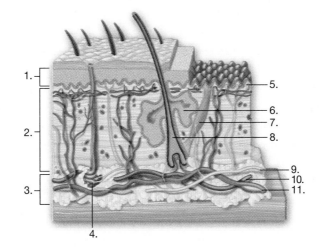

1._____   7._____

2._____   8._____

3._____   9._____

4._____   10._____

5._____   11._____

6._____

Build Medical Terms

Use each of the following word parts to build the indicated medical terms.

1. The suffix –**derma** means skin condition.
   a. dry skin condition _____
   b. red skin condition _____
   c. pus skin condition _____
   d. hard skin condition _____
   e. thick skin condition _____

2. The combining form **hidr/o** means sweat.
   a. sweat gland inflammation _____
   b. lack of sweat abnormal condition _____

3. The combining form **melan/o** means black.
   a. black cell _____
   b. black tumor _____

4. The combining form **dermat/o** means skin.
   a. skin disease _____
   b. skin surgical repair _____
   c. skin study of _____

5. The combining form **onych/o** means nail.
   a. nail softening _____
   b. nail fungus abnormal condition _____
   c. nail surgical removal _____

Spelling

Some of the following terms are misspelled. Identify the incorrect terms and spell them correctly in the blank provided.

1. empetigo _____

2. urticaria _____

3. wheel _____

4. psoriasis _____

5. fissure _____

6. tenia _____

7. peteckiae _____

8. gangreen _____

9. cauterization _____

10. necrowsis _____

Fill in the Blank

Fill in the blank to complete each of the following sentences.

1. A(n) _____ is a cracklike break in the skin while a(n) _____ is a jagged-edged skin wound.

2. Infection by the _____ virus causes painful blisters around the lips.

3. Ms. Branch had her acne scars removed with _____.

4. A diagnosis of _____ burn was made when the physician noted that the full thickness of skin was burned away.

5. A freckle is an example of a(n) _____.

6. The severe area of necrosis required _____ to remove the dead and damaged tissue.

7. An _____ is a typical black and blue bruise from trauma.

8. The physician performed a(n) _____ to obtain a sample of the infected tissue to examine under a microscope.

9. A raised skin lesion that is solid is a(n) _____, but if it contains pus, it is a(n) _____.

10. Unfortunately, the bedridden patient developed _____ from being in one position too long.

Abbreviation Matching

Match each abbreviation with its definition.

_____	**1.** bx	**A.**	skin graft
_____	**2.** MM	**B.**	basal cell carcinoma
_____	**3.** SQ	**C.**	intradermal
_____	**4.** SCC	**D.**	split thickness skin graft
_____	**5.** C&S	**E.**	biopsy
_____	**6.** BCC	**F.**	ointment
_____	**7.** SG	**G.**	squamous cell carcinoma
_____	**8.** STSG	**H.**	subcutaneous
_____	**9.** ung	**I.**	malignant melanoma
_____	**10.** ID	**J.**	culture and sensitivity

Medical Term Analysis

*Examine each of the following terms. Begin by dividing it into its word parts and writing them in the indicated blanks (**P = prefix**, **WR = word root**; **CF = combining form**; **S = suffix**). Follow with the definition of each word part and then finally the meaning of the full term.*

1. **adenomegaly**

   CF _____

   means _____

   S _____

   means _____

   Term meaning: _____
   _____

2. **adipocyte**

   CF _____

   means _____

   S _____

   means _____

   Term meaning: _____
   _____

3. **cyanosis**

   CF _____

   means _____

   S _____

   means _____

   Term meaning: _____
   _____

4. **hypodermic**

   P _____

   means _____

   WR _____

   means _____

   S _____

   means _____

   Term meaning: _____
   _____

5. **keratogenic**

   CF _____

   means _____

   S _____

   means _____

   Term meaning: _____
   _____

6. **lipectomy**

   WR _____

   means _____

   S _____

   means _____

   Term meaning: _____
   _____

7. pyorrhea

CF _____

means _____

S _____

means _____

Term meaning: _____

_____

8. erythroderma

CF _____

means _____

S _____

means _____

Term meaning: _____

_____

9. trichomycosis

CF _____

means _____

WR _____

means _____

S _____

means _____

Term meaning: _____

_____

10. subcutaneous

P _____

means _____

WR _____

means _____

S _____

means _____

Term meaning: _____

_____

Photomatch Challenge

Match each skin lesion with its picture.

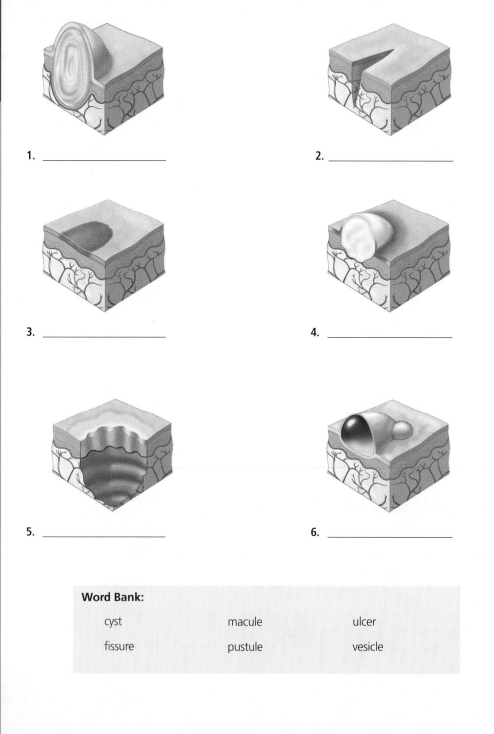

1. _____

2. _____

3. _____

4. _____

5. _____

6. _____

Word Bank:

cyst	macule	ulcer
fissure	pustule	vesicle

Crossword Puzzle

Use the definitions given to complete the crossword puzzle.

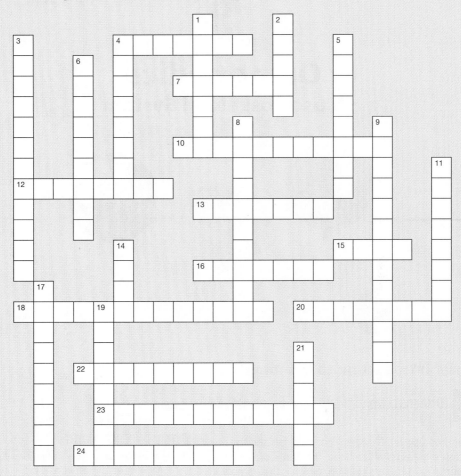

ACROSS

4 Localized collection of pus
7 Flat, discolored spot
10 Term meaning "surgical removal of nail"
12 Area of tissue death
13 Inflamed nail bed
15 Also called a furuncle
16 Cracklike break in the skin
18 Term meaning "one who studies the skin"
20 Term describing blue skin
22 Outer layer of the skin
23 Also called a chemical peel
24 Chicken pox

DOWN

1 Hard protein in hair and nails
2 Fungal skin disease
3 Term meaning "pertaining to under skin"
4 Term meaning "gland inflammation"
5 Term meaning "black tumor"
6 Term meaning "dry skin"
8 "Black and blue" bruise
9 Term meaning "abnormal condition of excessive sweat"
11 Severe itching
14 Fluid-filled sac under the skin
17 instrument used to cut skin
19 Baldness
21 Term meaning "resembling fat"

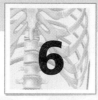

6

Orthopedics
Musculoskeletal System

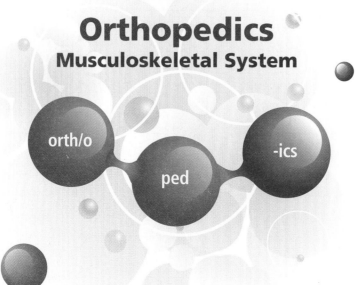

orth/o

ped

-ics

A Brief Introduction to Orthopedics

UNDERSTAND the function of the musculoskeletal system.

The musculoskeletal system consists of the **bones, muscles,** and **joints** of the body. The bones are joined by **ligaments** to form the **skeleton,** which is the framework of the body. The place where two bones meet is called a joint and provides flexibility for movement. Muscles, attached to the skeleton by **tendons,** cross over joints. These muscles contract to move the bones at each joint.

> **✚ TERMINOLOGY TIDBIT**
>
> The term *skeleton* comes from the Greek word *skeltos* meaning "dried up." It was originally used to refer to a dried-up mummified body, but over time came to be used for bones.

DESCRIBE the medical specialty of orthopedics.

   Orthopedics, or **orthopedic surgery,** is the medical specialty that treats disorders involving the musculoskeletal system. Physicians in this specialty, called **orthopedists** or **orthopedic surgeons,** use medical, surgical, and physical means to correct defects and improve the function of bones, joints, and muscles. Examples of conditions treated by orthopedists are:

- Birth defects such as spina bifida
- Trauma such as fractures
- Infections such as osteomyelitis

- Tumors such as osteogenic sarcoma
- Inflammatory conditions such as arthritis
- Muscular problems such as muscular dystrophy

 DEFINE orthopedic-related combining forms, prefixes, and suffixes.

Orthopedic Combining Forms

The following list presents new combining forms important for building and defining orthopedic terms.

arthr/o	joint		my/o	muscle
burs/o	bursa		myel/o	bone marrow
carp/o	carpals (wrist)		oste/o	bone
chondr/o	cartilage		patell/o	patella (knee cap)
clavicul/o	clavicle (collar bone)		phalang/o	phalanges (fingers and toes)
coccyg/o	coccyx (tailbone)		pub/o	pubis (part of pelvis)
cost/o	rib		radi/o	radius (part of forearm)
crani/o	skull		sacr/o	sacrum
femor/o	femur (thigh bone)		scapul/o	scapula (shoulder blade)
fibul/o	fibula (thinner lower leg bone)		spondyl/o	vertebra
humer/o	humerus (upper arm bone)		stern/o	sternum (breast bone)
ili/o	ilium (part of pelvis)		tars/o	tarsals (ankle)
ischi/o	ischium (part of pelvis)		ten/o	tendon
mandibul/o	mandible (lower jaw)		tendin/o	tendon
maxill/o	maxilla (upper jaw)		tibi/o	tibia (shin, larger lower leg bone)
metacarp/o	metacarpus (hand bones)		uln/o	ulna (part of forearm)
metatars/o	metatarsus (foot bones)		vertebr/o	vertebra
muscul/o	muscle			

The following list presents combining forms that are not specific to orthopedics but are also used for building and defining orthopedic terms.

cutane/o	skin		lord/o	bent backward
electr/o	electricity		orth/o	straight
fibr/o	fibrous		path/o	disease
kyph/o	hump		scoli/o	crooked, bent

Suffix Review

These suffixes and prefixes were introduced in Chapters 2 and 3. They are being reviewed in this chapter because they are especially important for building orthopedic terms.

-ac	pertaining to		-itis	inflammation
-al	pertaining to		-kinesia	movement
-algia	pain		-malacia	softening
-ar	pertaining to		-metry	process of measuring
-ary	pertaining to		-oma	tumor
-asthenia	weakness		-osis	abnormal condition
-centesis	puncture to withdraw fluid		-otomy	cutting into
-clasia	surgical breaking		-ous	pertaining to
-cyte	cell		-pathy	disease
-desis	surgical fixation		-plasty	surgical repair
-dynia	pain		-porosis	porous
-eal	pertaining to		-rrhaphy	suture
-ectomy	surgical removal		-rrhexis	rupture
-genic	producing		-scope	instrument for viewing
-gram	record		-scopy	process of visually examining
-graphy	process of recording		-tome	instrument to cut
-ic	pertaining to		-trophy	development

Prefix Review

a-	without		hyper-	excessive
brady-	slow		per-	through
dys-	difficult		sub-	under
inter-	between		supra-	above
intra-	within			

Organs Commonly Treated in Orthopedics

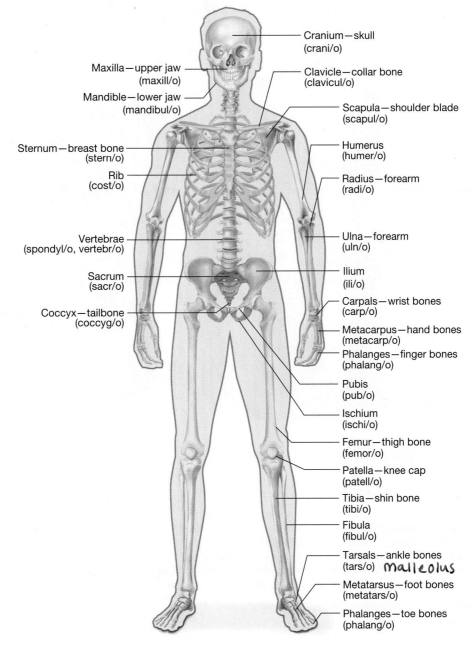

Cranium—skull
(crani/o)

Maxilla—upper jaw
(maxill/o)

Mandible—lower jaw
(mandibul/o)

Clavicle—collar bone
(clavicul/o)

Scapula—shoulder blade
(scapul/o)

Sternum—breast bone
(stern/o)

Humerus
(humer/o)

Rib
(cost/o)

Radius—forearm
(radi/o)

Vertebrae
(spondyl/o, vertebr/o)

Ulna—forearm
(uln/o)

Sacrum
(sacr/o)

Ilium
(ili/o)

Coccyx—tailbone
(coccyg/o)

Carpals—wrist bones
(carp/o)

Metacarpus—hand bones
(metacarp/o)

Phalanges—finger bones
(phalang/o)

Pubis
(pub/o)

Ischium
(ischi/o)

Femur—thigh bone
(femor/o)

Patella—knee cap
(patell/o)

Tibia—shin bone
(tibi/o)

Fibula
(fibul/o)

Tarsals—ankle bones
(tars/o) *malleolus*

Metatarsus—foot bones
(metatars/o)

Phalanges—toe bones
(phalang/o)

>6.1 The skeleton

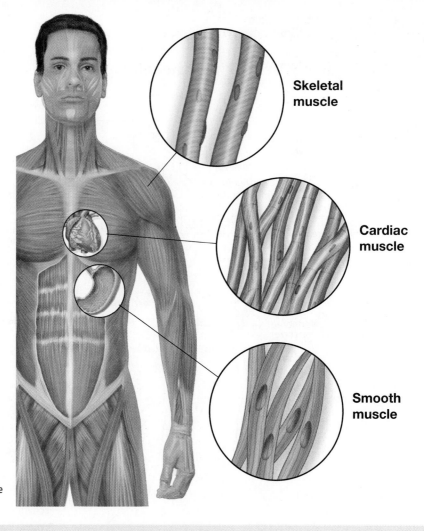

Skeletal muscle

Cardiac muscle

Smooth muscle

>6.2 Types of muscle tissue in the body

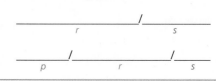 **BUILD** orthopedic medical terms from word parts.

Building Orthopedic Terms

This section presents word parts most often used to build orthopedic terms. Following the explanation of the term, you have the opportunity to begin building your own vocabulary. Read the meaning for each term and then fill in the blanks to build a single medical term. Use the slashes to divide prefixes, word roots, combining vowels, and suffixes. To help you out you will find a key to the word parts underneath the blanks: r for word roots, p for prefix, cv for combining vowel, and s for suffix. Remember that not every term will contain all these word parts; it's up to you to decide which to use. As you gain experience, this process becomes easier. Answers can be found at the back of the book.

1. **-ac**–suffix meaning **pertaining to**

   A suffix used to turn a combining form for a bone into an adjective

   a. pertaining to the ilium

   _____/_____
                           r   s

   b. pertaining to under the ilium

   _____/_____/_____
          p   r   s

2. **-al**–suffix meaning **pertaining to**

A suffix used to turn a combining form for a bone into an adjective

a. pertaining to the wrist

_____/_____
r   s

b. pertaining to the rib

_____/_____
r   s

c. pertaining to between the ribs

_____/_____/_____
p   r   s

d. pertaining to the femur

_____/_____
r   s

e. pertaining to the humerus

_____/_____
r   s

f. pertaining to the ischium

_____/_____
r   s

g. pertaining to the metacarpus

_____/_____
r   s

h. pertaining to the metatarsus

_____/_____
r   s

i. pertaining to the radius

_____/_____
r   s

j. pertaining to the sacrum

_____/_____
r   s

k. pertaining to the sternum

_____/_____
r   s

l. pertaining to under the sternum

_____/_____/_____
p   r   s

m. pertaining to the tarsus

_____/_____
r   s

n. pertaining to the tibia

_____/_____
r   s

o. pertaining to the vertebra

_____/_____
r   s

p. pertaining to between the vertebra

_____/_____/_____
p   r   s

---

3. **-ar**–suffix meaning **pertaining to**

A suffix used to turn a combining form for a bone into an adjective

a. pertaining to the clavicle

_____/_____
r   s

b. pertaining to the fibula

_____/_____
r   s

c. pertaining to the mandible

_____/_____
r   s

d. pertaining to under the mandible

_____/_____/_____
p   r   s

e. pertaining to the patella   _____/_____
                                              r   s

f. pertaining to the scapula   _____/_____
                                              r   s

g. pertaining to under the scapula   _____/_____/_____
                                                p   r   s

h. pertaining to the ulna   _____/_____
                                          r   s

---

4. **arthr/o**–combining form meaning **joint**

A joint is formed where two or more bones meet; also called an **articulation;** most joints in the body are freely moving called **synovial joints**

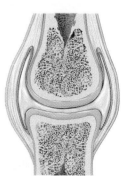

>6.3 Joints

a. puncture to withdraw fluid from a joint   _____/_____/_____
                                                         r   cv   s

b. surgically break a joint   _____/_____/_____
                                          r   cv   s

c. surgical fixation of a joint   _____/_____/_____
                                              r   cv   s

d. process of recording a joint   _____/_____/_____
                                              r   cv   s

e. record of a joint   ___arthr___/_o_/_gram_
                                 r   cv   s

f. joint inflammation   _____/_____
                                    r   s

g. process of visually examining a joint   _____/_____/_____
                                                       r   cv   s

h. instrument to visually examine a joint   _____/_____/_____
                                                        r   cv   s

i. surgical repair of a joint   _____/_____/_____
                                           r   cv   s

j. joint pain   _____/_____
                           r   s

---

5. **-ary**–suffix meaning **pertaining to**

A suffix used to turn a combining form for a bone into an adjective

a. pertaining to the maxilla   _____/_____
                                            r   s

b. pertaining to above the maxilla   _____/_____/_____
                                                p   r   s

---

6. **burs/o**–combining form meaning **bursa**

   A bursa is a fluid-filled sac found between tendon and bone to reduce friction

   a. pertaining to a bursa _____/_____
   r   s

   b. bursa inflammation _____/_____
   r   s

   c. surgical removal of a bursa _____/_____
   r   s

7. **chondr/o**–combining form meaning **cartilage**

   Cartilage is a tough, flexible connective tissue covers ends of bones in joint; serves as shock absorber

   a. pertaining to cartilage _____/_____
   r   s

   b. cartilage inflammation _____/_____
   r   s

   c. surgical removal of cartilage _____/_____
   r   s

   d. cartilage softening _____/____/_____
   r   cv   s

   e. cartilage tumor _____/_____
   r   s

   f. surgical repair of cartilage _____/____/_____
   r   cv   s

8. **crani/o**–combining form meaning **skull**

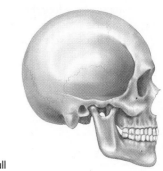

>6.4 Skull

   a. pertaining to the skull _____/_____
   r   s

   b. pertaining to within the skull _____/_____/____
   p   r   s

   c. cutting into the skull _____/_____
   r   s

   d. surgical repair of the skull _____crani____/_o_/_plasty_
   r   cv   s

9. **-eal**–suffix meaning **pertaining to**

A suffix used to turn a combining form for a bone into an adjective

a. pertaining to the coccyx

_____/_____
　　　　　　　　　r　　　　　　s

b. pertaining to the phalanges

_____/_____
　　　　　　　　　r　　　　　　s

10. **-ic**–suffix meaning **pertaining to**

A suffix used to turn a combining form for a bone into an adjective

a. pertaining to the pubis

_____/_____
　　　　　　　　　r　　　　　　s

b. pertaining to above the pubis

_____/_____/_____
　　　p　　　　　　　　r　　　　　s

11. **-kinesia**–suffix meaning **movement**

a. slow movement

_____/_____
　　　　　　　　　p　　　　　　s

b. difficult movement

_____/_____
　　　　　　　　　p　　　　　　s

c. excessive movement

_____/_____
　　　　　　　　　p　　　　　　s

12. **muscul/o**–combining form meaning **muscle**

Contraction of muscle tissue produces movement in the body; three types of muscles are found in the body: **skeletal muscle** moves the skeleton, **smooth muscle** produces movement of internal organs such as the stomach and bladder, **cardiac muscle** produces heartbeat

a. pertaining to muscle

_____/_____
　　　　　　　　　r　　　　　　s

b. pertaining to within muscle

_____/_____/_____
　　　p　　　　　　　　r　　　　　s

>6.5 Muscles

13. **myel/o**–combining form meaning **red bone marrow**

Red bone marrow is tissue found inside bones that produces blood cells

a. red bone marrow tumor

_____/_____
　　　　　　　　　r　　　　　　s

b. producing red bone marrow

_____/_____/_____
　　　　　　　　　r　　　cv　　　s

c. disease of red bone marrow

_____/_____/_____
　　　　　　　　　r　　　cv　　　s

14. **my/o**–combining form meaning **muscle**

   a. muscle pain   _____/_____
                                              r   s

   b. muscle weakness   _____/_____
                                              r   s

   c. record of muscle's electricity   _____/__/_____/__/___
                                       r   cv   r   cv   s

   d. process of recording muscle's electricity   _____/__/_____/__/___
                                       r   cv   r   cv   s

   e. muscle disease   _____/__/_____
                                         r   cv   s

   f. suture a muscle   _____/__/_____
                                         r   cv   s

   g. ruptured muscle   _____/__/_____
                                         r   cv   s

---

15. **oste/o**–combining form meaning **bone**

Bone is a hard, calcified connective tissue; functions include supporting and moving the body, providing vital protection to underlying organs such as heart, lungs, liver, and bladder, housing red bone marrow, which produces all blood cells, and serving as store house for important minerals such as calcium

   a. bone pain   _____/_____
                                             r   s

   b. bone cell   _oste_   / _o_ / _cyte_
                                       r   cv   s

   c. producing bone   _oste_   / _o_ / _gunic_
                                       r   cv   s

   d. bone and joint inflammation   _____/__/_____/_____
                                       r   cv   r   s

   e. bone and cartilage inflammation   _____/__/_____/_____
                                       r   cv   r   s

   f. bone and cartilage tumor   _____/__/_____/_____
                                       r   cv   r   s

   g. surgical breaking of a bone   _____/__/_____
                                       r   cv   s

   h. bone and red bone marrow inflammation   _____/__/_____/_____
                                       r   cv   r   s   >6.6 **Bone**

   i. bone disease   _oste_   / _o_ / _pathy_
                                     r   cv   s

   j. instrument to cut bone   _____/__/_____
                                       r   cv   s

k. bone softening

_____/____/_____
r   CV   s

l. porous bone

_____/____/_____
r   CV   s

---

16. spondyl/o–combining form meaning **vertebra**

a. abnormal condition of a vertebra

_____/_____
r   s

b. vertebra inflammation

_____/_____
r   s

---

17. ten/o–combining form meaning **tendon**
Tendons are strong bands of connective tissue that anchor muscles to bone

a. tendon pain

_____/_____
r   s

b. tendon pain

_____/____/_____
r   CV   s

c. surgical fixation of a tendon

_____/____/_____
r   CV   s

d. suture of a tendon

_____/____/_____
r   CV   s

---

18. tendin/o–combining form meaning **tendon**

a. pertaining to a tendon

_____/_____
r   s

b. tendon inflammation

_____/_____
r   s

c. surgical repair of a tendon

_____/____/_____
r   CV   s

d. abnormal condition of a tendon

_____/_____
r   s

EXPLAIN orthopedic medical terms.

Orthopedic Vocabulary

The orthopedic terms presented in this section include eponyms, modern English words, and those that contain Latin or Greek word parts but are not constructed solely from these word parts. When you recognize word parts within a term they will give you a hint about the word's meaning. In these instances, look for the word parts to follow the term.

Term	Explanation
bone graft	Surgical procedure that uses piece of bone to replace lost bone or to fuse two bones together
bone scan	Nuclear medicine scan using radioactive dye to visualize bones; especially useful for finding stress fractures and bone cancer

carpal tunnel syndrome (CTS)
carp/o = wrist
-al = pertaining to

Repetitive motion disorder caused by pressure on tendons and nerves as they pass through carpal tunnel of wrist

Inflamed median nerve

Tendons crossing the wrist

Carpal tunnel

Carpal bones

Blood vessel

>6.7 Nerves and blood vessels enclosed by carpal tunnel formed by wrist bones and tendons

closed fracture

Broken bone with no open skin wound; also called *simple fracture*

A

B

>6.8 (A) Closed (or simple) fracture and (B) compound (or open) fracture

comminuted fracture

Bone break where bone shatters into many small fragments

➕ **TERMINOLOGY TIDBIT**

The term *comminuted* comes from the Latin word *comminuere* meaning "to break into pieces."

compound fracture

Broken bone with open skin wound; also called *open fracture*

compression fracture

Bone break causing loss of height of vertebral body; may result from trauma, but in older persons, especially women, may occur in a bone weakened by osteoporosis

contracture

Abnormal shortening of muscle fibers, tendons, or connective tissue making it difficult to stretch muscle

Term	Explanation
creatine kinase (CK)	Muscle enzyme found in skeletal and cardiac muscle; elevated blood levels associated with heart attack, muscular dystrophy, and other skeletal muscle pathologies
deep tendon reflexes (DTR)	Involuntary muscle contraction in response to striking muscle tendon with reflex hammer; test used to determine whether muscles respond properly >6.9 Testing patellar reflex with a reflex hammer
dislocation	Occurs when bones in joint are displaced from normal alignment and ends of bones are no longer in contact with each other >6.10 The large bump on the top of the shoulder is caused by the upward dislocation of the humerus
dual-energy absorptiometry (DXA) **-metry** = process of measuring	Test using low-dose x-ray beams to measure bone density; used to diagnose osteoporosis
fibromyalgia fibr/o = fibrous my/o = muscle -algia = pain	Chronic condition with widespread aching and pain in the muscles and fibrous soft tissue
fixation	Procedure to stabilize fractured bone while it heals; *external fixation* includes casts, splints, and pins inserted through skin; *internal fixation* includes pins, plates, rods, screws, and wires that are put into place during surgical procedure called *open reduction*
fracture (FX, Fx)	Broken bone
greenstick fracture	Fracture with incomplete break; one side of the bone breaks and other side only bends; commonly seen in children because their bones are still pliable

+ TERMINOLOGY TIDBIT

The term *fracture* comes from the Latin word *fractura* meaning "to break."

Term	Explanation

herniated nucleus pulposus (HNP)

Protrusion of intervertebral disk between two vertebrae, which puts pressure on spinal nerves; also called *herniated disk* or *ruptured disk;* may require surgery

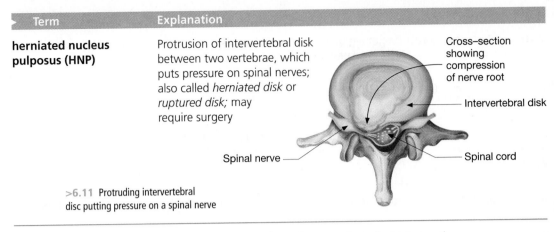

Cross–section showing compression of nerve root

Intervertebral disk

Spinal nerve

Spinal cord

>6.11 Protruding intervertebral disc putting pressure on a spinal nerve

---

impacted fracture

Fracture in which one bone fragment is pushed into another

---

kyphosis
 kyph/o = hump
 -osis = abnormal condition

Abnormal increase in normal outward curvature of thoracic spine; also called *hunchback* or *humpback*

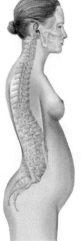
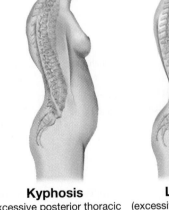
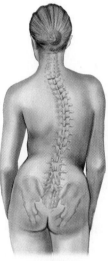

Kyphosis
(excessive posterior thoracic curvature—hunchback)

Lordosis
(excessive anterior lumbar curvature—swayback)

Scoliosis
(lateral curvature)

>6.12 Abnormal spinal curvatures: kyphosis, lordosis, and scoliosis

---

lordosis
 lord/o = bent backward
 -osis = abnormal condition

Abnormal increase in normal forward curvature of lumbar spine; also called *swayback* (see Figure 6.12>)

---

muscle atrophy
 a- = without
 -trophy = development

Loss of muscle bulk due to muscle disease, nervous system disease, or lack of use; commonly called *muscle wasting*

muscular dystrophy (MD)
muscul/o = muscle
-ar = pertaining to
dys- = difficult
-trophy = development

One of a group of inherited diseases involving progressive muscle degeneration, weakness, and atrophy

---

nonsteroidal anti-inflammatory drugs (NSAIDs)

Large group of drugs that provide mild pain relief and anti-inflammatory benefits for conditions such as arthritis

---

oblique fracture

Bone break in which fracture line runs along an angle to shaft of the bone

---

orthosis
orth/o = straight

Externally applied brace or splint used to prevent or correct deformities; *orthotist* is person skilled in making and adjusting orthoses

>6.13 A stroke patient with an orthotic brace on her right arm

---

osteoarthritis (OA)
oste/o = bone
arthr/o = joint
-itis = inflammation

Arthritis caused by loss of cartilage cushion covering bones in joint; most common in bearing weight joints; results in bone rubbing against bone

---

osteogenic sarcoma
oste/o = bone
-genic = producing
-oma = tumor

Most common type of bone cancer; usually begins in osteocytes found at ends of bones; most frequently occurs in persons 10–25 years old

---

pathologic fracture
path/o = disease

Broken bone caused by diseased or weakened bone, not trauma

---

percutaneous diskectomy
per- = through
cutane/o = skin
-ous = pertaining to
-ectomy = surgical removal

Use of a thin catheter tube inserted into intervertebral disk through skin to suck out pieces of herniated or ruptured disk; or laser is used to vaporize disk

prosthesis

Any artificial device used as substitute for body part that is either missing from birth or lost as the

> **+ TERMINOLOGY TIDBIT**
>
> The term *prosthesis* comes from the Greek word *prostithenai* meaning "an addition."

result of an accident or disease; example: artificial leg; *prosthetist* is person trained in making prostheses

---

radiography
 -graphy = process of recording

Diagnostic imaging procedure using x-rays to see internal structure of body; especially useful for visualizing bones and joints

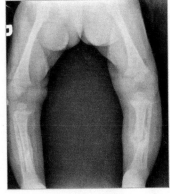

>6.14 X-ray of legs showing fractures in both tibias

---

reduction

Correcting fracture or dislocation by realigning bone; *closed reduction* moves bones externally;

> **+ TERMINOLOGY TIDBIT**
>
> The term *reduction* comes from the Latin word *reductio* meaning "to lead back."

open reduction manipulates bones through a surgical incision; open reduction usually performed before *internal fixation* of bony fragments

---

repetitive motion disorder

Group of chronic disorders with tendon, muscle, joint, and nerve damage caused by prolonged periods of pressure, vibration, or repetitive movements

---

rheumatoid arthritis (RA)
 arthr/o = joint
 -itis = inflammation

Arthritis with swelling, stiffness, pain, and degeneration of cartilage in joints caused by chronic soft tissue inflammation; may result in crippling deformities; an autoimmune disease

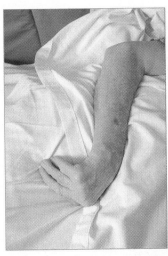

>6.15 Typical hand and wrist deformities of rheumatoid arthritis

scoliosis
  scoli/o = crooked
  -osis = abnormal condition

Abnormal lateral curvature of spine (see Figure 6.12>)

spasm

Sudden, involuntary, strong muscle contraction

spina bifida

Birth defect that occurs when vertebra fails to fully form around spinal cord; ranges from mild to severe; if spinal cord is damaged, paralysis results

spiral fracture

Bone break in which fracture line spirals around shaft of the bone; caused by twisting injury; often slower to heal than other types of fractures

sprain

Ligament injury from overstretching, but without joint dislocation or bone fracture

strain

Damage to the muscle or tendons from overuse or overstretching

stress fracture

A slight bone break caused by repetitive low-impact forces, such as running, rather than single forceful impact

total hip arthroplasty (THA)
  arthr/o = joint
  -plasty = surgical repair

Surgical reconstruction of hip with artificial hip joint; also called *total hip replacement (THR)*.

>6.16 A fractured femur (A) repaired with a total hip arthroplasty (B) **A**   **B**

total knee arthroplasty (TKA)
  arthr/o = joint
  -plasty = surgical repair

Surgical reconstruction of knee joint with artificial knee joint; also called *total knee replacement (TKR)*

transverse fracture

Bone break with fracture line straight across shaft of bone

Orthopedic Abbreviations

The following list presents common orthopedic abbreviations.

AE	above elbow	LE	lower extremity
AK	above knee	LLE	left lower extremity
BDT	bone density testing	LUE	left upper extremity
BE	below elbow	MD	muscular dystrophy
BK	below knee	NSAID	nonsteroidal anti-inflammatory drug
BMD	bone mineral density		
C1, C2, etc.	first cervical vertebra, second cervical vertebra, etc.	OA	osteoarthritis
		ORIF	open reduction–internal fixation
Ca	calcium	Orth, ortho	orthopedics
CK	creatine kinase	RA	rheumatoid arthritis
CTS	carpal tunnel syndrome	RLE	right lower extremity
DJD	degenerative joint disease	RUE	right upper extremity
DTR	deep tendon reflex	T1, T2, etc.	first thoracic vertebra, second thoracic vertebra, etc.
DXA	dual-energy absorptiometry		
EMG	electromyogram	THA	total hip arthroplasty
FX, Fx	fracture	THR	total hip replacement
HNP	herniated nucleus pulposus	TKA	total knee arthroplasty
IM	intramuscular	TKR	total knee replacement
JRA	juvenile rheumatoid arthritis	UE	upper extremity
L1, L2, etc.	first lumbar vertebra, second lumbar vertebra, etc.		

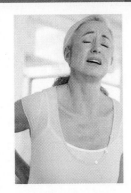

History of Present Illness

A 68-year-old female presents at the orthopedic clinic for an initial evaluation of severe low back pain that radiates into the posterior RLE and into her foot. Patient has experienced intermittent mild symptoms for the past 6 months. She states these symptoms typically last only one day and are gone when she wakes up the next morning. Current episode of severe pain began 2 days ago. She reports that there was no lifting or injury immediately preceding the pain but notes that both her husband and youngest son require physical assistance due to their medical conditions. She struggles to provide this assistance due to her history of carpal tunnel syndrome and compression fracture.

Past Medical History

Osteoporosis and compression fx of T10 four years ago, treated with an orthotic to support thoracic spine. She continues to take NSAIDs if experiences any thoracic back pain. Breast cancer, mastectomy, and chemotherapy with no reoccurrence in 12 years. Carpal tunnel syndrome requiring carpal tunnel release surgery when she was 52.

Family and Social History

Patient is married. Her husband, 85, has moderate Alzheimer's disease but is still able to remain at home. She was a line worker at a battery factory where she was required to lift 5-pound boxes of batteries at a rate of 60 per hour. She retired on disability following carpal tunnel release. Patient smoked cigarettes for 45 years, but quit 14 years ago. Father died at age 72 from myocardial infarction; mother died at 84 from renal failure; one sister is alive and well; three living children, no miscarriages, two children, oldest son and daughter are healthy, youngest son, 40, has spina bifida. He is confined to a wheelchair and lives at home with parents.

Physical Examination

Well-nourished, well-developed cooperative Caucasian female in obvious pain sitting on examination table. She has tenderness over lower spinal muscles on both sides of lumbar spine with right more tender than left. LE muscle strength is normal and there is no apparent muscle atrophy. DTR are normal on left and reduced on right.

Diagnostic Tests

Lumbar x-ray revealed mild spondylosis at L4-5 but no appreciable spinal arthritis. MRI confirms HNP at L45 level.

Diagnosis

L4-5 HNP

Plan of Treatment

1. Conservative treatment with physical therapy for pain relief, traction, and back-strengthening exercises
2. Consider percutaneous diskectomy if conservative treatment fails to improve symptoms
3. Meet with patient and family to plan alternative strategies so that she may avoid having to lift other family members

Critical Thinking Questions

Answer the following questions regarding this case study. Do not just copy words out of the case study; translate all medical terms. To answer some of these questions, you may need to look up information from another chapter of this text, in a medical dictionary, or online. Answers are found at the back of the book.

1. Use a medical reference source to give more information on osteoporosis. Why do you think that osteoporosis commonly leads to compression fractures?

   _____

   _____

2. Go to www.drugs.com and click on "Drugs by Condition." Then search for drugs that treat osteoporosis. Describe two different drugs that treat this condition.

   _____

   _____

3. List all abbreviations used and what each stands for.

   _____

   _____

4. Which of the following is NOT part of this patient's Previous Medical Diagnoses?
   a. collapse of 10th thoracic vertebra
   b. radiation treatment for cancer
   c. a repetitive motion disorder
   d. wearing a brace

5. Define the medical conditions of her parents, husband, and son. Use the index of your text to find these conditions.

_____

_____

6. List and describe the two diagnostic imaging procedures this patient underwent. What were their results?

_____

_____

7. What are the PT plans for this patient?

_____

_____

8. Describe the planned surgical treatment if the conservative treatment does not improve her symptoms.

_____

_____

Sound It Out

The following are some of the key terms from this chapter written as their phonetic spelling. Sound out each term and write it in the blank. Pronunciations for all terms are included in the audio glossary at www.mymedicalterminologylab.com <http://www.mymedicalterminologylab.com/>.

1. OSS-tee-oh-sight _____

2. figh-broh-my-AL-jee-ah _____

3. brad-ee-kih-NEE-see-ah _____

4. KON-droh-plas-tee _____

5. mack-sih-LAIR-ree _____

6. cock-eh-JEE-all _____

7. ee-lek-troh-MY-oh-gram _____

8. or-THO-sis _____

9. sin-OH-vee-al _____

10. FEM-or-all _____

11. HYOO-mer-us _____

12. SAY-crum _____

13. ar-thro-PLAS-tee _____

14. ILL-ee-ack _____

15. in-ter-VER-teh-bral _____

16. in-tra-MUSS-kew-lar _____

17. ki-FOH-sis _____

18. lor-DOH-sis _____

19. man-DIB-yoo-lar _____

20. fay-lan-JEE-all _____

21. ber-SIGH-tis _____

22. met-ah-CAR-pal _____

23. UHL-nar _____

24. FIB-yoo-lar _____

25. my-ah-LOH-mah _____

26. ar-thro-sen-TEE-sis _____

27. kray-nee-OTT-oh-mee _____

28. my-oh-REK-sis _____

29. oss-tee-oh-mi-ell-EYE-tis _____

30. skoh-lee-OH-sis _____

31. pa-TELL-ar _____

32. ten-NOR-ah-fee _____

33. pross-THEE-sis _____

34. ten-oh-DEE-sis _____

35. PYOO-bik _____

36. RAY-dee-all _____

37. met-ah-TAHR-sal _____

38. ISS-she-um _____

39. ray-dee-OG-rah-fee _____

40. SKAP-yoo-lah _____

41. spon-dih-LOW-sis _____

42. STER-num _____

43. CAR-tih-lij _____

44. kon-DROH-mah _____

45. TEN-din-oh-plas-tee _____

46. oss-tee-oh-por-ROH-sis _____

47. ten-oh-DIN-ee-ah _____

48. kon-TRACK-chur _____

49. PYOO-bis _____

50. TIB-ee-all _____

Transcription Practice

Each of the following sentences is written in common English. Underline any words or phrases that can be replaced by a medical term. Then rewrite the entire sentence using medical terms. Answers are found at the end of the book.

1. The shattered bone break required manipulation through a surgical incision and a surgical procedure to stabilize.

   _____

   _____

2. Diagnostic imaging procedure to visualize bones revealed a pertaining to the femur bone and cartilage tumor.

   _____

   _____

3. The patient's chronically inflamed bursa eventually required surgical removal of the bursa.

   _____

   _____

4. Mary's hand deformities from an autoimmune type of arthritis were improved by wearing an external brace or splint.

_____

_____

5. When Otto's loss of cartilage cushion arthritis in his knee prevented him from walking, he had a surgical reconstruction with an artificial knee.

_____

_____

6. What first appeared to be a fracture with an angled fracture line turned out to be a fracture that spirals down the bone shaft.

_____

_____

7. A nuclear medicine scan of the bone was necessary to identify the slight fracture caused by repetitive low-impact forces.

_____

_____

8. Jean's pertaining to the vertebrae porous bones was diagnosed by low dose x-ray beams that measure bone density.

_____

_____

9. The child's abnormal movements caused the physician to suspect an inherited disease with progressive muscle degeneration and weakness.

_____

_____

10. The ankle damage to the tendons from overstretching was severe enough to require surgical fixation of the tendon.

_____

_____

Labeling Exercise

Write the name of each bone on the numbered line. Also use this space to write the common name and combining form where appropriate.

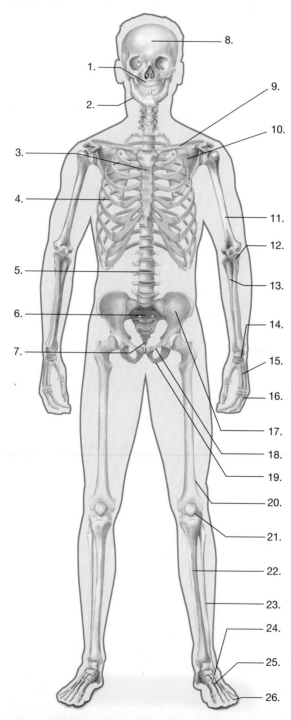

1.
2.
3.
4.
5.
6.
7.
8.
9.
10.
11.
12.
13.
14.
15.
16.
17.
18.
19.
20.
21.
22.
23.
24.
25.
26.

1._____

2._____

3._____

4._____

5._____

6._____

7._____

8._____

9._____

10._____

11._____

12._____

13._____

14._____

15._____

16._____

17._____

18._____

19._____

20._____

21._____

22._____

23._____

24._____

25._____

26._____

Build Medical Terms

Use each of the following word parts to build the indicated medical terms.

The combining form *arthr/o* means joint.

1. puncture to withdraw fluid from joint _____

2. joint inflammation _____

3. instrument to visually examine joint _____

4. joint surgical repair _____

5. process of recording joint _____

The combining form *my/o* means muscle.

6. muscle weakness _____

7. muscle suture _____

The suffix *-kinesia* means movement.

8. excessive movement _____

9. slow movement _____

The combining form *oste/o* means bone.

10. instrument to cut bone _____

11. bone porous _____

12. bone producing _____

The combining form *chondr/o* means cartilage.

13. cartilage softening _____

14. cartilage tumor _____

15. cartilage surgical repair _____

Fill in the Blank

Fill in the blank to complete each of the following sentences.

1. In a _____ fracture there is no open skin wound.

2. DXA is a diagnostic test for _____.

3. The common name for _____ is hunchback.

4. Braces and splints are examples of an _____.

5. _____ is an example of a repetitive motion disorder affecting the wrist.

6. A _____ is any medical device used to substitute for a body part.

7. _____ fractures are most commonly seen in children.

8. Bones are held together by _____, while _____ anchor muscles to bones.

9. Pins, plates, and rods are examples of _____.

10. A _____ is a sudden, strong, involuntary muscle contraction.

Abbreviation Matching

Match each abbreviation with its definition.

_____ **1.** LLE   **A.** rheumatoid arthritis

_____ **2.** OA   **B.** fracture

_____ **3.** MD   **C.** second lumbar vertebra

_____ **4.** CTS   **D.** left lower leg

_____ **5.** RA   **E.** total hip arthroplasty

_____ **6.** L2   **F.** muscular dystrophy

_____ **7.** ORIF   **G.** osteoarthritis

_____ **8.** Fx   **H.** intramuscular

_____ **9.** IM   **I.** open reduction, internal fixation

_____ **10.** THA   **J.** carpal tunnel syndrome

PEARSON mymedicalterminologylab

MyMedicalTerminologyLab is a premium online homework management system that includes a host of features to help you study. Registered users will find:

- Fun games and activities built within a virtual hospital
- Powerful tools that track and analyze your results—allowing you to create a personalized learning experience
- Videos, flashcards, and audio pronunciations to help enrich your progress
- Streaming lesson presentations and self-paced learning modules
- A space where you and your instructors can view and manage your assignments

Medical Term Analysis

Examine each of the following terms. Begin by dividing it into its word parts and writing them in the indicated blanks (P = prefix, WR = word root; CF = combining form; S = suffix). Follow with the definition of each word part and finally the meaning of the full term.

1. **arthrodesis**

   CF _____

   means _____

   S _____

   means _____

   Term Meaning: _____

   _____

2. **bursectomy**

   WR _____

   means _____

   S _____

   means _____

   Term Meaning: _____

   _____

3. **electromyogram**

   CF _____

   means _____

   CF _____

   means _____

   S _____

   means _____

   Term Meaning: _____

   _____

4. **intracranial**

   P _____

   means _____

   WR _____

   means _____

   S _____

   means _____

   Term Meaning: _____

   _____

5. **osteomyelitis**

   CF _____

   means _____

   WR _____

   means _____

   S _____

   means _____

   Term Meaning: _____

   _____

6. **tenalgia**

   WR _____

   means _____

   S _____

   means _____

   Term Meaning: _____

   _____

7. spondylosis

WR _____

means _____

S _____

means _____

Term Meaning: _____

_____

8. substernal

P _____

means _____

WR _____

means _____

S _____

means _____

Term Meaning: _____

_____

9. intervertebral

P _____

means _____

WR _____

means _____

S _____

means _____

Term Meaning: _____

_____

10. supramaxillary

P _____

means _____

WR _____

means _____

S _____

means _____

Term Meaning: _____

_____

Spelling

Some of the following terms are misspelled. Identify the incorrect terms and spell them correctly in the blank provided.

1. contracture _____

2. bursektomy _____

3. lordosis _____

4. nonsteroidal _____

5. orthosis _____

6. arthrocentesis _____

7. chondroectomy _____

8. coxygeal _____

9. diskinesia _____

10. spondilosis _____

Photomatch Challenge

Match each fracture with its name in the Word Bank.

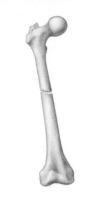

1. _____

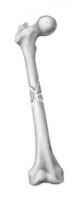

4. _____

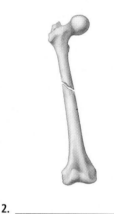

2. _____

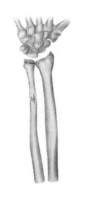

5. _____

Word Bank:

Transverse fracture

Oblique fracture

Spiral fracture

Comminuted fracture

Greenstick fracture

Compression fracture

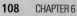

3. _____

6. _____

Crossword Puzzle

Use the definitions given to complete the crossword puzzle.

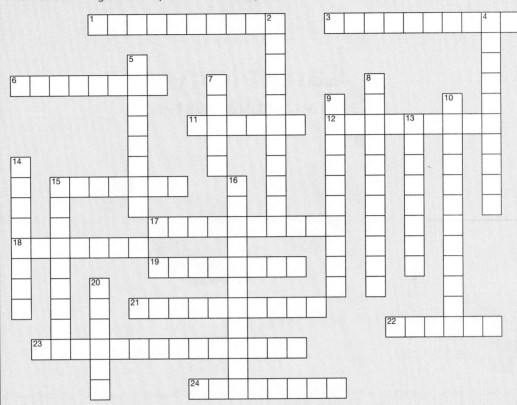

ACROSS

1 Fracture caused by diseased or weakened bone
3 Fracture with incomplete break
6 Medical term for hunchback
11 _____ tunnel syndrome, repetitive motion disorder
12 Procedure to correct fracture by realigning bone
15 Osteogenic _____, most common type of bone cancer
17 Fracture with line straight across shaft of bone
18 _____ fracture, fracture line runs on angle to bone shaft
19 Medical term for swayback
21 _____ arthritis is an autoimmune disease
22 Damage to the muscle or tendons from overstretching
23 Arthritis caused by loss of cartilage cushion covering bones
24 Anatomical name for the lower jaw

DOWN

2 Abnormal shortening of muscle fibers
4 Fracture with shattered bone
5 Procedure to stabilize fracture bone
7 Sudden, involuntary, strong muscle contraction
8 Imaging procedure using x-rays
9 Artificial device used to substitute for missing body part
10 Chronic condition with widespread muscle aching and pain
13 Fracture in which broken bone causes open skin wound
14 Externally applied brace or splint
15 Abnormal lateral curvature of the spine
16 Joint is displaced from normal alignment
20 Slight fracture caused by repetitive low-impact forces

7

Cardiology
Cardiovascular System

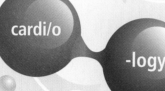

cardi/o

-logy

A Brief Introduction to Cardiology

UNDERSTAND the functions of the cardiovascular system.

The cardiovascular system consists of the **heart** and **blood vessels.** The heart, composed of cardiac muscle tissue, contracts to push blood through the blood vessels to transport substances such as oxygen, nutrients, and waste products to all areas of the body. The three types of blood vessels are the **arteries, veins, and capillaries.** Blood is carried from the heart by arteries, and then it enters capillary beds. Capillaries are the narrowest blood vessels and the location to which oxygen and nutrients are delivered and wastes are picked up. The blood travels back to the heart through veins.

DESCRIBE the medical specialty of cardiology.

   Cardiology is the diagnosis and treatment of diseases and conditions affecting the cardiovascular system. **Cardiologists** are responsible for treating conditions such as coronary artery disease, cardiac arrhythmias, hypertension, heart valve disease, congenital heart defects, cardiomyopathy, congestive heart failure, myocardial infarction, heart transplants, and peripheral vascular diseases.

   Cardiovascular technologists are allied health professionals who work alongside the cardiologist. These technologists perform a variety of diagnostic and therapeutic procedures including electrocardiography, echocardiography, exercise stress testing, and cardiac catheterization.

Cardiology Combining Forms

The following list presents new combining forms important for building and defining cardiology terms.

angi/o	vessel		**steth/o**	chest
aort/o	aorta		**thromb/o**	clot
arteri/o	artery		**valv/o**	valve
arteriol/o	arteriole		**valvul/o**	valve
ather/o	fatty substance, plaque		**varic/o**	dilated vein
atri/o	atrium		**vascul/o**	blood vessel
cardi/o	heart		**vas/o**	blood vessel
coron/o	heart		**ven/o**	vein
embol/o	plug		**ventricul/o**	ventricle
isch/o	to keep back		**venul/o**	venule
phleb/o	vein			

The following list presents combining forms that are not specific to the cardiovascular system but are also used for building and defining cardiology terms.

cutane/o	skin		**pulmon/o**	lung
electr/o	electricity		**son/o**	sound
esophag/o	esophagus		**sphygm/o**	pulse
my/o	muscle			

Suffix Review

These suffixes and prefixes were introduced in Chapters 2 and 3. They are being reviewed in this chapter because they are especially important for building cardiology terms.

-ac	pertaining to		**-graphy**	process of recording
-al	pertaining to		**-ia**	condition
-ar	pertaining to		**-ic**	pertaining to
-ary	pertaining to		**-ism**	condition
-dynia	pain		**-itis**	inflammation
-eal	pertaining to		**-logist**	one who studies
-ectomy	surgical removal		**-logy**	study of
-emia	blood condition		**-lysis**	destruction
-genic	producing		**-lytic**	destruction
-gram	record		**-manometer**	instrument to measure pressure

-megaly	enlarged		-rrhaphy	suture
-ole	small		-rrhexis	rupture
-oma	tumor		-sclerosis	hardening
-ose	pertaining to		-scope	instrument for viewing
-osis	abnormal condition		-spasm	involuntary muscle contraction
-otomy	cutting into		-stenosis	narrowing
-ous	pertaining to		-tic	pertaining to
-pathy	disease		-ule	small
-plasty	surgical repair			

Prefix Review

a-	without		per-	through
brady-	slow		peri-	around
endo-	within		poly-	many
hyper-	excessive		tachy-	fast
hypo-	insufficient		trans-	across
inter-	between		ultra-	excess
intra-	within			

Organs Commonly Treated in Cardiology

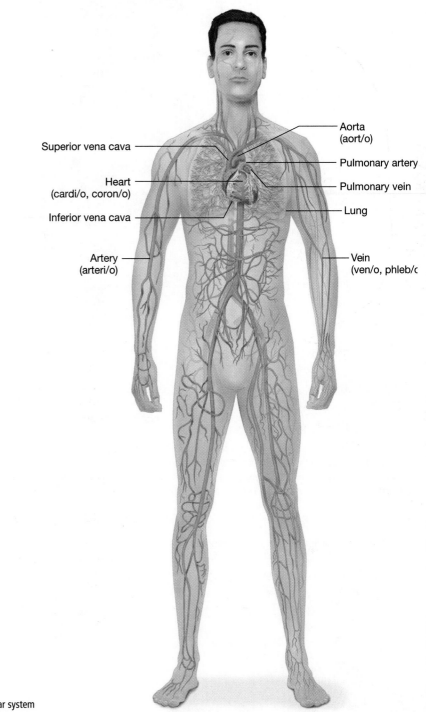

Superior vena cava

Heart
(cardi/o, coron/o)

Inferior vena cava

Artery
(arteri/o)

Aorta
(aort/o)

Pulmonary artery

Pulmonary vein

Lung

Vein
(ven/o, phleb/o)

>7.1 The cardiovascular system

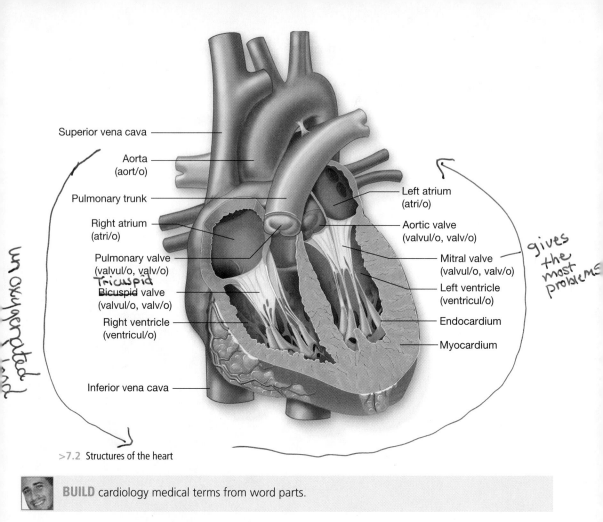

Superior vena cava

Aorta
(aort/o)

Pulmonary trunk

Right atrium
(atri/o)

Pulmonary valve
(valvul/o, valv/o)

Tricuspid

Bicuspid valve
(valvul/o, valv/o)

Right ventricle
(ventricul/o)

Inferior vena cava

Left atrium
(atri/o)

Aortic valve
(valvul/o, valv/o)

Mitral valve
(valvul/o, valv/o)

Left ventricle
(ventricul/o)

Endocardium

Myocardium

unoxygenated blood

gives the most problems

>7.2 **Structures of the heart**

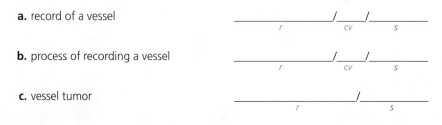

BUILD cardiology medical terms from word parts.

Building Cardiology Terms

This section presents word parts most often used to build cardiology terms. Following the explanation of the term, you have the opportunity to begin building your own vocabulary. Read the meaning for each term and then fill in the blanks to build a single medical term. Use the slashes to divide prefixes, word roots, combining vowels, and suffixes. To help you out you will find a key to the word parts underneath the blanks: r for word roots, p for prefix, cv for combining vowel, and s for suffix. Remember that not every term will contain all these word parts; it's up to you to decide which to use. As you gain experience, this process becomes easier. Answers can be found at the back of the book.

1. **angi/o**–combining form meaning **vessel**

    This combining form may be used to refer to either blood vessels or lymph vessels; it does not indicate what type of blood vessel, artery, vein, or capillary

    a. record of a vessel

    _____/_____/_____
    　　　　　　　r　　　　cv　　　s

    b. process of recording a vessel

    _____/_____/_____
    　　　　　　　r　　　　cv　　　s

    c. vessel tumor

    _____/_____
    　　　　　　　　r　　　　　s

d. surgical repair of a vessel

_____/____/_____
r   CV   S

e. involuntary muscle spasm in a vessel

_____/____/_____
r   CV   S

f. inflammation of many vessels

_____/_____/____
p   r   S

---

2. aort/o–combining form meaning **aorta**

The aorta is the largest artery in the body; carries oxygenated blood from left ventricle to body

a. pertaining to the aorta

_____/_____
r   S

b. surgical repair of the aorta

_____/____/_____
r   CV   S

---

3. arteri/o–combining form meaning **artery**

Arteries are blood vessels that carry blood away from the heart and toward a capillary bed; arteries to the lungs carry deoxygenated blood and arteries to the body carry oxygenated blood

>7.3 Artery

a. pertaining to an artery

_____/_____
r   S

b. record of an artery

_____/____/_____
r   CV   S

c. process of recording an artery

_____/____/_____
r   CV   S

d. suture of an artery

_____/____/_____
r   CV   S

e. ruptured artery

_____/____/_____
r   CV   S

f. narrowing of an artery

_____/____/_____
r   CV   S

g. small artery

_____/_____
r   S

---

4. arteriol/o–combining form meaning **arteriole**

Arterioles are the smallest arteries; carry blood from artery to capillary bed

a. pertaining to an arteriole

_____/_____
r   S

5. ather/o–combining form meaning **fatty substance, plaque**

This combining form refers to the soft, yellow, fatty deposits that build up along inner wall of blood vessels; this deposits is referred to as *plaque*

a. hardening of plaque

_____/____/_____
r   CV   S

b. surgical removal of plaque

_____/_____
r   S

---

6. atri/o–combining form meaning **atrium**

Atria are the upper chambers of the heart; receive blood returning to the heart; left atrium receives oxygenated blood from lungs and right atrium receives deoxygenated blood from body

a. pertaining to the atrium

_____/_____
r   S

b. pertaining to between the atria

_____/_____/_____
p   r   S

c. pertaining to the atrium and ventricle

_____/____/_____/____
r   CV   r   S

---

7. cardi/o–combining form meaning **heart**

The heart is composed of cardiac muscle tissue called the myocardium that contracts to develop the pressure needed to push blood through blood vessels; divided into left and right halves by **septum;** upper chambers are **atria** that receive blood returning to heart; lower chambers are **ventricles** that contract to force blood out of heart and into arteries

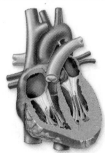

>7.4 **Heart**

a. pertaining to the heart

_____/_____
r   S

b. heart pain

_____/____/_____
r   CV   S

c. record of heart's electricity

_____/____/_____/____/____
r   CV   r   CV   S

d. process of recording heart's electricity

_____/____/_____/____/____
r   CV   r   CV   S

e. one who studies the heart

_____/____/_____
r   CV   S

f. study of the heart

_____/____/_____
r   CV   S

g. enlarged heart

_____/____/_____
r   CV   S

h. disease of the heart muscle

_____/____/_____/____/____
r   CV   r   CV   S

i. ruptured heart

_____/____/_____
r   cv   s

j. involuntary heart muscle spasm

_____/____/_____
r   cv   s

k. pertaining to around the heart

_____/_____/_____
p   r   s

l. pertaining to within the heart

_____/_____/_____
p   r   s

m. pertaining to heart muscle

_____/____/_____/____
r   cv   r   s

---

8. coron/o–combining form meaning **heart**

> ✚ **TERMINOLOGY TIDBIT:**
>
> The term _coronary_ comes from the Latin word _coronarius_ meaning "like a crown." This describes how the great vessels encircle the heart as they emerge from the top of the heart.

a. pertaining to the heart

_____/_____
r   s

---

9. embol/o–combining form meaning **plug, embolus**

An embolus is a piece broken off from a clot, mass of fat, or bacteria that floats through blood vessels until it plugs up small blood vessel, blocking blood flow

a. surgical removal of an embolus

_____/_____
r   s

b. condition of having an embolus

_____/_____
r   s

---

10. isch/o–combining form meaning **to hold back**

To hold back means to stop, as in blood flow

a. condition of blood being held back

_____/_____
r   s

---

11. phleb/o–combining form meaning **vein**

Veins are blood vessels that carry blood back to the heart from capillary beds; veins from body carry deoxygenated blood and veins from lungs carry oxygenated blood

>7.5 **Vein**

a. vein inflammation

_____/_____
r   s

b. cutting into a vein

_____/____/_____
r   cv   s

c. record of a vein

_____/_____/_____
r   CV   s

d. process of recording a vein

_____/_____/_____
r   CV   s

12. -sclerosis–suffix meaning **hardening**

This suffix is used in the cardiovascular system indicates blood vessel becoming hard and inflexible due to buildup of cholesterol plaques along vessel wall

a. hardening of an artery

_____/_____/_____
r   CV   s

13. steth/o–combining form meaning **chest**

a. instrument to view the chest

_____/_____/_____
r   CV   s

14. thromb/o–combining form meaning **blood clot, thrombus**

This suffix refers to a blood clot forming in blood vessel; if large enough, it will partially or completely block blood flow through blood vessel

a. pertaining to a clot

_____/_____/_____
r   CV   s

b. abnormal condition of having clots

_____/_____
r   s

c. vessel inflammation with clots

_____/_____/_____/____
r   CV   r   s

d. inflammation of vein with clots

_____/_____/_____/____
r   CV   r   s

e. producing a clot

_____/_____/_____
r   CV   s

f. destruction of a clot

_____/_____/_____
r   CV   s

15. valv/o–combining form meaning **valve** ~ cusps

Valves are flaplike structures that close tightly to prevent backflow of blood; ensures that blood always flows in forward direction; there are four valves in heart (**tricuspid, mitral, pulmonary,** and **aortic**) and many valves in veins

a. surgical repair of a valve

_____/_____/_____
r   CV   s

b. cutting into a valve

_____/_____/_____
r   CV   s

c. small valve

_____/_____
r   s

16. valvul/o–combining form meaning **valve**

a. pertaining to a valve

_____/_____
r   s

b. inflammation of a valve

_____/_____
r   s

17. varic/o–combining form meaning **dilated vein, varicosity**

Condition in which a vein becomes dilated due to ineffective valves; blood flow through varicosity becomes very slow and sluggish

a. abnormal condition of having a varicosity

_____/_____
                   _r_   _s_

b. pertaining to a varicosity

_____/_____
                   _r_   _s_

---

18. vascul/o–combining form meaning **blood vessel**

a. pertaining to a blood vessel

_____/_____
                   _r_   _s_

b. pertaining to the heart and blood vessels

_____/____/_____/____
      _r_   _cv_   _r_   _s_

---

19. vas/o–combining form meaning **blood vessel**

a. involuntary muscle contraction of a blood vessel

_____/____/_____
      _r_   _cv_   _s_

---

20. ven/o–combining form meaning **vein**

a. pertaining to a vein

_____/_____
                   _r_   _s_

b. record of a vein

_____/____/_____
      _r_   _cv_   _s_

c. process of recording a vein

_____/____/_____
      _r_   _cv_   _s_

d. pertaining to within a vein

_____/_____/____
      _p_   _r_   _s_

e. small vein

_____/_____
                   _r_   _s_

---

21. ventricul/o–combining form meaning **ventricle**

The ventricles are large, very muscular pumping chambers of the heart; left ventricle pumps oxygenated blood to body and right ventricle pumps deoxygenated blood to lungs

✚ TERMINOLOGY TIDBIT:

The term _ventricle_ comes from the Latin term _venter_, meaning "little belly." Although it originally referred to the abdomen and then the stomach, it came to stand for any hollow region inside an organ.

a. pertaining to a ventricle

_____/_____
                   _r_   _s_

b. pertaining to between the ventricles

_____/_____/_____
      _p_   _r_   _s_

---

22. venul/o–combining form meaning **venule**

Venules are the smallest veins; receive blood from capillaries and carry it to larger veins

a. pertaining to a venule

_____/_____
                   _r_   _s_

Cardiology Vocabulary

The cardiology terms presented in this section include eponyms, modern English words, and those that contain Latin or Greek word parts but are not constructed solely from these word parts. When you recognize word parts within a term they will give you a hint about the word's meaning. In these instances, look for the word parts to follow the term.

Term	Explanation
aneurysm	Localized widening of artery due to weakness in arterial wall; may develop in any artery, but common sites are abdominal aorta and cerebral arteries

Right kidney

Abdominal aorta

Aneurysm

Inferior vena cava

>7.6 Illustration of a large aneurysm in the abdominal aorta that has ruptured

angina pectoris	Severe chest pain caused by myocardial ischemia

➕ **TERMINOLOGY TIDBIT:**

The term *angina* comes from the Greek word *ankhone* meaning "strangling." This describes the sensation that occurs during angina pectoris.

arrhythmia a- = without	Irregular heart beat

auscultation	Listening to sounds within body, such as heart or lungs, by using *stethoscope*

➕ **TERMINOLOGY TIDBIT:**

The term *auscultation* comes from the Latin word *auscultare* meaning "to listen to."

bacterial endocarditis endo- = inner cardi/o = heart -itis = inflammation	Inflammation of inner lining of heart (the endocardium) caused by bacteria; may result in visible accumulation of bacteria called *vegetation*
blood pressure (BP)	Measurement of pressure exerted by blood against walls of blood vessel

bradycardia
 brady- = slow
 cardi/o = heart
 -ia = condition

Abnormally slow heart rate below 60 beats per minute (bpm)

cardiac arrest
 cardi/o = heart
 -ac = pertaining to

Complete stoppage of all heart activity, both electrical signals and muscle contractions

cardiac catheterization (CC)
 cardi/o = heart
 -ac = pertaining to

Passage of thin tube (catheter) through veins or arteries leading into heart; used to detect heart abnormalities, to collect cardiac blood samples, and to determine pressure within heart

cardiac enzymes
 cardi/o = heart
 -ac = pertaining to

Complex proteins released by heart muscle when it is damaged; taken by blood sample to determine amount of heart disease or damage; most common cardiac enzymes are creatine kinase (CK), glutamic oxaloacetic transaminase (GOT), and lactate dehydrogenase (LDH)

cardiopulmonary resuscitation (CPR)
 cardi/o = heart
 pulmon/o = lungs
 -ary = pertaining to

Applying external compressions to rib cage in order to maintain blood flow and air movement in and out of lungs during cardiac and respiratory arrest

congenital septal defect (CSD)

Birth defect in wall separating two chambers of heart allowing blood to pass between two chambers; there can be atrial septal defect (ASD) or ventricular septal defect (VSD)

+ TERMINOLOGY TIDBIT:

The term *congenital* comes from the Latin word *congenitus* meaning "born with."

congestive heart failure (CHF)

Condition that develops when heart muscle is not able to pump blood forcefully enough, reducing blood flow to body; results in weakness, dyspnea, and edema

coronary artery bypass graft (CABG)

coron/o = heart
-ary = pertaining to

Open-heart surgery in which blood vessel, often leg vein, is grafted to route blood around occluded coronary artery

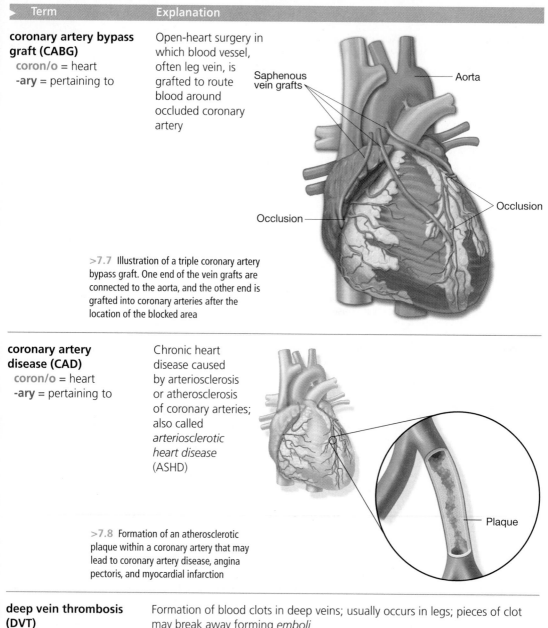

Saphenous vein grafts

Aorta

Occlusion

Occlusion

>7.7 Illustration of a triple coronary artery bypass graft. One end of the vein grafts are connected to the aorta, and the other end is grafted into coronary arteries after the location of the blocked area

coronary artery disease (CAD)

coron/o = heart
-ary = pertaining to

Chronic heart disease caused by arteriosclerosis or atherosclerosis of coronary arteries; also called *arteriosclerotic heart disease* (ASHD)

Plaque

>7.8 Formation of an atherosclerotic plaque within a coronary artery that may lead to coronary artery disease, angina pectoris, and myocardial infarction

deep vein thrombosis (DVT)

thromb/o = clot
-osis = abnormal condition

Formation of blood clots in deep veins; usually occurs in legs; pieces of clot may break away forming *emboli*

Term	Explanation
defibrillation	Using instrument called *defibrillator* to give electrical shock to heart for purpose of converting arrhythmia back to normal heart beat; also called *cardioversion* >7.9 An emergency medical technician positions defibrillator paddles on the chest of a supine male patient
Doppler ultrasonography **ultra-** = excess **son/o** = sound **-graphy** = process of recording	Imaging technique using ultrasound to create moving image; utilized to evaluate blood flow through blood vessels, movement of heart valves, and movement of heart muscle during contraction
electrocardiography **electr/o** = electricity **cardi/o** = heart **-graphy** = process of recording	Diagnostic procedure that records electrical activity of heart; used to diagnose damage to heart tissue from coronary heart disease or myocardial infarction
endarterectomy **endo-** = within **arteri/o** = artery **-ectomy** = surgical removal	Surgical removal of inner lining of artery in order to remove plaques
fibrillation	Abnormal quivering or contractions of heart fibers; occurrence within fibers of ventricle of heart result in cardiac arrest and death; emergency equipment to defibrillate, or convert heart to normal beat, is necessary
heart murmur	Abnormal heart sound such as soft blowing sound or harsh click; they may be soft and heard only with stethoscope or so loud they can be heard several feet away
heart transplantation	Replacement of diseased or malfunctioning heart with donor's heart
heart valve prolapse	Cusps or flaps of heart valve are too loose and fail to shut tightly, allowing blood to flow backwards (regurgitation) through valve when heart chamber contracts; most commonly occurs in mitral valve, but may affect any heart valve
heart valve stenosis **-stenosis** = narrowing	Cusps or flaps of heart valve are too stiff and unable to open fully, making it difficult for blood to flow through; condition may affect any of heart valves but most often affects mitral valve

Holter monitor

Portable ECG monitor worn by patient for period of few hours to few days to assess heart and pulse activity as person goes through activities of daily living; used to assess patient who experiences chest pain and unusual heart activity during exercise and normal activities

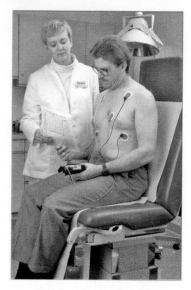

>7.10 Patient being set up with Holter monitor. Electrodes placed on chest are connected to small monitor that he will wear

hypertension (HTN)
 hyper- = excessive

Blood pressure above normal range; usually systolic pressure above 140 mmHg or diastolic pressure above 90 mmHg

hypotension
 hypo- = insufficient

Decrease in blood pressure; can occur in shock, infection, cancer, anemia, or as death approaches

implantable cardioverter defibrillator (ICD)
 cardi/o = heart

Electrical device implanted in chest cavity with electrodes to heart; applies shock to heart to stop potentially life-threatening arrhythmias such as fibrillation

infarct

Area of tissue necrosis that develops from ischemia

intravascular thrombolytic therapy
 intra- = within
 vascul/o = blood vessel
 -ar = pertaining to
 thromb/o = clot
 -lytic = destruction

Treatment for clots occluding blood vessel; drugs, such as streptokinase (SK) or tissue-type plasminogen activator (tPA), are injected into blood vessels to chemically dissolve clots; commonly referred to as *clot-busters*

Term	Explanation

myocardial infarction (MI)
 my/o = muscle
 cardi/o = heart
 -al = pertaining to

Infarct of heart muscle caused by occlusion of one or more of coronary arteries; symptoms include angina pectoris and shortness of breath; also referred to as *heart attack*

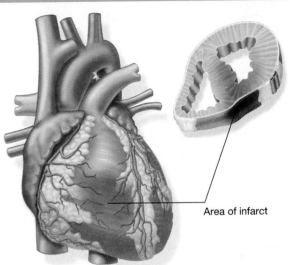

Area of infarct

>7.11 External and cross-sectional view of an infarct caused by a myocardial infarction

---

myocardial ischemia
 my/o = muscle
 cardi/o = heart
 -al = pertaining to
 isch/o = hold back
 -emia = blood condition

Loss of blood supply to heart muscle tissue of myocardium due to occlusion of coronary artery; may cause angina pectoris or myocardial infarction

---

occlusion

Blockage of blood vessel or other hollow structure; may be caused by thrombus, plaque, or embolus

Artery

Embolus

>7.12 Illustration of an embolus floating in an artery. The embolus will eventually lodge in an artery that is smaller than it is, resulting in occlusion of that artery

Term	Explanation

pacemaker

Electrical device that artificially stimulates contraction of heart muscle; treatment for bradycardia

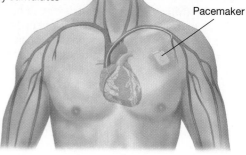

Pacemaker

>7.13 Placement of a pacemaker under the skin between the heart and shoulder. Electrode wires then run to the heart muscle

---

percutaneous transluminal coronary angioplasty (PTCA)
  per- = through
  cutane/o = skin
  -ous = pertaining to
  trans- = across
  coron/o = heart
  -ary = pertaining to
  angi/o = vessel
  -plasty = surgical repair

Method for treating coronary artery narrowing; balloon catheter is inserted into coronary artery and inflated to dilate narrow blood vessel

---

peripheral vascular disease (PVD)
  vascul/o = blood vessel
  -ar = pertaining to

Disease of blood vessels away from central region of body, most typically in legs; symptoms include pain, numbness, and impaired circulation

---

sphygmomanometer
  sphygm/o = pulse
  -manometer = instrument to measure pressure

Instrument for measuring blood pressure; also referred to as *blood pressure cuff*

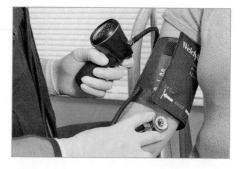

>7.14 Using a sphygmomanometer to measure blood pressure

Term	Explanation

stent

Stainless steel tube placed within blood vessel or duct to widen lumen; may be placed in coronary artery to treat myocardial ischemia due to atherosclerosis

>7.15 The process of placing a stent in a blood vessel. (A) Catheter is used to place a collapsed stent next to an atherosclerotic plaque; (B) stent is expanded; (C) catheter is removed, leaving the expanded stent behind

A　　**B**　　**C**

stress test

Method for evaluating cardiovascular fitness; patient is placed on treadmill or a bicycle and then subjected to steadily increasing levels of work; EKG and oxygen levels are taken while patient exercises; test is stopped if abnormalities occur on EKG

tachycardia
　tachy- = fast
　cardi/o = heart
　-ia = condition

Abnormally fast heart rate more than 100 beats per minute (bpm)

transesophageal echocardiography (TEE)
　trans- = across
　esophag/o = esophagus
　-eal = pertaining to
　cardi/o = heart
　-graphy = process of recording

Specialized echocardiography procedure in which patient swallows ultrasound head in order to better visualize internal cardiac structures, especially cardiac valves

varicose veins
　varic/o = dilated vein

Swollen and distended veins, most commonly in legs

Normal vein—competent valves

Open

Closed

Varicose veins

Dilated vein—incompetent valves

+ TERMINOLOGY TIDBIT:

The term *varicose* comes from the Latin word *varix* meaning "dilated vein."

>7.16 Varicose veins develop when their valves fail to control blood flow, which allows more than the normal amount of blood to collect in superficial leg veins

Term	Explanation
venipuncture ven/o = vein	Puncture into vein to withdraw blood or inject medication or fluids

 USE cardiology abbreviations.

Cardiology Abbreviations

The following list presents common cardiology abbreviations.

ACG	angiocardiography	**HTN**	hypertension
AF	atrial fibrillation	**ICD**	implantable cardioverter defibrillator
AS	aortic stenosis, arteriosclerosis	**ICU**	intensive care unit
ASCVD	arteriosclerotic cardiovascular disease	**IV**	intravenous
ASD	atrial septal defect	**LDH**	lactate dehydrogenase
ASHD	arteriosclerotic heart disease	**LVH**	left ventricular hypertrophy
AV, A-V	atrioventricular	**MI**	myocardial infarction
BP	blood pressure	**mmHg**	millimeters of mercury
bpm	beats per minute	**MS**	mitral stenosis
CABG	coronary artery bypass graft	**MVP**	mitral valve prolapse
CAD	coronary artery disease	**NSR**	normal sinus rhythm
cath	catheterization	**P**	pulse
CC	cardiac catheterization	**PTCA**	percutaneous transluminal coronary angioplasty
CCU	coronary care unit		
CHD	congestive heart disease	**PVC**	premature ventricular contraction
CHF	congestive heart failure	**PVD**	peripheral vascular disease
CK	creatine kinase	**SA, S-A**	sinoatrial
CP	chest pain	**SGOT**	serum glutamic oxaloacetic transaminase
CPR	cardiopulmonary resuscitation		
CSD	congenital septal defect	**SK**	streptokinase
CV	cardiovascular	**SOB**	shortness of breath
DVT	deep vein thrombosis	**TEE**	transesophageal echocardiogram
ECG	electrocardiogram	**tPA**	tissue-type plasminogen activator
ECHO	echocardiogram	**VFib**	ventricular fibrillation
EKG	electrocardiogram	**VSD**	ventricular septal defect
GOT	glutamic oxaloacetic transaminase	**VT, V-tach**	ventricular tachycardia
HR	heart rate		

History of Present Illness

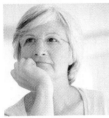

Patient is a 56-year-old female, referred to the cardiology clinic by her family physician for increasingly severe SOB. She denies angina pectoris. Symptoms first appeared 5 years ago following an acute episode of viral bronchitis. At that time, the SOB was attributed to the lung infection. However, symptoms continued to gradually worsen rather than improve. Adult-onset asthma and emphysema have been ruled out by a pulmonologist. At this time, the patient is experiencing severe SOB with mild activity. She has recently noticed swelling in her feet, and her family physician has now diagnosed CHF, prescribed digoxin, and referred her for further diagnosis and treatment.

Past Medical History

Appendectomy at age 8. Rheumatic fever at age 16. Three pregnancies, all children delivered vaginally and are healthy. Left breast lumpectomy at age 45 with no reoccurrence of malignancy.

Family and Social History

Patient drinks 1–2 alcoholic beverages weekly. She has not ever smoked, but husband smokes one pack/day. She is a school teacher. No exposure to environmental toxins. Family history is negative for heart disease. Mother died at age 26 from complications of childbirth. Father died at age 60 from lung cancer. She has one sister, age 60, who is healthy except for rheumatoid arthritis.

Physical Examination

Pt is mildly SOB sitting in exam room. HR is 153 bpm, rhythm is normal. BP is 180/90 in left arm while sitting. No cyanosis is noted. Weight is within normal range, but she does have noticeable edema in bilateral feet but not in her hands or face. Abdomen is mildly distended with fluid, but no organomegaly is palpated. Chest auscultation reveals a clearly audible heart murmur during ventricular contraction.

Diagnostic Tests

EKG: tachycardia at rate of 153 bpm but normal rhythm and no evidence of an MI. Transesophageal echocardiography is consistent with mitral prolapse with regurgitation of blood into left atrium from left ventricle.

Diagnosis

Mitral valve prolapse and CHF secondary to rheumatic heart disease.

Plan of Treatment

1. Schedule patient for mitral valvoplasty with prosthetic valve

Critical Thinking Questions

Answer the following questions regarding this case study. Do not just copy words out of the case study, translate all medical terms. To answer some of these questions, you may need to look up information from another chapter of this text, in a medical dictionary, or online. Answers are found at the back of the book.

1. Name and define the symptom that brought this patient to the cardiologist. Name and define the symptoms that the patient denies having.

2. Name and describe the family physician's diagnosis. What new symptom led this physician to make this diagnosis?

   _____

   _____

3. This patient takes digoxin. Look this up, and describe why it is prescribed.

   _____

   _____

4. Explain the results of the EKG.

   _____

   _____

5. What is edema? Where does and does not this patient have edema?

   _____

   _____

6. *Cyanosis* means:
   a. an abnormal breath sound
   b. blue color to the skin
   c. dizziness
   d. yellow color to the whites of the eyes

7. Explain the final diagnosis. What diagnostic test best supported this diagnosis? Justify your conclusion.

   _____

   _____

   _____

8. Explain the treatment planned for this patient.

   _____

   _____

Sound It Out

The following are some of the key terms from this chapter written as their phonetic spelling. Sound out each term and write it in the blank. Pronunciations for all terms are included in the audio glossary at www.mymedicalterminologylab.com <http://www.mymedicalterminologylab.com/>.

1. VAY-zoh-spazm _____

2. AN-jee-oh-plas-tee _____

3. in-trah-VEE-nus _____

4. car-dee-oh-my-OP-ah-thee _____

5. ah-RITH-mee-ah _____

6. ar-TEE-ree-oh-GRAH-fee _____

7. ath-er-oh-skleh-ROH-sis _____

8. ay-tree-oh-ven-TRIK-yoo-lar _____

9. AY-tree-um _____

10. brad-ee-CAR-dee-ah _____

11. VEN-yoo-lar _____

12. CAR-dee-ak _____

13. MY-tral _____

14. CAR-dee-oh-VAS-kyoo-lar _____

15. ay-OR-tik _____

16. KOR-ah-nair-ee _____

17. dee-fib-rih-LAY-shun _____

18. ee-lek-troh-car-dee-OG-rah-fee _____

19. ul-trah-son-OG-rah-fee _____

20. is-KEYH-mee-ah _____

21. em-boh-LIZ-em _____

22. an-jee-OH-mah _____

23. end-ar-teh-REK-toh-mee _____

24. fih-brill-AY-shun _____

25. pair-ih-CAR-dee-all _____

26. oss-kul-TAY-shun _____

27. high-per-TEN-shun _____

28. card-dee-oh-REK-sis _____

29. high-poh-TEN-shun _____

30. IN-farkt _____

31. VEE-nus _____

32. my-oh-CAR-dee-all _____

33. fleh-BYE-tis _____

34. en-doh-car-DYE-tis _____

35. FLEE-boh-gram _____

36. SEP-tum _____

37. VEN-ih-PUNK-true _____

38. sfig-moh-mah-NOM-eh-ter _____

39. tak-ee-CAR-dee-ah _____

40. in-ter-ven-TRIK-yoo-lar _____

41. throm-boh-LYE-sis _____

42. VAL-view-lar _____

43. VAIR-ih-kohs _____

44. AN-yoo-rizm _____

45. plak _____

46. car-dee-oh-MEG-ah-lee _____

47. pol-ee-an-jee-EYE-tis _____

48. ven-TRIK-yoo-lar _____

49. throm-BOH-sis _____

50. STETH-oh-scope _____

Transcription Practice

Each of the following sentences is written in common English. Underline any words or phrases that can be replaced by a medical term. Then rewrite the entire sentence using medical terms. Answers are found at the end of the book.

1. Dr. Jones suspected his patient had had a heart attack, so he ordered a record of the heart's electricity and a blood test to look for proteins released into the blood by damaged heart muscle.

   _____

   _____

2. The paramedics applied an electrical shock to the patient's heart because abnormal quivering was detected.

   _____

   _____

3. The patient developed an abnormally slow heart beat and required surgery to implant an electrical device to artificially stimulate the heart to beat.

   _____

   _____

4. Susan wore a portable ECG monitor for 24 hours to further evaluate her severe chest pain caused by myocardial ischemia.

   _____

   _____

5. The patient had an ultrasound imaging technique to create a moving image of her heart valves to assess whether she had heart valves that were too loose and failed to shut tightly or heart valves that were too stiff and unable to open fully.

   _____

   _____

6. During listening to the sounds within the body, the nurse detected an abnormal heart sound caused by mitral valve flaps that are too loose.

   _____

   _____

7. The patient suffered tissue necrosis because of an area losing its blood supply when a floating clot broke off a soft, yellow, fatty deposit.

   _____

   _____

8. A procedure to pass a thin tube through veins leading into the heart was ordered to determine whether the patient requires a balloon procedure to widen a narrow coronary artery.

_____

_____

9. The patient experiences severe chest pain due to severe hardening of the coronary arteries.

_____

_____

10. This patient's high blood pressure eventually caused him to develop a condition in which the heart muscle is not able to pump forcefully enough.

_____

_____

Spelling

Some of the following terms are misspelled. Identify the incorrect terms and spell them correctly in the blank provided.

1. tackycardia _____

2. arrhythmia _____

3. phlebotomy _____

4. awscultation _____

5. atheriosclerosis _____

6. defibrillation _____

7. thrombophlebitis _____

8. anurysm _____

9. angiohma _____

10. occlusion _____

Labeling Exercise

Write the name of each structure on the numbered line. Also use this space to write the combining form where appropriate.

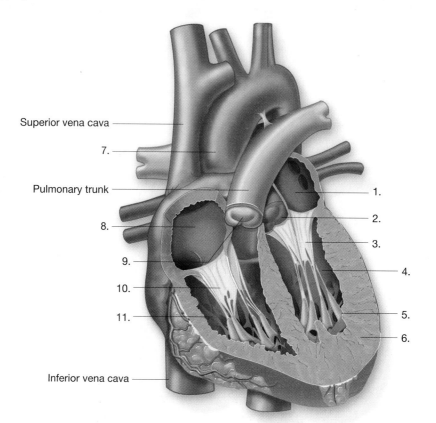

Superior vena cava

7.

Pulmonary trunk

8.

9.

10.

11.

Inferior vena cava

1.

2.

3.

4.

5.

6.

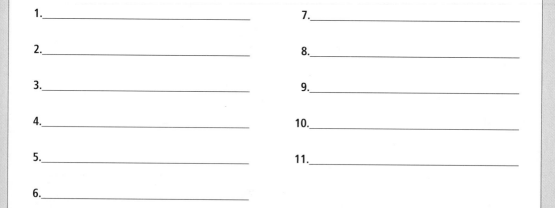

1._____

2._____

3._____

4._____

5._____

6._____

7._____

8._____

9._____

10._____

11._____

Build Medical Terms

Use each of the following word part to build the indicated medical terms.

The combining form *cardi/o* **means heart.**

1. heart study of _____

2. heart enlarged _____

3. heart rupture _____

4. heart record _____

The combining form *valv/o* **means valve.**

5. valve surgical repair _____

6. valve cutting into _____

The suffix *-sclerosis* **means hardening.**

7. artery hardening _____

8. plaque hardening _____

The combining form *angi/o* **means blood vessel.**

9. blood vessel tumor _____

10. blood vessel involuntary muscle spasm _____

The combining form *arteri/o* **means artery.**

11. artery suture _____

12. artery pertaining to _____

13. artery process of recording _____

The combining form *thromb/o* **means clot.**

14. clot vein inflammation _____

15. clot destruction _____

Fill in the Blank

Fill in the blank to complete each of the following sentences.

1. An _____ is a localized wide spot in an artery.

2. Complete stoppage of all heart activity is called _____.

3. Auscultation uses an instrument called a(n) _____.

4. A _____ is a portable EKG monitor worn by a person for several hours to a few days.

5. A baby born with a(n) _____ has a birth defect in the wall separating the two chambers of the heart.

6. A(n) _____ is performed to withdraw blood or inject medication into a vein.

7. Endocarditis may result in the visible growth of bacteria called _____.

8. Drugs such as streptokinase are commonly called _____.

9. A _____ is an abnormal heart sound such as soft blowing or harsh clicking.

10. The paramedics performed _____ by compressing the rib cage to maintain blood flow.

Abbreviation Matching

Match each abbreviation with its definition.

_____ 1. ASHD   **A.** coronary artery disease

_____ 2. ACG   **B.** electrocardiogram

_____ 3. HTN   **C.** myocardial infarction

_____ 4. EKG   **D.** arteriosclerotic heart disease

_____ 5. VSD   **E.** chest pain

_____ 6. CHF   **F.** hypertension

_____ 7. CAD   **G.** ventricular septal defect

_____ 8. PVC   **H.** angiocardiography

_____ 9. CP   **I.** congestive heart failure

_____10. MI   **J.** premature ventricular contraction

Medical Term Analysis

Examine each of the following terms. Begin by dividing it into its word parts and writing them in the indicated blanks (P = prefix, WR = word root, CF = combining form, S = suffix). Follow with the definition of each word part and then finally the meaning of the full term.

1. **aortoplasty**

   CF _____

   means _____

   S _____

   means _____

   Term Meaning: _____

   _____

2. **embolectomy**

   WR _____

   means _____

   S _____

   means _____

   Term Meaning: _____

   _____

3. **cardiomyopathy**

   CF _____

   means _____

   CF _____

   means _____

   S _____

   means _____

   Term Meaning: _____

   _____

4. **endocardial**

   P _____

   means _____

   WR _____

   means _____

   S _____

   means _____

   Term Meaning: _____

   _____

5. **thromboangiitis**

   CF _____

   means _____

   WR _____

   means _____

   S _____

   means _____

   Term Meaning: _____

   _____

6. **atherosclerosis**

   CF _____

   means _____

   S _____

   means _____

   Term Meaning: _____

   _____

7. valvulotomy

WR _____

means _____

S _____

means _____

Term Meaning: _____

_____

8. interventricular

P _____

means _____

WR _____

means _____

S _____

means _____

Term Meaning: _____

_____

9. cardiovascular

CF _____

means _____

WR _____

means _____

S _____

means _____

Term Meaning: _____

_____

10. stethoscope

CF _____

means _____

S _____

means _____

Term Meaning: _____

_____

PEARSON
mymedicalterminologylab

MyMedicalTerminologyLab is a premium online homework management system that includes a host of features to help you study. Registered users will find:

- Fun games and activities built within a virtual hospital
- Powerful tools that track and analyze your results—allowing you to create a personalized learning experience
- Videos, flashcards, and audio pronunciations to help enrich your progress
- Streaming lesson presentations and self-paced learning modules
- A space where you and your instructors can view and manage your assignments

Photomatch Challenge

Match each procedure illustrated below with its name in Word Bank.

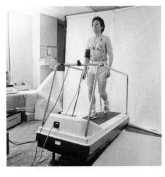

1. _____

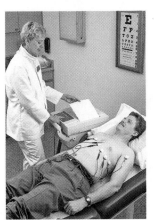

Source: © Dorling Kindersley,
Dorling Kindersley Media Library

3. _____

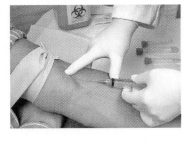

2. _____

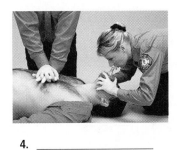

4. _____

Prefixes can help you tell apart these two EKG strips.

One is bradycardia and the other is tachycardia.

A

B

5. What does the prefix **brady-** mean, and which strip is bradycardia?

_____

6. What does the prefix **tachy-** mean, and which strip is tachycardia?

_____

Crossword Puzzle

Use the definitions given to complete the crossword puzzle.

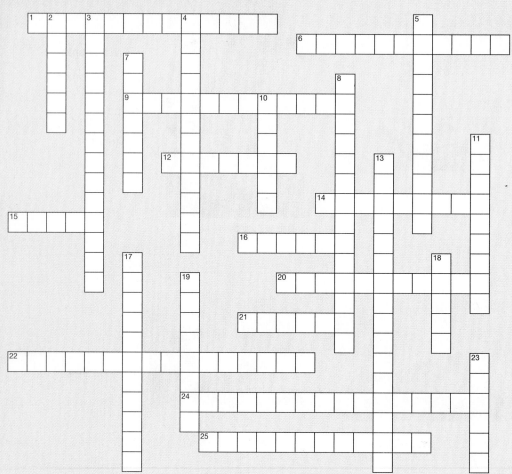

ACROSS

1 Term meaning ruptured heart
6 Slow heart beat
9 Quivering of heart fibers
12 Cardiac _____ are released by damaged heart muscle
14 Pumping heart chamber
15 Stainless steel tube placed in a vessel
16 Term meaning small vein
20 Instrument used to listen to body sounds
21 Heart divided into halves by the _____
22 Term meaning pertaining to between ventricles
24 Blood pressure cuff
25 Listening to body sounds such as heart sounds

DOWN

2 Heart chamber that receives blood
3 Also called cardioversion
4 High blood pressure
5 Abnormally fast heart rate
7 Area of tissue necrosis from ischemia
8 Removal of inner lining of artery
10 Blood vessel carries blood away from heart
11 Electrical device to stimulate heart
13 Term meaning hardening of an artery
17 Low blood pressure
18 Largest artery in the body
19 Widening of artery due to weak arterial wall
23 Abnormal heart sound

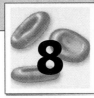

Hematology

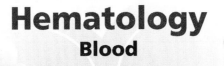
Blood

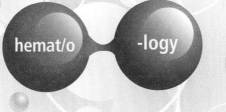

hemat/o   -logy

A Brief Introduction to Hematology

 UNDERSTAND the function of blood.

Blood is the fluid found inside of blood vessels. Approximately 55% of blood is a watery fluid called **plasma.** Many important substances such as **glucose, amino acids, hormones,** and **electrolytes** are transported as dissolutions in the plasma. The remaining 45% of blood consists of the **formed elements,** which are cells (or cell fragments), floating in the plasma. The formed elements include **erythrocytes** (red blood cells), **leukocytes** (white blood cells), and **platelets** (formerly called *thrombocytes*). Erythrocytes contain **hemoglobin** (protein that transports oxygen); leukocytes provide protection against pathogens (there are five specialized types: **neutrophils, basophils, eosinophils, monocytes, lymphocytes**); platelets are small platelike fragments of a larger cell and initiate **hemostasis** (blood-clotting process). All of the formed elements are produced in red bone marrow by a process called **hematopoiesis.**

 DESCRIBE the medical specialty of hematology.

Hematology is the diagnosis and treatment of disorders of the blood and blood-forming tissues. A **hematologist** specializes in the treatment of bleeding disorders, cancers of the blood-forming tissues, and anemia as well as in interpreting blood tests and the science of blood transfusions.

Hematology Combining Forms

The following list presents new combining forms important for building and defining hematology. terms

bas/o	base		**hemat/o**	blood
coagul/o	clotting		**lymph/o**	lymph
eosin/o	rosy red		**leuk/o**	white
erythr/o	red		**neutr/o**	neutral
hem/o	blood		**thromb/o**	clot

The following list presents combining forms that are not specific to hematology but are also used for building and defining hematology terms.

cyt/o	cell		**path/o**	disease
embol/o	plug		**phleb/o**	vein
glyc/o	sugar		**septic/o**	infection
lip/o	fat			

Suffix Review

These suffixes and prefixes were introduced in Chapters 2 and 3. They are being reviewed in this chapter because they are especially important for building hematology terms.

-cyte	cell		**-metry**	process of measuring
-cytosis	abnormal cell condition (too many)		**-oma**	mass
-ectomy	surgical removal		**-osis**	abnormal condition
-emia	blood condition		**-otomy**	cutting into
-globin	protein		**-penia**	too few
-ia	condition		**-phil**	attracted to
-ic	pertaining to		**-plasm**	formation
-logist	one who studies		**-poiesis**	formation
-logy	study of		**-rrhage**	bursting forth
-lysis	destruction		**-stasis**	stopping
-lytic	destruction		**-tic**	pertaining to
-meter	instrument for measuring			

Prefix Review

a-	without		**hypo-**	insufficient
an-	without		**mono-**	one
anti-	against		**pan-**	all
auto-	self		**poly-**	many
hyper-	excessive			

Components of Blood

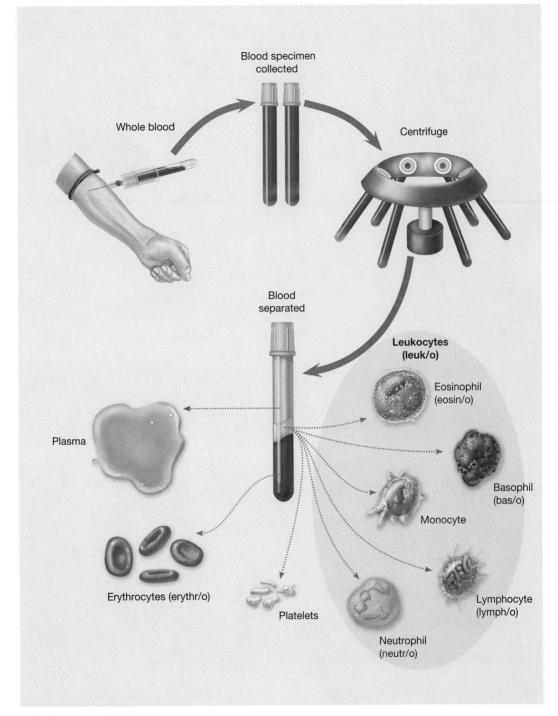

Blood specimen
collected

Whole blood

Centrifuge

Blood
separated

Plasma

**Leukocytes
(leuk/o)**

Eosinophil
(eosin/o)

Basophil
(bas/o)

Monocyte

Erythrocytes (erythr/o)

Platelets

Lymphocyte
(lymph/o)

Neutrophil
(neutr/o)

>8.1 Components of whole blood

Building Hematology Terms

This section presents word parts most often used to build hematology terms. Following the explanation of the term, you have the opportunity to begin building your own vocabulary. Read the meaning for each term and then fill in the blanks to build a single medical term. Use the slashes to divide prefixes, word roots, combining vowels, and suffixes. To help you out you will find a key to the word parts underneath the blanks: r for word roots, p for prefix, cv for combining vowel, and s for suffix. Remember that not every term will contain all these word parts; it's up to you to decide which to use. As you gain experience, this process becomes easier. Answers can be found at the back of the book.

1. **-cyte**–suffix meaning **cell**

   This suffix is used to refer to formed elements

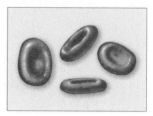

>8.2 Erythrocytes

   a. red cell
   _____/____/_____
   　　　　　　　　r　　　　cv　　s

   b. white cell
   _____/____/_____
   　　　　　　　　r　　　　cv　　s

   c. clotting cell
   _____/____/_____
   　　　　　　　　r　　　　cv　　s

   d. one cell
   _____/_____
   　　　　　　　　p　　　　　　s

   e. lymph cell
   _____/____/_____
   　　　　　　　　r　　　　cv　　s

2. **-cytosis**–suffix meaning **abnormal cell condition**

   This suffix is typically used to indicate abnormal increase in cell numbers

   a. abnormal condition in red cells
   _____/____/_____
   　　　　　　　　r　　　　cv　　s

   b. abnormal condition in white cells
   _____/____/_____
   　　　　　　　　r　　　　cv　　s

   c. abnormal condition in clotting cells
   _____/____/_____
   　　　　　　　　r　　　　cv　　s

3. **-emia**–suffix meaning **blood condition**

   a. condition of being without blood
   _____/_____
   　　　　　　　　p　　　　　　s

   b. blood condition with excessive sugar
   _____/_____/_____
   　　　　　　　p　　　　　　r　　　　s

   c. blood condition with insufficient sugar
   _____/_____/_____
   　　　　　　　p　　　　　　r　　　　s

   d. blood condition with excessive fat
   _____/_____/_____
   　　　　　　　p　　　　　　r　　　　s

4. **hemat/o**–combining form meaning **blood**

   a. study of blood

                     _____ / ____ / _____
                               r   *CV*   *s*

   b. one who studies blood

                     _____ / ____ / _____
                               r   *CV*   *s*

   c. pertaining to blood

                     _____ / _____
                               r   *s*

   d. blood mass

                     _____ / _____
                               r   *s*

   e. study of blood diseases

                     _____ / ____ / _____ / ____ / ____
                            r   *CV*   *r*   *CV*   *s*

   f. too few blood cells

                     _____ / ____ / _____ / ____ / ____
                            r   *CV*   *r*   *CV*   *s*

   g. blood formation

                     _____ / ____ / _____
                               r   *CV*   *s*

5. **hem/o**–combining form meaning **blood**

   a. blood cell

   b. blood protein

   c. stopping of blood

   d. bursting forth of blood

   e. blood destruction

   f. blood cell destruction

   g. blood cell mass

   h. instrument for measuring blood cells

   i. process of measuring blood cells

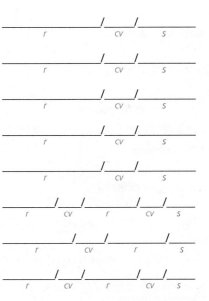

6. **-penia**–suffix meaning **too few**

   This suffix is typically used to indicate that there are too few cells

   a. too few red (cells)

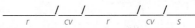

   b. too few white (cells)

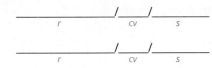

c. too few clotting cells

_____/___/_____/___/_____
r   cv   r   cv   s

d. too few of all cells

_____/_____/___/_____
p   r   cv   s

e. too few rosy red (cells)

_____/_____/_____
r   cv   s

f. too few neutral (cells)

_____/_____/_____
r   cv   s

---

7. -phil–suffix meaning **attracted to**

This suffix is used to name three types of white blood cells based on type of stain they attract (chemically bind with)

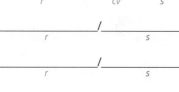

>8.3 Eosinophil

a. attracted to rosy red

_____/_____/_____
r   cv   s

b. attracted to basic

_____/_____/_____
r   cv   s

c. attracted to neutral

_____/_____/_____
r   cv   s

---

8. -poiesis–suffix meaning **formation**

This suffix is used to indicate process that produces new blood cells

a. formation of red (cells)

_____/_____/_____
r   cv   s

b. formation of white (cells)

_____/_____/_____
r   cv   s

c. formation of clotting (cells)

_____/_____/_____
r   cv   s

---

9. thromb/o–combining form meaning **clot**

A clot is a hard collection of fibrin, blood cells, and tissue debris that is end result of hemostasis or blood-clotting process

a. destruction of a clot

_____/_____/_____
r   cv   s

b. surgical removal of a clot

_____/_____
r   s

c. abnormal condition of clots

_____/_____
r   s

Hematology Vocabulary

The hematology terms presented in this section include eponyms, modern English words, and those that contain Latin or Greek word parts but are not constructed solely from these word parts. When you recognize word parts within a term they will give you a hint about the word's meaning. In these instances, look for the word parts to follow the term.

Term	Explanation
anemia an- = without **-emia** = blood condition	Group of blood disorders involving either a reduction in number of circulating erythrocytes or amount of hemoglobin in red blood cells; results in decreased oxygen delivery to tissues
anticoagulant anti- = against **coagul/o** = clotting	Any substance that prevents clot formation
aplastic anemia a- = without **-plasm** = formation **-tic** = pertaining to an- = without **-emia** = blood condition	Severe form of anemia caused by loss of functioning red bone marrow; results in decrease in number of all blood cells; may require bone marrow transplant
autotransfusion auto- = self	Collecting and storing one's own blood to use to replace blood lost during surgery
blood culture and sensitivity (C&S)	Blood specimen incubated to check for bacterial growth; if bacteria are present, they are identified and best antibiotic treatment is determined
blood transfusion	Transfer of blood from one person to another

TERMINOLOGY TIDBIT

The term *anemia* is built by combining the Greek prefix *an-* meaning "without" and *haima* meaning "blood." The *h* has been lost over time.

TERMINOLOGY TIDBIT

The term *culture* comes from the Latin word *cultura* meaning "to grow or cultivate." This part of a lab test involves growing bacteria from an infection

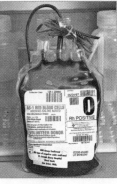

>8.4 A blood bag prepared for a transfusion. Bag is clearly labeled with blood type and identification number

bone marrow aspiration

Removal of small sample of bone marrow by needle and examined for diseases such as leukemia or aplastic anemia

>8.5 Bone marrow is being aspirated from leg of an infant to test for leukemia

bone marrow transplant (BMT)

Patient receives red bone marrow donation after own bone marrow is destroyed by radiation or chemotherapy

coagulate
  coagul/o = clotting

Formation of blood clot

➕ **TERMINOLOGY TIDBIT**

The term *coagulate* comes from the Latin word *coagulare* meaning "to curdle."

complete blood count (CBC)

Comprehensive blood test that includes red blood cell count (RBC), white blood cell count (WBC), hemoglobin (Hgb), hematocrit (Hct), white blood cell differential, and platelet count *blood volume*

embolus
  embol/o = plug

Commonly called *floating clot;* usually piece of thrombus breaks away and floats through bloodstream until it lodges in a smaller blood vessel and blocks blood flow

erythrocyte sedimentation rate (ESR, sed rate)
  erythr/o = red
  -cyte = cell

Blood test that measures rate at which red blood cells settle out of blood to form sediment in bottom of test tube; indicates presence of inflammatory disease

hematocrit (HCT, Hct, crit)
  hemat/o = blood

Blood test that measures volume of red blood cells within total volume of blood

hematoma
  hemat/o = blood
  -oma = mass

Blood collection under skin by escaping into tissue from damaged blood vessel; commonly called *bruise*

➕ **TERMINOLOGY TIDBIT**

The term *hematoma* can be confusing. Its simple translation is "blood tumor"; however, it is used to refer to blood that has leaked out of a blood vessel and pooled in the tissues. For example, a bruise is a type of hematoma.

>8.6 A large hematoma on the forehead of a young man

Term	Explanation
hemoglobin (Hgb, hb) hem/o = blood -globin = protein	Blood test that measures amount of hemoglobin present in given volume of blood
hemophilia hem/o = blood -phil = attraction	Inherited lack of a vital clotting factor; results in almost complete inability to stop bleeding
iron-deficiency anemia an- = without -emia = blood condition	Anemia resulting when there is not enough iron to build hemoglobin for red blood cells
leukemia leuk/o = white -emia = blood condition	Cancer of leukocyte-forming red bone marrow; patient has large number of abnormal and immature leukocytes circulating in blood
pernicious anemia (PA) an- = without -emia = blood condition	Anemia resulting when digestive system absorbs insufficient amount of vitamin B_{12}; vitamin B_{12} is necessary for erythrocyte production

＋ TERMINOLOGY TIDBIT

The term *pernicious* comes from the Latin word *perniciosus* meaning "destructive."

[handwritten: Small intestine] *[handwritten: IM injections about 1 x mont]*

Term	Explanation
phlebotomy phleb/o = vein -otomy = cutting into	Removal of blood specimen from vein for laboratory tests; also called *venipuncture*
platelet count	Blood test that determines number of platelets in given volume of blood
polycythemia vera poly- = many cyt/o = cell hem/o = blood -ia = condition	Condition characterized by too many erythrocytes; blood becomes too thick to flow easily through blood vessels
prothrombin time (Pro time, PT)	Blood test that measures how long it takes for clot to form after prothrombin, a blood clotting protein, is activated
red blood cell count (RBC)	Blood test that determines number of erythrocytes in volume of blood; decrease may indicate anemia; increase may indicate polycythemia vera
septicemia septic/o = infection -emia = blood condition	Presence of bacteria or their toxins in bloodstream; commonly called *blood poisoning*

Term	Explanation
sequential multiple analyzer computer (SMAC)	Machine that performs multiple blood chemistry tests automatically
serum	Blood that has had formed elements and clotting factors removed

sickle cell anemia
  an- = without
  -emia = blood condition
	Inherited blood cell disorder in which erythrocytes take on an abnormal curved or "sickle" shape; cells are fragile and easily damaged resulting in anemia; occurs almost exclusively in persons of African descent

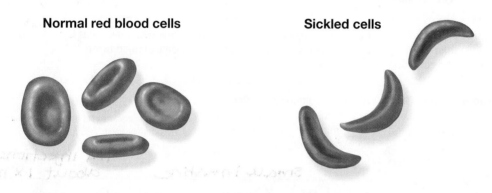

Normal red blood cells   Sickled cells

>8.7 Comparison of normal-shaped and abnormal sickle-shaped red blood cells

Term	Explanation	
thalassemia **-emia** = blood condition	Inherited blood disorder in which body is unable to correctly make hemoglobin, resulting in anemia	**➕ TERMINOLOGY TIDBIT** The term *thalassemia* comes from the Greek word *thalassa* meaning "sea." This name came about because this condition was first known around the Mediterranean Sea.

thrombolytic therapy
  thromb/o = clot
  -lytic = destruction
	Administering medication to dissolve blood clot and restore normal circulation	

white blood cell count (WBC)	Blood test that determines number of leukocytes in volume of blood; increase may indicate infection or leukemia; decrease may be caused by some diseases, radiation therapy, or chemotherapy	
white blood cell differential (diff)	Blood test determines number of each type of leukocyte	

Hematology Abbreviations

The following list presents common hematology abbreviations.

basos	basophils	**PMN, polys**	polymorphonuclear
BMT	bone marrow transplant		neutrophil
CBC	complete blood count	**PT, pro-time**	prothrombin time
diff	differential	**RBC**	red blood cell, red blood
eosins, eos	eosinophils		count
ESR, SR, sed rate	erythrocyte sedimentation	**Rh+**	Rh-positive
	rate	**Rh-**	Rh-negative
HCT, Hct, crit	hematocrit	**segs**	segmented neutrophils
Hgb, Hb, HGB	hemoglobin	**SMAC**	sequential multiple analyzer
lymphs	lymphocytes		computer
monos	monocytes	**WBC**	white blood cell, white
PA	pernicious anemia		blood count

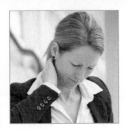

History of Present Illness

A 42-year-old woman is referred to the hematology clinic by her family physician. She reports experiencing increasing fatigue and dyspnea. It was initially associated only with intense physical activity, but now she cannot walk up a flight of stairs without becoming short of breath. She has had three episodes of sinusitis and pharyngitis in the last six months. She has noticed that she bruises more easily than usual and in the last week has had two spontaneous episodes of epistaxis. A CBC performed by her family physician reveals marked pancytopenia prompting the hematology referral.

Past Medical History

Past medical history is unremarkable. She had an appendectomy at age 12 and cholecystectomy at age 35. She has been pregnant three times and has two healthy children and had one miscarriage. She reports normal and regular menstrual periods, no signs of menopause. Patient currently takes no regular medications.

Family and Social History

Patient is married. She works as a chemical researcher for a company producing pesticides. She has no travel outside the country. Parents are alive. Father has hypertension; mother is healthy. Patient is an only child.

Physical Examination

Patient is a thin but well-nourished female who appears older than her stated age. She appears pale and has multiple dime-sized bruises scattered across her arms and lower legs. Respiratory rate is 22 breaths/minute, heart rate is 102 bpm, and blood pressure is 140/78.

(continued)

CASE STUDY

Laboratory Findings

Due to already established pancytopenia, a bone marrow aspiration was performed for a bone marrow biopsy. Results of biopsy revealed that bone marrow contained fewer of all cell types than normal. The cells that are present are normal, no evidence of cancer.

Diagnosis

Aplastic anemia

Plan of Treatment

1. Blood transfusion to restore normal erythrocyte and platelet counts and relieve current symptoms
2. Long-term antibiotics to prevent recurring infection
3. Bone marrow–stimulating medication
4. If cell counts do not improve following bone marrow–stimulating medication or if cell counts continue to drop, patient will need a bone marrow transplant
5. Patient is advised to avoid strenuous exercise, refrain from contact sports, to practice good hand washing, and to avoid sick people

Critical Thinking Questions

Answer the following questions regarding this case study. Do not just copy words out of the case study; translate all medical terms. To answer some of these questions, you may need to look up information from another chapter of this text, in a medical dictionary, or online. Answers are found at the back of the book.

1. Summarize the complaints that brought this patient to her family physician. Look up and define all medical terms used to describe her symptoms.

   _____

   _____

2. What test did the family physician perform? What does this test entail?

   _____

   _____

3. What was the result of the CBC? How does this explain each of the patient's symptoms?

   _____

   _____

4. What is this patient's medical history in nonmedical terms?

   _____

   _____

5. Carefully review the patient's family and social history. Is there some factor that might be the cause of her bone marrow dysfunction?

   _____

   _____

6. What are the patient's respiratory rate and heart rate? Measure your own breathing rate and pulse and compare them with the patient's results. Go to National Institutes of Health Medline Plus Medical Encyclopedia at http://www.nlm.nih.gov/medlineplus/encyclopedia.html. Click on V, and scroll down the list and click on Vital Signs. Are her values high, low, or normal?

_____

_____

7. What is a biopsy? What tissue was biopsied in this patient? Summarize the results.

_____

_____

8. List the treatments planned for this patient and indicate which treats her current symptoms and which treat the underlying cause of her condition.

_____

_____

Sound It Out

The following are some of the key terms from this chapter written as their phonetic spelling. Sound out each term and write it in the blank. Pronunciations for all terms are included in the audio glossary at www.mymedicalterminologylab.com <http://www.mymedicalterminologylab.com/>.

1. hee-MAT-oh-krit _____

2. an-tih-koh-AG-yoo-lant _____

3. loo-koh-poy-EE-sis _____

4. koh-ag-YOO-late _____

5. EM-boh-lus _____

6. hee-moe-sigh-TOM-eh-ter _____

7. EE-oh-sin-oh-PEE-nee-ah _____

8. hee-MAT-ik _____

9. an-NEE-mee-ah _____

10. hee-mat-oh-path-ALL-oh-jee _____

11. BASE-oh-fill _____

12. hee-mah-toh-poy-EE-sis _____

13. eh-RITH-roh-sight _____

14. HEE-moe-sigh-toh-LYE-sis _____

15. throm-boh-LYE-sis _____

16. hee-moh-GLOH-bin _____

17. AW-toh-trans-FYOO-zhun _____

18. hee-MALL-ih-sis _____

19. ee-RITH-row-PEE-nee-ah _____

20. HYE-per-lih-PEE-me-ah _____

21. loo-KEE-mee-ah _____

22. ee-RITH-row-sigh-toe-sis _____

23. LOO-koh-sight _____

24. hee-mah-TALL-oh-jist _____

25. LOO-koh-sigh-toh-sis _____

26. hee-moe-sigh-TOH-mah _____

27. throm-BOH-sis _____

28. hee-moh-STAY-sis _____

29. LIM-foh-sight _____

30. MON-oh-sight _____

31. hee-moe-sigh-TOM-eh-tree _____

32. ee-oh-SIN-oh-fill _____

33. NOO-troh-fill _____

34. PAN-sigh-toe-PEE-nee-ah _____

35. hee-mah-TOH-mah _____

36. fleh-BOT-oh-mee _____

37. eh-rith-roh-poy-EE-sis _____

38. PLAZ-mah _____

39. HEM-er-rij _____

40. PLAYT-lets _____

41. sep-tih-SEE-mee-ah _____

42. thal-ah-SEE-mee-ah _____

43. HIGH-poh-gly-SEE-me-ah _____

44. throm-BEK-toh-me _____

45. noo-troh-PEE-nee-ah _____

46. THROM-boh-sight _____

47. throm-boh-sigh-TOH-sis _____

48. hee-moh-FILL-ee-ah _____

49. LOO-koh-PEE-nee-ah _____

50. throm-boh-poy-EE-sis _____

Transcription Practice

Each of the following sentences is written in common English. Underline any words or phrases that can be replaced by a medical term. Then rewrite the entire sentence using medical terms. Answers are found at the end of this book.

1. The formed elements of blood are red blood cells, white blood cells, and clotting cells.

   _____

   _____

2. The patient had a small sample of bone marrow removed to determine whether she had cancer of the white cell that forms bone marrow.

   _____

   _____

3. The blood vessel was blocked by a floating clot.

_____

_____

4. Elena received medication to dissolve a blood clot during her heart attack.

_____

_____

5. Because he had diabetes, Ted monitored his blood for excessive sugar blood condition.

_____

_____

6. The patient suffered bursting forth of blood and a blood mass as a result of the auto accident.

_____

_____

7. The blood specialist determined that Genevieve had developed anemia due to vitamin B_{12} deficiency.

_____

_____

8. Following heart surgery, Tran received a blood transfusion of his own blood.

_____

_____

9. A comprehensive blood test including six different tests revealed that Marco had too few of all cells.

_____

_____

10. Because blood poisoning was suspected, a test to check for bacteria growth in the blood was ordered.

_____

_____

Abbreviation Matching

Match each abbreviation with its definition.

_____ **1.** ESR   **A.** red blood cell

_____ **2.** PT   **B.** hemoglobin

_____ **3.** CBC   **C.** pernicious anemia

_____ **4.** RBC   **D.** bone marrow transplant

_____ **5.** diff   **E.** complete blood count

_____ **6.** HCT   **F.** sequential multiple analyzer computer

_____ **7.** BMT   **G.** erythrocyte sedimentation rate

_____ **8.** Hgb   **H.** hematocrit

_____ **9.** SMAC   **I.** differential

_____ **10.** PA   **J.** prothrombin time

Fill in the Blank

Fill in the blank to complete each of the following sentences.

1. _____ anemia is caused by loss of functioning red bone marrow.

2. The medical term for *floating clot* is _____.

3. Receiving medication to dissolve a blood clot is called _____ therapy.

4. Polycythemia vera is a condition marked by _____ erythrocytes.

5. Another term for *phlebotomy* is _____.

6. A blood _____ is a test to check for bacterial growth.

7. A(n) _____ is a test that measures the volume of red blood cells.

8. Cancer of the leukocyte-forming bone marrow is called _____.

9. Pernicious anemia is caused by insufficient _____.

10. Septicemia is commonly called _____.

Labeling Exercise

Write the name of each blood cell on the numbered line. Also use this space to write the combining form where appropriate.

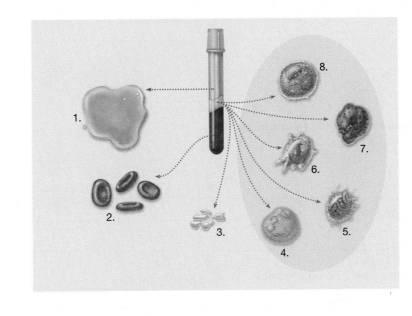

1._____   5._____

2._____   6._____

3._____   7._____

4._____   8._____

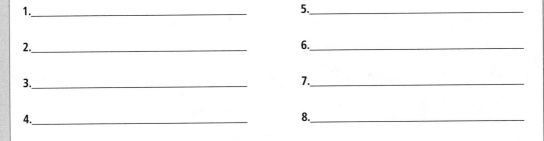

PEARSON mymedicalterminologylab

MyMedicalTerminologyLab is a premium online homework management system that includes a host of features to help you study. Registered users will find:

- Fun games and activities built within a virtual hospital
- Powerful tools that track and analyze your results—allowing you to create a personalized learning experience
- Videos, flashcards, and audio pronunciations to help enrich your progress
- Streaming lesson presentations and self-paced learning modules
- A space where you and your instructors can view and manage your assignments

Build Medical Terms

Use each of the following word parts to build the indicated medical terms.

The combining form *cyt/o* means cell.

1. red cell _____

2. white cell _____

3. clotting cell _____

The combining form *hemat/o* means blood.

4. study of blood _____

5. blood formation _____

6. pertaining to blood _____

7. blood mass _____

The suffix *-emia* means blood condition.

8. excessive sugar blood condition _____

9. without blood condition _____

The combining form *hem/o* means blood.

10. blood stopping _____

11. blood bursting forth _____

12. blood destruction _____

The suffix *-phil* means attracted to.

13. rosy red attracted to _____

14. basic attracted to _____

15. neutral attracted to _____

Medical Term Analysis

Examine each of the following terms. Begin by dividing it into its word parts and writing them in the indicated blanks (P = prefix, WR = word root; CF = combining form; S = suffix). Follow with the definition of each word part and then finally the meaning of the full term.

1. **erythrocytosis**

   CF _____

   means _____

   S _____

   means _____

   Term Meaning: _____

   _____

2. **hematologist**

   CF _____

   means _____

   S _____

   means _____

   Term Meaning: _____

   _____

3. **hematopathology**

   CF _____

   means _____

   CF _____

   means _____

   S _____

   means _____

   Term Meaning: _____

   _____

4. **hyperlipemia**

   P _____

   means _____

   WR _____

   means _____

   S _____

   means _____

   Term Meaning: _____

   _____

5. **hemocytometer**

   CF _____

   means _____

   CF _____

   means _____

   S _____

   means _____

   Term Meaning: _____

   _____

6. **leukopoiesis**

   CF _____

   means _____

   S _____

   means _____

   Term Meaning: _____

   _____

7. lymphocyte

CF _____

means _____

S _____

means _____

Term Meaning: _____

_____

8. hemoglobin

CF _____

means _____

S _____

means _____

Term Meaning: _____

_____

9. pancytopenia

P _____

means _____

CF _____

means _____

S _____

means _____

Term Meaning: _____

_____

10. thrombectomy

WR _____

means _____

S _____

means _____

Term Meaning: _____

_____

Spelling

Some of the following terms are misspelled. Identify the incorrect terms and spell them correctly in the blank provided.

1. hypoglysemia _____

2. pernicious _____

3. anticoagulant _____

4. septecemia _____

5. thalassemia _____

6. platlet _____

7. polycytemia vera _____

8. phlebotomy _____

9. thrombocytopenia _____

10. eyrthropoiesis _____

Photomatch Challenge

Put the following phlebotomy photos in order by placing the appropriate letter beside the corresponding number in the blanks below.

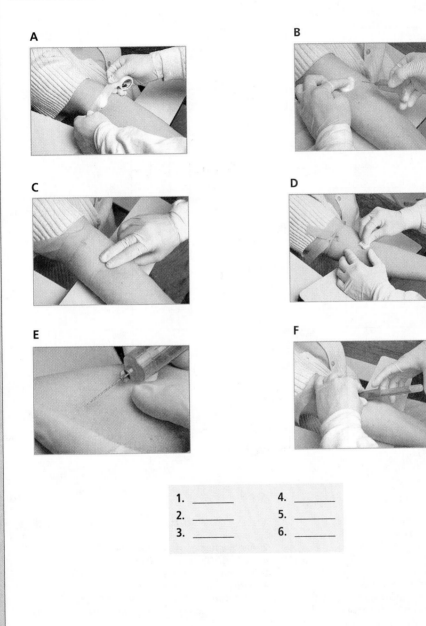

A

B

C

D

E

F

1. _____   4. _____

2. _____   5. _____

3. _____   6. _____

Crossword Puzzle

Use the definitions given to complete the crossword puzzle.

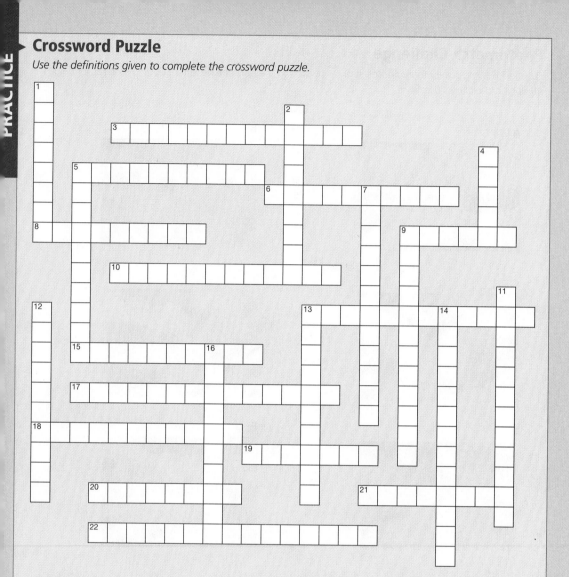

ACROSS

3 Substance that prevents clot formation
5 Protein that transports oxygen
6 Inherited lack of vital clotting factor
8 Formation of a blood clot
9 Fluid portion of blood
10 Term for abnormal increase in number of white cells
13 _____ vera, too many erythrocytes
15 Term meaning "clot abnormal condition"
17 Term meaning "formation of red cells"
18 Inherited blood disorder, unable to correctly make hemoglobin
19 A floating clot
20 Commonly called a bruise
21 Cancer of leukocyte-forming bone marrow
22 Receiving one's own blood to replace lost blood

DOWN

1 _____ anemia, caused by loss of functioning bone marrow
2 Another name for thrombocytes
4 Plasma with clotting factors deactivated
5 Test that measures volume of red blood cells
7 Term meaning low blood sugar
9 Term meaning "too few of all cells"
11 Test determines number of each type of leukocyte
12 Venipuncture
13 _____ anemia, results from B12 deficiency
14 Term for instrument for measuring blood cells
16 Blood poisoning

Immunology
Immune Systems

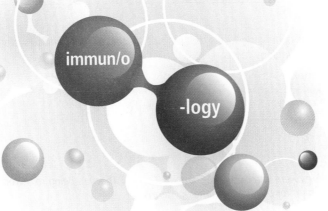

immun/o

-logy

A Brief Introduction to Immunology

 UNDERSTAND the function of the immune and lymphatic systems.

The **immune system** is a network of cells, tissues, and organs throughout the body that work together to protect the body against **pathogens,** anything that can damage the body including viruses, bacteria, toxins, or cancerous cells. Many of the functions of the immune system are carried out by white blood cells called **lymphocytes.** These cells are concentrated throughout the body in the organs of the **lymphatic system:** lymph nodes, tonsils, thymus gland, and spleen.

DESCRIBE the medical specialty of immunology.

   Immunology is the branch of medicine that diagnoses and treats conditions involving the immune system. Conditions that **immunologists** often treat include allergies, immunodeficiency disorders, autoimmune diseases, and cancers of the immune system. An **allergist** is an immunologist who has specialized training in treating allergies.

Immunology Combining Forms

The following list presents new combining forms important for building and defining immunology terms.

adenoid/o	adenoids		path/o	disease
immun/o	protection		phag/o	eating
lymph/o	lymph		splen/o	spleen
lymphaden/o	lymph node		thym/o	thymus
lymphangi/o	lymph vessel		tonsill/o	tonsils

The following list presents combining forms that are not specific to the immune system but are also used for building and defining immunology terms.

cortic/o	cortex
cyt/o	cell
system/o	system

Suffix Review

These suffixes and prefixes were introduced in Chapters 2 and 3. They are being reviewed in this chapter because they are especially important for building immunology terms.

-ar	pertaining to		-logist	one who studies
-atic	pertaining to		-logy	study of
-cyte	cell		-malacia	softening
-ectasis	dilated		-megaly	enlarged
-ectomy	surgical removal		-oid	resembling
-edema	swelling		-oma	tumor
-gen	that which produces		-osis	abnormal condition
-genic	producing		-pathy	disease
-globulin	protein		-pexy	surgical fixation
-gram	record		-plasty	surgical repair
-graphy	process of recording		-rrhaphy	suture
-iasis	abnormal condition		-stasis	stopping
-ic	pertaining to		-therapy	treatment
-ist	specialist		-toxic	poison
-itis	inflammation			

Prefix Review

anti-	against
auto-	self
mono-	one

Organs Commonly Treated in Immunology

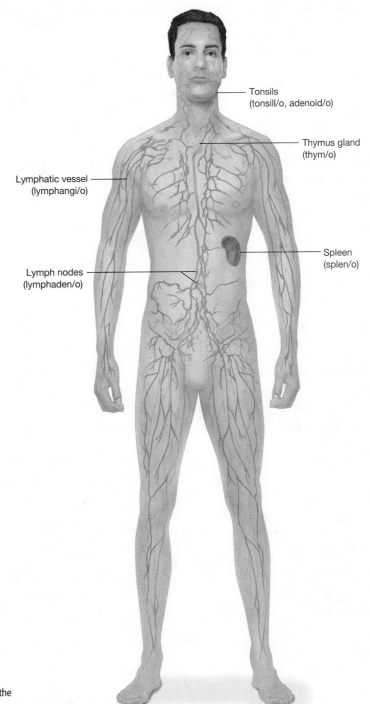

Tonsils
(tonsill/o, adenoid/o)

Thymus gland
(thym/o)

Lymphatic vessel
(lymphangi/o)

Spleen
(splen/o)

Lymph nodes
(lymphaden/o)

>9.1 Organs of the
lymphatic system

BUILD immunology medical terms from word parts.

Building Immunology Terms

This section presents word parts most often used to build immunology terms. Following the explanation of the term, you have the opportunity to begin building your own vocabulary. Read the meaning for each term and then fill in the blanks to build a single medical term. Use the slashes to divide prefixes, word roots, combining vowels, and suffixes. To help you out you will find a key to the word parts underneath the blanks: r for word roots, p for prefix, cv for combining vowel, and s for suffix. Remember that not every term will contain all these word parts; it's up to you to decide which to use. As you gain experience, this process becomes easier. Answers can be found at the back of the book.

1. **adenoid/o**–combining form meaning **adenoids**

    Adenoids is the commonly used term for **pharyngeal tonsils,** located on back wall of upper throat

    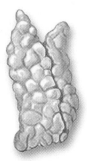

    >9.2 Adenoid

    a. surgical removal of adenoids   _____/_____
                                              r   s

    b. inflammation of adenoids   _____/_____
                                          r   s

2. **immun/o**–combining form meaning **protection, immunity**

    The immune system is responsible for protecting body against pathogens and removing damaged cells

    a. one who studies immunity   _____/_____/_____
                                          r   cv   s

    b. study of immunity   _____/_____/_____
                                   r   cv   s

    c. protection protein   _____/_____/_____
                                    r   cv   s

    d. producing protection   _____/_____/_____
                                      r   cv   s

    e. immunity treatment   _____/_____/_____
                                    r   cv   s

3. **lymph/o**–combining form meaning **lymph**

Lymph is the clear fluid collected from tissues of body by lymphatic vessels; flows through vessels to be returned to venous circulation

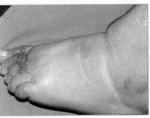

+ TERMINOLOGY TIDBIT

The term *lymph* comes from the Latin word *lympha*, which means "clear spring water."

>9.3 Lymphedema very commonly occurs in the lower leg

a. pertaining to lymph

_____/_____
          r   s

b. lymph tumor

_____/_____
          r   s

c. lymph swelling

_____/_____
          r   s

d. lymph cell

_____/____/_____
       r   cv   s

e. pertaining to a lymph cell

_____/____/_____/____
    r   cv   r   s

f. lymph cell tumor

_____/____/_____/____
    r   cv   r   s

g. producing lymph

_____/____/_____
       r   cv   s

h. resembling lymph

_____/_____
          r   s

i. stopping lymph

_____/____/_____
       r   cv   s

4. **lymphaden/o**–combining form meaning **lymph node**

The simple translation of this combining form is "lymph gland," however these organs are not actually glands; lymph nodes are small roundish organs located along the path of lymphatic vessels that house lymphocytes and other white blood cells; as lymph passes through the lymph nodes its cells are able to remove pathogens and damaged cells

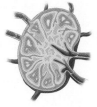

>9.4 Lymph node

a. surgical removal of a lymph node

_____/_____
          r   s

b. disease of lymph nodes

_____/____/_____
       r   cv   s

c. process of recording lymph nodes

_____/____/_____
       r   cv   s

d. record of lymph nodes

_____/____/_____
       r   cv   s

e. lymph node inflammation

_____/_____
          r   s

f. abnormal condition of the lymph nodes

_____/_____
          r   s

5. **lymphangi/o**–combining form meaning **lymph vessel**

    Vessels that pick up excess fluid from tissues and return it to circulatory system

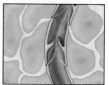

>9.5 Lymphatic vessel

   a. lymph vessel inflammation   _____/_____
                                                 r   s

   b. disease of lymph vessel   _____/____/_____
                                              r   cv   s

   c. lymph vessel tumor   _____/_____
                                         r   s

   d. process of recording lymph vessels   _____/____/_____
                                                        r   cv   s

   e. record of a lymph vessel   _____/____/_____
                                             r   cv   s

   f. surgical removal of a lymph vessel   _____/_____
                                                       r   s

   g. dilated lymph vessel   _____/_____
                                          r   s

   h. surgical repair of a lymph vessel   _____/____/_____
                                                      r   cv   s

6. **path/o**–combining form meaning **disease**

   a. disease producing   _____/____/_____
                                      r   cv   s

   b. that which produces disease   _____/____/_____
                                               r   cv   s

   c. study of disease   _____/____/_____
                                     r   cv   s

   d. one who studies disease   _____/____/_____
                                           r   cv   s

7. **phag/o**–combining form meaning **eating**

    Some leukocytes, such as **monocytes,** are important to immune system because they are able to engulf or "eat" pathogens or damaged cells

   a. eating cell   _____/____/_____
                                r   cv   s

   b. pertaining to an eating cell   _____/____/_____/____
                                                r   cv   r   s

8. **splen/o**–combining form meaning **spleen**

The spleen is an organ in the lymphatic system; located on left side of upper abdomen; houses leukocytes responsible for filtering blood and destroying worn-out red blood cells

>9.6 Spleen

a. pertaining to the spleen

_____/_____
r   s

b. spleen inflammation

_____/_____
r   s

c. resembling the spleen

_____/_____
r   s

d. spleen tumor

_____/_____
r   s

e. surgical removal of the spleen

_____/_____
r   s

f. enlarged spleen

_____/_____/_____
r   CV   s

g. softening of the spleen

_____/_____/_____
r   CV   s

h. surgical fixation of the spleen

_____/_____/_____
r   CV   s

i. suture of the spleen

_____/_____/_____
r   CV   s

9. **thym/o**–combining form meaning **thymus gland**

The thymus gland is located in mediastinum behind sternum; in early life is necessary for proper development of immune system; by puberty has begun to shrink

⊞ **TERMINOLOGY TIDBIT**

The Greek term *thymos*, meaning "warty," was used to describe the bumpy appearance of the thymus gland.

>9.7 Thymus gland

a. pertaining to the thymus gland

_____/_____
r   s

b. surgical removal of the thymus gland

_____/_____
r   s

c. thymus gland tumor

_____/_____
r   s

10. **tonsill/o**–combining form meaning **tonsils**

The three sets of tonsils are located in throat: palatine, pharyngeal, and lingual; contain lymphatic tissue that protects body from pathogens in air breathed and food eaten

a. pertaining to the tonsils

_____/_____
r   s

b. surgical removal of the tonsils

_____/_____
r   s

c. tonsils inflammation

_____/_____
r   s

EXPLAIN immunology medical terms.

Immunology Vocabulary

The immunology terms presented in this section include eponyms, modern English words, and those that contain Latin or Greek word parts but are not constructed solely from these word parts. When you recognize word parts within a term they will give you a hint about the word's meaning. In these instances, look for the word parts to follow the term.

Term	Explanation
AIDS-related complex (ARC)	Early stage of human immunodeficiency virus (HIV) infection in which mild symptoms of infection are present, including lymphadenopathy, fatigue, fever, night sweats, weight loss, and diarrhea
acquired immunodeficiency syndrome (AIDS) immun/o = protection	Later stage of human immunodeficiency virus (HIV) infection when the cells of the immune system lose their ability to fight off infection; patients become unable to resist opportunistic infections such as *Pneumocystis carinii* pneumonia and Kaposi sarcoma
allergist -ist = specialist	Physician specializing in diagnosis and treatment of allergies
allergy	Hypersensitivity to a common substance in environment (such as pollen), to food, or to medication
anaphylactic shock	Life-threatening condition resulting from severe allergic reaction causing cardio-vascular and respiratory problems; may be triggered by bee stings, medications, or certain foods; also called *anaphylaxis*
antihistamine anti- = against	Medication that blocks effects of histamine released by body during allergic reactions
antinuclear antibody titer (ANA) anti- = against	Blood test that determines number of antibodies against cell nuclei present in bloodstream; elevated in autoimmune conditions
autoimmune disease auto- = self	Disease resulting from body's immune system attacking its own cells as if they were pathogens; examples include systemic lupus erythematosus and sarcoidosis
corticosteroids cortic/o = cortex	Hormones produced by adrenal cortex; used as medication to treat autoimmune diseases due to their very strong anti-inflammatory properties

Term	Explanation

cytotoxic cells
 cyt/o = cell
 -toxic = poison

Cells capable of physically attacking and killing pathogens or diseased cells

elephantiasis
 -iasis = abnormal condition

Results from blockage of lymphatic vessels that causes extreme tissue edema

+ **TERMINOLOGY TIDBIT**

Elephantiasis causes so much swelling in the leg that the knee and ankle disappear making it look like an elephant's leg.

Blocked lymphatic vessel

Swollen lymphatic vessel

>9.8 Elephantiasis. Note how a blocked lymphatic vessel causes fluid to collect in the leg

enzyme-linked immunosorbent assay (ELISA)

Blood test for antibody to acquired immunodeficiency syndrome (AIDS) virus; positive result means the person has been exposed to virus

hives

Common name for appearance of wheals during allergic reaction

Hodgkin disease (HD)

Cancer of lymphatic cells found in lymph nodes; also called *Hodgkin lymphoma*

immunodeficiency
 immun/o = protection

Having an immune system that is unable to respond properly to pathogens; also called *immunocompromised*

immunosuppressant
 immun/o = protection

Medication to block certain actions of immune system; used to prevent rejection of transplanted organ

inflammation

Tissue response to injury; characterized by redness, pain, swelling, and feeling hot to touch

>9.9 Inflammation as illustrated by cellulitis of the forearm. Note that the area is red and swollen. It is also painful and hot to touch

Kaposi sarcoma (KS)
  -oma = tumor

Type of skin cancer often seen in patients with AIDS; consists of brownish-purple papules that begin in skin and spread to internal organs

>9.10 Skin lesions characteristic of Kaposi sarcoma

mononucleosis (mono)
  mono- = one
  -osis = abnormal condition

Acute viral infection of lymphoid tissue with large number of abnormal white blood cells circulating in bloodstream

non-Hodgkin lymphoma (NHL)
  lymph/o = lymph
  -oma = tumor

Cancer of the lymphatic tissues other than Hodgkin lymphoma

>9.11 Lymphoma

opportunistic infections

Infections seen in patients with compromised immune systems

***Pneumocystis carinii* pneumonia (PCP)**

Opportunistic infection common in immunodeficient persons

sarcoidosis
  -osis = abnormal condition

Autoimmune disease with fibrous lesions forming in lymph nodes, liver, skin, lungs, spleen, eyes, and small bones of hands and feet

scratch test

Type of allergy testing in which body is exposed to allergens through a light scratch in skin

Term	Explanation
severe combined immunodeficiency syndrome (SCIDS) immun/o = protection	Genetic condition of children born with nonfunctioning immune system who often forced to live in sealed sterile rooms
systemic lupus erythematosus (SLE) system/o = systems -ic = pertaining to	Autoimmune disease in which immune system attacks connective tissue throughout body such as in joints and skin
urticaria	Severe itching associated with hives, usually seen in allergic reactions to food, stress, or medications
vaccination	Exposure to weakened pathogen to stimulate immune response and antibody production to give future protection against full-blown disease; also called *immunization*
Western blot test	Blood test to detect various antibodies in bloodstream such as HIV antibodies; considered more precise than ELISA

+ TERMINOLOGY TIDBIT

The first vaccine was to provide protection against smallpox; it was made from the drainage from cowpox sores, a condition closely related to smallpox. The term *vaccination* comes from the Latin word *vaccinus*, meaning "relating to a cow."

 USE Use immunology abbreviations.

Immunology Abbreviations

The following list presents common immunology abbreviations.

AIDS	acquired immunodeficiency syndrome	**KS**	Kaposi sarcoma
ANA	antinuclear antibody titer	**mono**	mononucleosis
ARC	AIDS-related complex	**NHL**	non-Hodgkin lymphoma
ELISA	enzyme-linked immunosorbent assay	**PCP**	*Pneumocystis carinii* pneumonia
HD	Hodgkin disease	**SCIDS**	severe combined immunodeficiency syndrome
HIV	human immunodeficiency virus (causes AIDS)	**T&A**	tonsillectomy and adenoidectomy
Ig	immunoglobulins (IgA, IgD, IgE, IgG, IgM)		

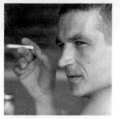

History of Present Illness

Patient is a 39-year-old male referred to the AIDS Clinic by the family physician. Patient was seen three weeks ago by family physician when he noticed he had white spots on his tongue and throat and had difficulty swallowing. Review of his physician's chart noted that this patient has had a 30-lb weight loss and several episodes of sinusitis and bronchitis over the past two years. When questioned, patient admitted that he was having regular bouts of diarrhea, night sweats, extreme fatigue, and unexplained fevers. Because of patient's past drug abuse history and current symptoms, he was referred to this clinic for evaluation.

Past Medical History

Patient is a recovering heroin abuser currently receiving treatment with methadone. Patient is on no other medication.

Family and Social History

Patient was a house painter but is becoming physically unable to perform the duties of his job. He is not married. Patient's parents are both alive and well.

Physical Examination

Patient appears older than his stated age, lethargic, and with muscular wasting. Temperature is 102°F, and the cervical and inguinal lymph nodes are enlarged.

Diagnostic Tests

ELISA was positive for HIV.

Diagnosis

AIDS-related complex

Plan of Treatment

1. Oral antifungal medication for treatment of thrush
2. Started on HIV drug regimen of Zidovudine (AZT), Epivir, and Viracept
3. Order Western blot to verify HIV infection
4. Monitor CD4 count

Critical Thinking Questions

Answer the following questions regarding this case study. Do not just copy words out of the case study; translate all medical terms. In order to answer some of these questions, you may need to look up information from another chapter of this text, in a medical dictionary, or online. Answers are found at the back of the book.

1. How was this patient probably infected by HIV? List two other ways in which persons may become exposed to HIV.

   _____

   _____

2. The white spots in the mouth of this patient are thrush. What causes this infection?

   _____

   _____

3. Read the entire case study carefully and list all of this patient's symptoms.

_____

_____

4. What is the first test used to diagnosis HIV infection, and why was a follow-up test ordered?

_____

_____

5. At this point, the patient is diagnosed with AIDS-related complex. What is the difference between ARC and AIDS?

_____

_____

6. What is an opportunistic infection? Name two that are commonly seen in AIDS patients.

_____

_____

7. This patient was started on an HIV drug regimen of three different medications. Use a website such as www.drugs.com or www.webmd.com/drugs to look up these drugs and briefly describe how they work.

_____

_____

8. A CD4 count was ordered for this patient. This is a count of a specific type of white blood cell targeted by HIV. Why do you think this piece of information is important for following this patient's progress?

_____

_____

Sound It Out

The following are some of the key terms from this chapter written as their phonetic spelling. Sound out each term and write it in the blank. Pronunciations for all terms are included in the audio glossary at www.mymedicalterminologylab.com <http://www.mymedicalterminologylab.com/>.

1. lim-FOH-mah _____

2. AL-er-jee _____

3. im-you-noh-JEN-ik _____

4. lim-fad-eh-NOP-ah-thee _____

5. im-yoo-noh-GLOB-yoo-lin _____

6. path-OL-oh-gee _____

7. lim-FAT-ik _____

8. IM-yoo-noh-thair-ah-pee _____

9. in-flah-MA-shun _____

10. LIMF _____

11. splen-oh-MEG-ah-lee _____

12. lim-fad-eh-NEK-toh-mee _____

13. an-tih-HIST-ah-meen _____

14. lim-fad-en-EYE-tis _____

15. core-tih-koh-STARE-royds _____

16. lim-fad-eh-NOG-rah-fee _____

17. ADD-eh-noy-DEK-toh-mee _____

18. LIM-fan-jee-EK-toh-me _____

19. LIM-fan-jee-EYE-tis _____

20. lim-FAN-jee-oh-gram _____

21. splen-OH-mah _____

22. lim-fan-jee-OH-mah _____

23. sar-koyd-OH-sis _____

24. lim-foh-SIT-ik _____

25. THIGH-mik _____

26. LIM-foyd _____

27. lim-foh-STAY-sis _____

28. mon-oh-nook-lee-OH-sis _____

29. PATH-oh-jen _____

30. SPLEN-oyd _____

31. path-oh-JEN-ik _____

32. FAY-go-sight _____

33. lim-foh-sigh-TOE-mah _____

34. er-tih-KAY-ree-ah _____

35. FAY-go-SIT-ik _____

36. splen-EK-toh-mee _____

37. ton-sih-LEK-toh-mee _____

38. splen-EYE-tis _____

39. im-yoo-NALL-oh-jist _____

40. SPLEN-oh-mah-LAY-shee-ah _____

41. el-eh-fan-TYE-ah-sis _____

42. limf-eh-DEE-mah _____

43. SPLEN-oh-PEKS-ee _____

44. thigh-MEK-toh-mee _____

45. TON-sih-lar _____

46. vak-sih-NAY-shun _____

47. thigh-MOH-mah _____

48. ADD-eh-noy-DYE-tis _____

49. lim-foh-JEN-ik _____

50. TON-sils _____

mymedicalterminologylab

PEARSON

MyMedicalTerminologyLab is a premium online homework management system that includes a host of features to help you study. Registered users will find:

- Fun games and activities built within a virtual hospital
- Powerful tools that track and analyze your results—allowing you to create a personalized learning experience
- Videos, flashcards, and audio pronunciations to help enrich your progress
- Streaming lesson presentations and self-paced learning modules
- A space where you and your instructors can view and manage your assignments

Transcription Practice

Each of the following sentences is written in common English. Underline any words or phrases that can be replaced by a medical term. Then rewrite the entire sentence using medical terms. Answers are found at the end of the book.

1. Marcie's repeated bouts of tonsil inflammation required her to have the tonsils surgically and adenoids surgically removed.

   _____

   _____

2. The lymph vessel record revealed a lymph vessel tumor.

   _____

   _____

3. The one who studies immunity is a physician who treats diseases in which the body's immune system attacks itself.

   _____

   _____

4. Jamar had a history of a life-threatening allergic reaction in response to a bee sting.

   _____

   _____

5. Mykos had to take medication to prevent transplant rejection after his kidney transplant.

   _____

   _____

6. Joyce's hypersensitivity to pollen was treated with medication that blocks the effects of histamine.

   _____

   _____

7. The patient in the late stages of HIV infection developed an opportunistic type of pneumonia.

   _____

   _____

8. Jennifer's allergic reactions consisted of wheals appearing and severe itching.

   _____

   _____

9. Shona's hand pain turned out to be caused by an autoimmune disease in which the immune system attacks connective tissue of her joints.

_____

_____

10. Carlos' lymph node disease turned out to be cancer of the lymphatic cells in the lymph nodes.

_____

_____

Build Medical Terms

Use each of the following word parts to build the indicated medical terms.

The combining form *lymphaden/o* means lymph node.

1. surgical removal of lymph node _____

2. lymph node record _____

3. lymph node disease _____

The combining form *immun/o* means protection or immunity.

4. protection protein _____

5. one who studies immunity _____

The combining form *splen/o* means spleen.

6. enlarged spleen _____

7. spleen resembling _____

8. pertaining to the spleen _____

The combining form *tonsill/o* means tonsils.

9. tonsil inflammation _____

10. tonsil surgical removal _____

11. pertaining to tonsils _____

The combining form *lymphangi/o* means lymph vessel.

12. lymph vessel inflammation _____

13. lymph vessel surgical repair _____

14. lymph vessel process of recording _____

15. lymph vessel tumor _____

Labeling Exercise

Write the name of each structure on the numbered line. Also use this space to write the combining form where appropriate.

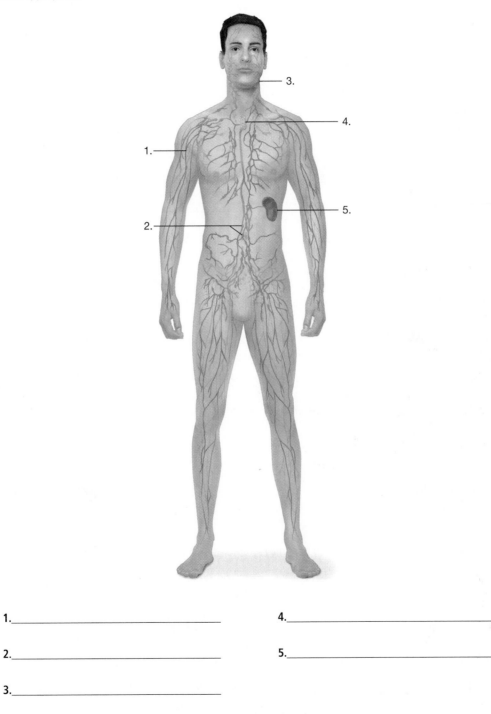

1._____

2._____

3._____

4._____

5._____

Spelling

Some of the following terms are misspelled. Identify the incorrect terms and spell them correctly in the blank provided.

1. urticoria _____

2. sarcoidosis _____

3. corticosteroids _____

4. anaphylactic _____

5. lymphadanosis _____

6. immunosuppressents _____

7. splenomalasia _____

8. tonsilitis _____

9. mononucleosis _____

10. antihistamine _____

Fill in the Blank

Fill in the blank to complete each of the following sentences.

1. The _____ is a physician specializing in treating allergies.

2. A(n) _____ disease results when the body's own immune system attacks itself.

3. Elephantiasis occurs when _____ become blocked causing extreme tissue _____.

4. Hives are the common name for _____ that appear during an allergic reaction.

5. _____ are hormones that can be used to treat autoimmune diseases.

6. The early stage of an HIV infection with mild symptoms is called _____.

7. Vaccinations may also be called _____.

8. Kaposi sarcoma is a type of _____ cancer seen in AIDS patients.

9. _____ is a life-threatening severe allergic reaction.

10. The _____ is considered more sensitive than an ELISA.

Abbreviation Matching

Match each abbreviation with its definition.

_____ **1.** T&A   **A.** severe combined immunodeficiency syndrome

_____ **2.** PCP   **B.** acquired immunodeficiency syndrome

_____ **3.** HD   **C.** *Pneumocystis carinii* pneumonia

_____ **4.** Ig   **D.** mononucleosis

_____ **5.** mono   **E.** non-Hodgkin lymphoma

_____ **6.** SCIDS   **F.** enzyme-linked immunosorbent assay

_____ **7.** NHL   **G.** tonsillectomy and adenoidectomy

_____ **8.** KS   **H.** immunoglobulin

_____ **9.** AIDS   **I.** Kaposi sarcoma

_____**10.** ELISA   **J.** Hodgkin disease

Medical Term Analysis

Examine each of the following terms. Begin by dividing it into its word parts and writing them in the indicated blanks (**P = prefix**, **WR = word root**; **CF = combining form**; **S = suffix**). Follow with the definition of each word part and then finally the meaning of the full term.

1. **adenoiditis**

    WR _____

    means _____

    S _____

    means _____

    Term Meaning: _____

    _____

2. **lymphogenic**

    CF _____

    means _____

    S _____

    means _____

    Term Meaning: _____

    _____

3. **immunotherapy**

    CF _____

    means _____

    S _____

    means _____

    Term Meaning: _____

    _____

4. **lymphocytoma**

CF _____

means _____

WR _____

means _____

S _____

means _____

Term Meaning: _____

_____

5. **phagocytic**

CF _____

means _____

WR _____

means _____

S _____

means _____

Term Meaning: _____

_____

6. **lymphadenopathy**

CF _____

means _____

S _____

means _____

Term Meaning: _____

_____

7. **pathology**

CF _____

means _____

S _____

means _____

Term Meaning: _____

_____

8. **lymphangiectasis**

WR _____

means _____

S _____

means _____

Term Meaning: _____

_____

9. **thymectomy**

WR _____

means _____

S _____

means _____

Term Meaning: _____

_____

10. **lymphedema**

WR _____

means _____

S _____

means _____

Term Meaning: _____

_____

Photomatch Challenge

The following figure illustrates what happens when inflammation occurs. The letters represent the order of events. The events listed are out of order. Your challenge is to match each letter on the figure with its description.

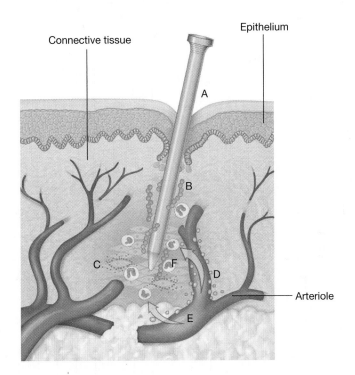

_____ 1. Bacteria enter and multiply

_____ 2. Arterioles dilate and become leaky

_____ 3. Dirty nail punctures skin

_____ 4. Injured cells release chemicals

_____ 5. Materials are released into damaged tissue to begin repairs

_____ 6. White blood cells destroy the bacteria

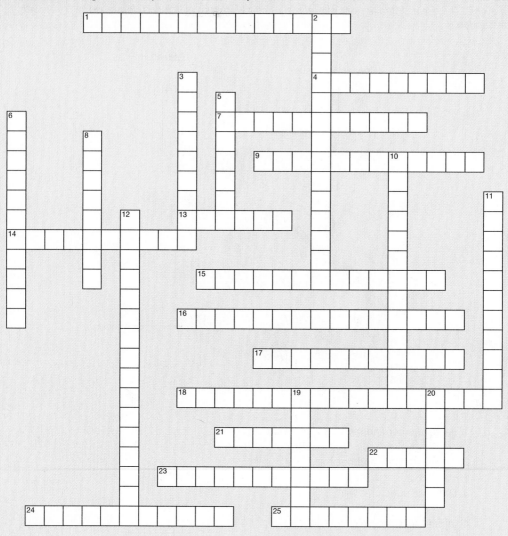

Crossword Puzzle

Use the definitions given to complete the crossword puzzle.

ACROSS

1 Medication used to treat autoimmune diseases
4 Severe itching with hives
7 Important white blood cells for immune system
9 Red, pain, hot, swollen issue response to injury
13 Gland necessary for development of immune system
14 SLE is a type of _____ disease
15 Condition results from blockage of lymphatic vessels
16 Term meaning lymphatic vessel disease
17 Term meaning tonsil inflammation
18 Medication to block immune system
21 Hypersensitivity to common substances
22 Appearance of wheals
23 Autoimmune disease with fibrous lesions
24 Another term for anaphylactic shock
25 Term for anything that can damage the body

DOWN

2 Term meaning protective protein
3 Term meaning cell that eats
5 Scratch test is a type of _____test
6 Also called immunization
8 Common name for pharyngeal tonsils
10 Medication to block effects of histamine
11 Term meaning one who studies disease
12 Another term for immunocompromised
19 Kaposi _____, skin cancer seen in AIDS patients
20 Organ that removes damaged red blood cells

10

Pulmonology
Respiratory System

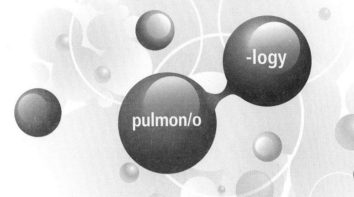

-logy

pulmon/o

A Brief Introduction to Pulmonology

 UNDERSTAND the functions of the respiratory system.

All cells of the body must have a constant supply of **oxygen** (O_2) in order to produce energy for cell work. The respiratory system is responsible for bringing fresh oxygen into the lungs where it is loaded into the bloodstream for distribution throughout the body. In addition, the blood has picked up **carbon dioxide** (CO_2), the waste product of energy production, from the cells and returned it to the lungs where it moves into the air sacs and is exhaled.

DESCRIBE the medical specialty of pulmonology.

   Pulmonology is the diagnosis and treatment of diseases and conditions affecting the lower respiratory system and chest cavity including the following organs: **trachea, bronchi, lungs,** and **pleura.** Therefore, it is most involved with the structures responsible for the exchange of oxygen and carbon dioxide between the air sacs of the lungs and the bloodstream. Conditions often treated by **pulmonologists** include cancer, infections, obstructive lung diseases, injuries, respiratory failure, environmental and occupational lung diseases, and disorders of the pleura. A **thoracic surgeon** performs surgical treatment of lung and thoracic cavity conditions. This subspecialty of surgery involves performing surgery on the lungs, trachea, esophagus, chest wall, heart, and other structures in the chest.

   Another health care provider intimately involved in respiratory care is the **respiratory therapist** whose duties include administering oxygen therapy, measuring lung capacity, monitoring blood concentrations of oxygen and carbon dioxide, administering breathing treatments, and providing care for ventilator patients.

Pulmonology Combining Forms

The following list presents new combining forms important for building and defining pulmonology terms.

alveol/o	alveolus; air sac		**ox/i**	oxygen
bronch/o	bronchus		**pleur/o**	pleura
bronchi/o	bronchus		**pneum/o**	lung, air
bronchiol/o	bronchiole		**pneumon/o**	lung
coni/o	dust		**pulmon/o**	lung
cyan/o	blue		**spir/o**	breathing
lob/o	lobe		**thorac/o**	chest
mediastin/o	mediastinum		**trache/o**	trachea, windpipe

The following list presents combining forms that are not specific to the respiratory system but are also used for building and defining pulmonology terms.

angi/o	vessel		**embol/o**	plug
arteri/o	artery		**fibr/o**	fibrous
atel/o	incomplete		**hem/o**	blood
carcin/o	cancer		**orth/o**	straight
cardi/o	heart		**py/o**	pus
cyt/o	cell			

Suffix Review

These suffixes and prefixes were introduced in Chapters 2 and 3. They are being reviewed in this chapter because they are especially important for building pulmonology terms.

-al	pertaining to		**-logy**	study of
-algia	pain		**-meter**	instrument to measure
-ar	pertaining to		**-metry**	process of measuring
-ary	pertaining to		**-ole**	small
-centesis	puncture to withdraw fluid		**-oma**	tumor
-dynia	pain		**-osis**	abnormal condition
-ectasis	dilated, expansion		**-ostomy**	create a new opening
-ectomy	surgical removal		**-otomy**	cutting into
-genic	producing		**-oxia**	oxygen
-gram	record		**-plasty**	surgical repair
-graph	instrument for recording		**-pnea**	breathing
-graphy	process of recording		**-ptysis**	spitting
-ia	state of		**-scope**	instrument for viewing
-ic	pertaining to		**-scopy**	process of visually examining
-itis	inflammation		**-spasm**	involuntary, strong muscle contraction
-logist	one who studies		**-thorax**	chest

Prefix Review

a-	without	eu-	normal
an-	without	hyper-	excessive
brady-	slow	hypo-	insufficient
dys-	abnormal, labored	tachy-	fast
endo-	within		

 IDENTIFY the organs treated in pulmonology.

Organs Commonly Treated in Pulmonary Disease

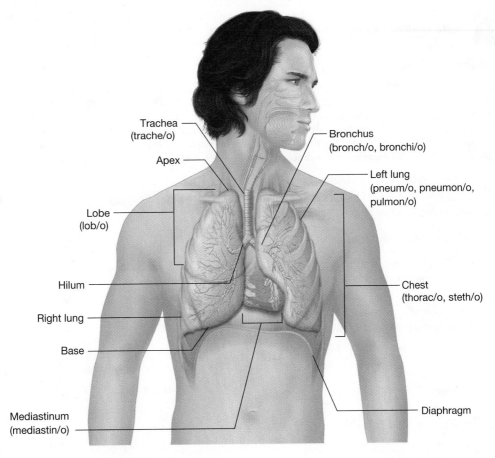

Trachea (trache/o)

Apex

Lobe (lob/o)

Hilum

Right lung

Base

Mediastinum (mediastin/o)

Bronchus (bronch/o, bronchi/o)

Left lung (pneum/o, pneumon/o, pulmon/o)

Chest (thorac/o, steth/o)

Diaphragm

>10.1 Respiratory organs in the thoracic cavity

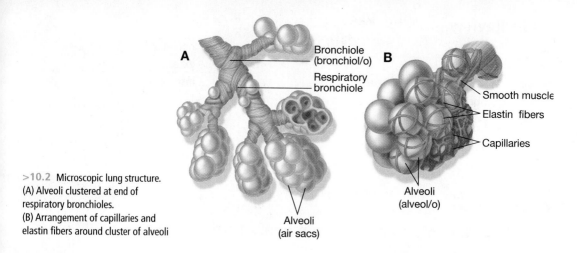

A

Bronchiole
(bronchiol/o)

Respiratory
bronchiole

B

Smooth muscle

Elastin fibers

Capillaries

>10.2 Microscopic lung structure.
(A) Alveoli clustered at end of
respiratory bronchioles.
(B) Arrangement of capillaries and
elastin fibers around cluster of alveoli

Alveoli
(air sacs)

Alveoli
(alveol/o)

BUILD pulmonology medical terms from word parts.

Building Pulmonology Terms

This section presents word parts most often used to build pulmonology terms. Following the explanation of the term, you have the opportunity to begin building your own vocabulary. Read the meaning for each term and then fill in the blanks to build a single medical term. Use the slashes to divide prefixes, word roots, combining vowels, and suffixes. To help you out you will find a key to the word parts underneath the blanks: r for word roots, p for prefix, cv for combining vowel, and s for suffix. Remember that not every term will contain all these word parts; it's up to you to decide which to use. As you gain experience, this process becomes easier. Answers can be found at the back of the book.

1. **alveol/o**–combining form meaning **alveolus**

    Alveoli are thin-walled air sacs at end of bronchioles; exchange of oxygen takes place between air in alveoli and capillary blood supply surrounding them

    a. pertaining to the alveolus

    _____/_____
    　　　　　　r　　　　　　　　s

2. **bronchi/o**–combining form meaning **bronchus**

    The bronchi are the two main divisions of trachea that carry air into each lung; they subdivide into more narrow bronchi and eventually become the narrowest bronchioles

    >10.3 Bronchus

    a. pertaining to the bronchus

    _____/_____
    　　　　　　r　　　　　　　　s

    b. small bronchus

    _____/_____
    　　　　　　r　　　　　　　　s

    c. dilated bronchus

    _____/_____
    　　　　　　r　　　　　　　　s

3. **bronchiol/o**–combining form meaning **bronchioles**

    Bronchioles are the narrowest airway tubes; carry air from bronchi to alveoli

    a. pertaining to a bronchiole

    _____ / _____
     r   s

4. **bronch/o**–combining form meaning **bronchus**

Cross-Section of Scope

Eye piece — Viewing channel
— Light source
Biopsy forceps and instrument channel
Flexible bronchoscopic tube

>10.4 Illustration of a physician using a bronchoscope to inspect the patient's bronchial tubes

a. record of the bronchus

_____ / ____ / _____
 r   CV   s

b. process of recording the bronchus

_____ / ____ / _____
 r   CV   s

c. bronchus inflammation

_____ / _____
 r   s

d. instrument for viewing the bronchus

_____ / ____ / _____
 r   CV   s

e. process of visually examining the bronchus

_____ / ____ / _____
 r   CV   s

f. involuntary muscle contraction of the bronchus

_____ / ____ / _____
 r   CV   s

g. bronchus producing

_____ / ____ / _____
 r   CV   s

5. **coni/o**–combining form meaning **dust**

    This combining form is used to refer to particles inhaled into lungs

    a. abnormal condition of dust in the lung

    _____ / ____ / _____ / _____
     r   CV   r   s

6. **cyan/o**–combining form meaning **blue**

    a. abnormal condition of being blue

    _____ / _____
     r   s

7. **lob/o**–combining form meaning **lobe**

Each lung subdivided into **lobes;** right lung has three lobes, left lung has two

a. pertaining to a lobe

_____ / _____
 r s

b. surgical removal of a lobe

_____ / _____
 r s

8. **mediastin/o**–combining form meaning **mediastinum**

The mediastinum is the central region of thoracic cavity between the lungs; contains trachea, heart, aorta, esophagus, lymph nodes and thymus gland

a. pertaining to the mediastinum

_____ / _____
 r s

b. cutting into the mediastinum

_____ / _____
 r s

9. **orth/o**–combining form meaning **straight**

This combining form is primarily used to refer to bone or skeleton terms; in pulmonology, it is used to indicate sitting straight up; people who have difficulty breathing often feel they can breathe easier if they are sitting up rather than lying down

a. breathing (sitting up) straight

_____ / _____ / _____
 r cv s

10. **-oxia**–suffix meaning **oxygen**

Oxygen is a gas required by every cell of body for its metabolism; main function of lungs is to inhale oxygen

a. without oxygen

_____ / _____
 p s

11. **ox/i**–combining form meaning **oxygen**

a. instrument for measuring oxygen

_____ / _____ / _____
 r cv s

b. process of measuring oxygen

_____ / _____ / _____
 r cv s

12. **pleur/o**–combining form meaning **pleura**

The pleura is a double layered membrane that forms protective sac around lungs; outer layer called **parietal pleura** and lines thoracic cavity; inner layer called **visceral pleura** and covers lungs; space formed by folded pleura is called **pleural cavity**

a. pertaining to the pleura

_____ / _____
 r s

b. puncture pleura to withdraw fluid

_____ / _____ / _____
 r cv s

c. pleura pain

_____ / _____ / _____
 r cv s

d. pleura pain

_____ / _____
 r s

e. pleura inflammation

_____ / _____
 r s

13. -pnea–suffix meaning **breathing**

A prefix is placed before this suffix to indicate what is happening with person's breathing pattern

a. without breathing

_____/_____
p   s

b. difficult breathing

_____/_____
p   s

c. normal breathing

_____/_____
p   s

d. excessive (deep) breathing

_____/_____
p   s

e. insufficient (shallow) breathing

_____/_____
p   s

f. slow breathing

_____/_____
p   s

g. fast breathing

_____/_____
p   s

14. pneum/o–combining form meaning **lung** or **air**

Lungs are paired organs found in thoracic cavity; each consists of tubelike airways that carry air to and from **alveoli,** or air sacs; gas exchange between outside air and bloodstream takes place in alveoli

>10.5 Lungs

a. record of a lung

_____/____/_____
r   CV   s

b. instrument to record the lung

_____/____/_____
r   CV   s

c. process of recording the lung

_____/____/_____
r   CV   s

d. air in the chest

_____/____/_____
r   CV   s

15. pneumon/o–combining form meaning **lung**

a. lung pertaining to

_____/_____
r   s

b. lung puncture to withdraw fluid

_____/____/_____
r   CV   s

c. lung surgical removal

_____/_____
r   s

d. lung cutting into

_____/_____
r   s

16. pulmon/o–combining form meaning **lung**

    a. pertaining to a lung

        _____ / _____
                 r   s

    b. study of the lung

        _____ / ____ / _____
                 r   cv   s

    c. one who studies lungs

        _____ / ____ / _____
                 r   cv   s

---

17. -ptysis–suffix meaning **spitting**

The main medical term built using this suffix means coughing up and spitting out of blood coming from lungs or bronchi

    a. spitting (up) blood

        _____ / ____ / _____
                 r   cv   s

---

18. spir/o–combining form meaning **breathing**

    a. record of breathing

        _____ / ____ / _____
                 r   cv   s

    b. instrument to measure breathing

        _____ / ____ / _____
                 r   cv   s

    c. process of measuring breathing

        _____ / ____ / _____
                 r   cv   s

---

19. thorac/o–combining form meaning **chest**

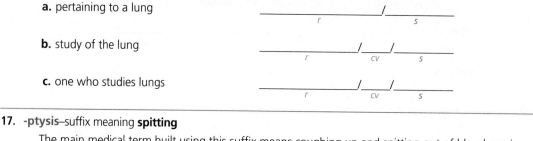

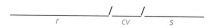

>10.6 Thoracentesis. A needle is inserted between the ribs to withdraw fluid from the pleural sac at the base of the left lung

Needle inserted into pleural space to withdraw fluid

    a. chest pain

        _____ / _____
                 r   s

    b. chest pain

        _____ / ____ / _____
                 r   cv   s

    c. pertaining to the chest

        _____ / _____
                 r   s

    d. cutting into the chest

        _____ / _____
                 r   s

    e. puncture chest to withdraw fluid

        _____ / ____ / _____
                 r   cv   s

    f. surgically create new opening in the chest   _____ / _____
                                                   r   s

20. -thorax–suffix meaning **chest**

This suffix is used to indicate presence of substance in chest

a. blood in the chest

_____ _/____/_____
    r   CV   S

b. pus in the chest

_____ _/____/_____
    r   CV   S

c. air in the chest

_____ _/____/_____
    r   CV   S

---

21. trache/o–combining form meaning **trachea**

The trachea is the tube that carries air from throat down into chest cavity; splits into two main bronchi; commonly called *windpipe*

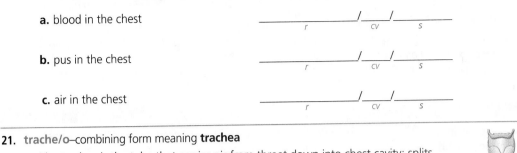

a. pertaining to the trachea

_____ _/_____
      r   S

b. surgical repair of trachea

_____ _/____/_____
    r   CV   S

c. surgically create an opening in trachea

_____ _/_____
      r   S

>10.7 Trachea

d. cutting into the trachea

_____ _/_____
      r   S

e. trachea inflammation

_____ _/_____
      r   S

f. pertaining to inside the trachea

_____ _/_____ _/_____
    p   r   S

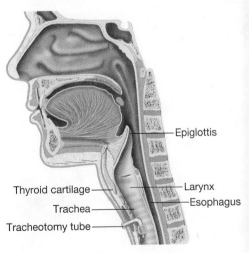

>10.8 A tracheotomy tube in place, inserted through an opening in the front of the neck and anchored within the trachea

Thyroid cartilage

Trachea

Tracheotomy tube

Epiglottis

Larynx

Esophagus

Pulmonology Vocabulary

The pulmonology terms presented in this section include eponyms, modern English words, and those that contain Latin or Greek word parts but are not constructed solely from these word parts. When you recognize word parts within a term they will give you a hint about the word's meaning. In these instances, look for the word parts to follow the term.

Term	Explanation
adult respiratory distress syndrome (ARDS)	Acute respiratory failure in adults characterized by tachypnea, dyspnea, cyanosis, tachycardia, and hypoxia
arterial blood gases (ABGs) **arteri/o** = artery **-al** = pertaining to	Laboratory test for levels of oxygen and carbon dioxide present in blood
asphyxia, asphyxiation	Lack of oxygen that can lead to unconsciousness and death if not corrected immediately; some common causes are drowning, foreign body in respiratory tract, poisoning, and electric shock; also called *suffocation*
aspirate	Inhaling fluid or foreign object into airways
asthma	Disease caused by various conditions, such as allergies, and resulting in bronchospasm, excessive mucus production, inflammation, airway constriction, wheezing, and coughing

➕ TERMINOLOGY TIDBIT

The term *aspirate* is built from the Latin prefix *a-* meaning "without" and *spiro* meaning "breathing." A person who has inhaled an object that blocks the airways is not able to breath.

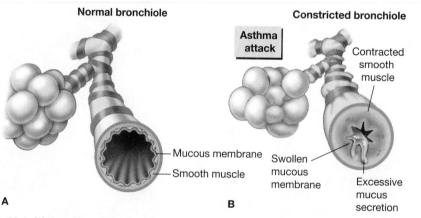

>10.9 (A) Normal bronchiole tube. (B) Bronchospasms and excessive mucus production associated with an asthma attack

atelectasis
  atel/o = incomplete
  -ectasis = dilation

Condition in which lung tissue collapses, preventing respiratory exchange of oxygen and carbon dioxide

＋TERMINOLOGY TIDBIT

The term *atelectasis* is built from the Greek terms *atelos* meaning "incomplete" and *ektasis* meaning "expansion." When *incomplete* modifies expansion, the term means *unexpanded* or, in other words, *collapsed*.

---

bronchodilator
  bronch/o = bronchus

Any medication that causes bronchi to dilate

---

bronchogenic carcinoma
  bronch/o = **bronchus**
  -genic = producing
  carcin/o = cancer
  -oma = tumor

Malignant lung tumor that originates in bronchi; often associated with a history of cigarette smoking

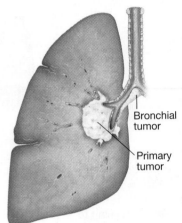

Bronchial tumor

Primary tumor

＋TERMINOLOGY TIDBIT

The best known meaning of the Greek term *karkinos* is "cancer," as in the zodiac sign. However, the term also meant a sore that won't heal, which is one of the warning signs of cancer.

>10.10 Illustration of a lung with two tumors growing out of the bronchial wall

---

cardiopulmonary resuscitation (CPR)
  cardi/o = heart
  pulmon/o = lung
  -ary = pertaining to

Applying external compressions to rib cage to maintain blood flow and air movement in and out of lungs during cardiac and respiratory arrest

---

chronic obstructive pulmonary disease (COPD)
  pulmon/o = lung
  -ary = pertaining to

Progressive, chronic, and usually irreversible condition in which air flow to and from lungs is decreased; patient can have severe dyspnea with exertion and cough; also called *chronic obstructive lung disease (COLD)*

---

croup

Acute viral infection in infants and children; symptoms include dyspnea and a characteristic harsh cough

＋TERMINOLOGY TIDBIT

This term is unusual because its origin is not Latin or Greek. *Croup* comes from the Anglo-Saxon word *kropan*, which means to "cry aloud" or "croak."

---

cystic fibrosis (CF)
  fibr/o = fibrous
  -osis = abnormal condition

Genetic condition that causes patient to produce very thick mucus resulting in severe congestion within lungs and digestive system

---

emphysema

Pulmonary condition resulting from destruction of alveolar walls leading to overinflated alveoli;
can occur as result of long-term heavy smoking or exposure to air pollution; characterized by dyspnea on exertion

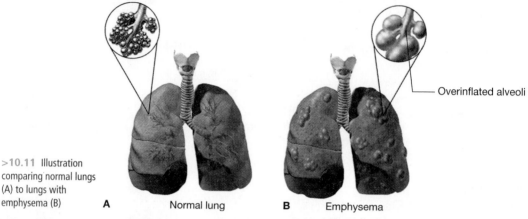

Overinflated alveoli

>10.11 Illustration comparing normal lungs (A) to lungs with emphysema (B)

A Normal lung **B** Emphysema

---

endotracheal (ET) intubation
  endo- = within
  trache/o = trachea
  -al = pertaining to

Placing tube through mouth and into trachea to maintain open airway and facilitate artificial ventilation

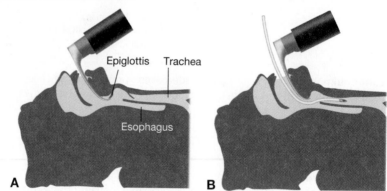

Epiglottis Trachea

Esophagus

A **B**

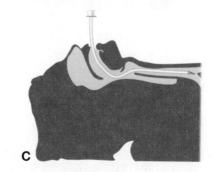

>10.12 Endotracheal intubation. (A) A lighted scope is used to identify the trachea from the esophagus. (B) The tube is placed through the pharynx and into the trachea. (C) The scope is removed, leaving the tube in place

C

Term	Explanation
hyperventilation **hyper-** = excessive	To breath too quickly (tachypnea) and too deeply (hyperpnea)
hypoventilation **hypo-** = insufficient	To breath too slowly (bradypnea) and too shallowly (hypopnea)
hypoxia **hypo-** = insufficient **-oxia** = oxygen	Having insufficient amount of oxygen in body
infant respiratory distress syndrome (IRDS)	Condition seen in premature infants whose lungs have not had time to fully develop; lungs are not able to expand fully, causing extreme difficulty in breathing and can result in death; also known as *hyaline membrane disease (HMD)*
influenza (flu)	Acute viral infection of airways; usually highly contagious; symptoms include chills, fever, body aches, and dry cough
intermittent positive pressure breathing (IPPB)	Method of artificial ventilation using mask connected to machine that produces pressure to assist air to fill lungs >10.13 Patient receiving assistance to breathe with an intermittent positive pressure breathing machine
phlegm	Thick mucus secreted by mucous membranes lining respiratory tract; phlegm is coughed through mouth is called *sputum*
pleural effusion **pleur/o** = pleura **-al** = pertaining to	Abnormal presence of fluid or gas in pleural cavity; presence of this fluid can be detected by tapping chest (percussion) or listening with stethoscope (auscultation)
pleurisy **pleur/o** = pleura	Inflammation of pleura
pneumonia **pneumon/o** = lung **-ia** = state of	Acute inflammatory condition of lung, which can be caused by bacterial and viral infections, diseases, and chemicals; severe dyspnea and death can result when alveoli fill with fluid (pulmonary infiltrate)

Term	Explanation

pneumothorax
pneum/o = air
-thorax = chest

Collection of air or gas in pleural cavity, which can result in collapse of lung

Torn pleura
Outside air enterir pleural cavity
Collapsed left lur
Inspiration
Diaphragm

>10.14 Illustration showing how outside air entering pleural cavity results in collapsed lung of pneumothorax

---

postural drainage

Drainage of secretions from bronchi by placing patient in position that uses gravity to promote drainage; used for treatment of cystic fibrosis and bronchiectasis

---

pulmonary angiography
pulmon/o = lung
-ary = pertaining to
angi/o = vessel
-graphy = process of recording

Injecting dye into blood vessel for purpose of taking x-ray of arteries and veins of lungs; test for pulmonary embolism

---

pulmonary edema
pulmon/o = lung
-ary = pertaining to

Condition in which lung tissue retains excessive amount of fluid; results in dyspnea

---

pulmonary embolism (PE)
pulmon/o = lung
-ary = pertaining to
embol/o = plug

Blood clot or air bubble in pulmonary artery or one of its branches; results in infarct of lung tissue

---

pulmonary function test (PFT)
pulmon/o = lung
-ary = pertaining to

Diagnostic procedure to assess respiratory function by using spirometer to measure air flow and lung volumes; often performed by respiratory therapists

>10.15 Patient breathing into a spirometer during a pulmonary function test

purulent	Containing pus, as in purulent sputum
rales	Abnormal "crackling" sound made during inhalation; caused by mucus or fluid in airways **⊞ TERMINOLOGY TIDBIT** The term *rales* is a French word meaning "rattle."
respiratory rate (RR)	Number of breaths per minute; one of vital signs (respiratory rate, heart rate, temperature, blood pressure)
rhonchi	Whistling sound that can be heard during either inhalation or exhalation; caused by narrowing of bronchi as in asthma or infection; also called *wheezing* **⊞ TERMINOLOGY TIDBIT** The term *rhonchi* comes from the Greek word *rhenchos* meaning "snoring."
severe acute respiratory syndrome (SARS)	Severe and highly contagious viral lung infection with high fever; threatened worldwide epidemic in 2003
sputum	Mucus or phlegm coughed up and spit out from respiratory tract
sputum culture and sensitivity (C&S)	Testing sputum by placing it on culture medium and observing any bacterial growth; specimen tested to determine selection of effective antibiotic
sputum cytology **cyt/o** = cell **-logy** = study of	Examination of sputum for malignant cells
sudden infant death syndrome (SIDS)	Unexpected and unexplained death of apparently well infant; sleep apnea, airway spasms, and failure of nerves to stimulate diaphragm have been studied as possible causes
sweat test	Diagnostic test for cystic fibrosis; children with this disease lose excessive amount of salt in their sweat

tuberculin skin tests (TB test)

Diagnostic test for exposure to tuberculosis bacteria by applying chemical agent (Tine or Mantoux tests) under surface of skin and evaluating site for reaction

0.1 ml tuberculin injected just under skin surface of forearm. Pale elevation results. Needle bevel directed upward to prevent too deep penetration.

Test read in 48 to 72 hours. Extent of induration determined by direct observation and palpation; limits marked. Area of erythema has no significance.

Diameter of marked indurated area measured in transverse plane. Reactions over 9 mm in diameter are regarded as positive; those 5 to 9 mm are questionable, and test may be repeated after 7 or more days to obtain booster effect. Less than 5 mm of induration is regarded as negative.

>10.16 Steps of a TB skin test

---

tuberculosis (TB)

Infectious disease caused by tubercle bacillus, *Mycobacterium tuberculosis;* most commonly affects respiratory system and causes inflammation and calcification in lungs

---

ventilation-perfusion scan

Nuclear medicine image particularly useful in diagnosing pulmonary emboli; involves inhalation of radioactive tagged air to evaluate air movement (ventilation) and injection of radioactive tagged dye into blood stream to evaluate blood flow (perfusion) to lungs

---

ventilator

Mechanical device to assist patient to breathe; also called *respirator*

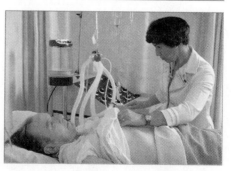

>10.17 Male patient breathing with the assistance of a ventilator attached to a tracheotomy tube

Pulmonology Abbreviations

The following list presents common pulmonaryy abbreviations.

ABGs	arterial blood gases	**IRDS**	infant respiratory distress syndrome
ARF	acute respiratory failure	**LLL**	left lower lobe
AP view	anteroposterior view in radiology	**LUL**	left upper lobe
ARD	acute respiratory disease	**O₂**	oxygen
ARDS	adult respiratory distress syndrome	**PA view**	posteroanterior view in radiology
Broncho	bronchoscopy	**PE**	pulmonary embolus
BS	breath sounds	**PFT**	pulmonary function test
CF	cystic fibrosis	**PPD**	purified protein derivative (tuberculin test)
CO₂	carbon dioxide	**R**	respirations
COLD	chronic obstructive lung disease	**RD**	respiratory disease
COPD	chronic obstructive pulmonary disease	**RDS**	respiratory distress syndrome
CPR	cardiopulmonary resuscitation	**RLL**	right lower lobe
C&S	sputum culture and sensitivity	**RML**	right middle lobe
CTA	clear to auscultation	**RR**	respiratory rate
CXR	chest x-ray	**RUL**	right upper lobe
DOE	dyspnea upon exertion	**SARS**	severe acute respiratory syndrome
ET	endotracheal	**SIDS**	sudden infant death syndrome
flu	influenza	**SOB**	shortness of breath
HMD	hyaline membrane disease	**TB**	tuberculosis
IPPB	intermittent positive pressure breathing	**TPR**	temperature, pulse, and respiration

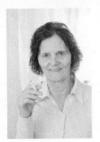

History of Present Illness

Female who is 72 years old complaining of increasing level of dyspnea with activity over the past 6 months. She now has a frequent harsh cough producing thick sputum and occasional hemoptysis.

Past Medical History

Patient has had hysterectomy for endometriosis at age 45, cholecystectomy for cholelithiasis at age 62, and recent compression fracture of lumbar spine secondary to osteoporosis. Patient takes only calcium supplement for osteoporosis.

Family and Social History

Patient began smoking at age 15 and currently smokes two packs a day. Denies use of alcohol. She is a retired school teacher who lives at home with her husband. She continues to drive a car, do light housework, and shop. Children are alive and well. She has one brother with hypertension. Mother died at age 60 from cerebrovascular accident. Father died at age 82 from complications of diabetes mellitus. There is no family history of asthma or emphysema.

Physical Examination

Patient is thin and short of stature. She has mild kyphosis. She is alert and answers all questions appropriately. She is not SOB sitting in examination room. Auscultation of chest reveals marked rales but no rhonchi. She has a persistent cough, and sputum was collected for a sputum culture and sensitivity and a sputum cytology.

(continued)

CASE STUDY

Radiology Findings
Chest radiograph, AP view, revealed a suspicious cloudy area in right lung. Follow-up with CT scan of the bronchial tree confirmed the presence of a mass in the right lung.

Laboratory Findings
Sputum C&S was negative for the presence of bacteria. Sputum cytology contained malignant cells, indicating presence of cancerous tumor in the lungs.

Diagnosis
Bronchogenic carcinoma

Plan of Treatment
1. Refer patient to thoracic surgeon for consultation regarding thoracotomy and lobectomy
2. Following surgery, she will be referred to oncologist for chemotherapy and to determine whether the tumor has metastasized

Critical Thinking Questions

Answer the following questions regarding this case study. Do not just copy words out of the case study; translate all medical terms. To answer some of these questions, you may need to look up information from another chapter of this text, in a medical dictionary, or online. Answers are found at the back of the book.

1. Which of the following is NOT a feature of this patient's history of the present illness?
   a. spitting up blood
   b. difficulty getting her breath when she is active
   c. coughing up mucus
   d. pain in the chest region

2. This patient's history is significant for three previous health problems. List and describe each health problem and the surgical treatment she received for two of them.
   _____
   _____

3. Is this patient's family history important to her current illness? Justify your answer.
   _____
   _____

4. What did the physician hear when listening to this patient's chest?
   _____
   _____

5. Two laboratory tests were performed. Explain the difference between the two tests. What were the results of each test?
   _____
   _____

6. List and describe the difference in the two types of x-ray procedures this patient underwent.
   _____
   _____

7. Explain why this patient was referred to two different physicians.
   _____
   _____

Sound It Out

The following are some of the key terms from this chapter written as their phonetic spelling. Sound out each term and write it in the blank. Pronunciations for all terms are included in the audio glossary at www.mymedicalterminologylab.com <http://www.mymedicalterminologylab.com/>.

1. tray-kee-OTT-oh-mee _____
2. AP-nee-ah _____
3. VENT-ih-later _____
4. AZ-mah _____
5. bray-DIP-nee-ah _____
6. BRONG-key-OHL-are _____
7. brong-KIGH-tis _____
8. BRONG-koh-dye-late-or _____
9. hee-moh-THOH-raks _____
10. al-vee-OH-lar _____
11. brong-koh-JEN-ik _____
12. noo-mon-EK-toe-me _____
13. BRONG-koh-scope _____
14. as-FIK-see-ah _____
15. BRONG-koh-spazm _____
16. sigh-ah-NO-sis _____
17. DISP-nee-ah _____
18. em-fih-SEE-mah _____
19. OX-sih-jen _____
20. at-eh-LEK-tah-sis _____
21. yoop-NEE-ah _____
22. hee-MOP-tih-sis _____
23. HYE-per-vent-ill-a-shun _____
24. FLEM _____
25. PULL-mon-air-ee _____
26. NOO-moe-graf _____
27. in-floo-EN-za _____
28. low-BEK-toh-mee _____
29. mee-dee-ASS-tih-nal _____
30. en-doh-TRAY-kee-al _____
31. ox-IM-eh-ter _____
32. KROOP _____
33. AS-peer-ate _____
34. PLOO-ral _____
35. brong-KOG-rah-fee _____
36. PLOOR-ih-see _____
37. pull-mon-ALL-oh-jee _____
38. noo-moe-sin-TEE-sis _____
39. noo-moh-koh-nee-OH-sis _____
40. new-moh-THOH-raks _____
41. too-ber-kyoo-LOH-sis _____
42. PURE-you-lent _____

43. tho-RASS-ik _____

47. ploor-oh-sen-TEE-sis _____

44. pye-oh-THOH-raks _____

48. ah-NOK-see-ah _____

45. spy-ROM-eh-tree _____

49. thor-ah-KOT-oh-mee _____

46. SPEW-tum _____

50. TRAY-kee-oh-plas-tee _____

Transcription Practice

Each of the following sentences is written in common English. Underline any words or phrases that can be replaced by a medical term. Then rewrite the entire sentence using medical terms. Answers can be found at the end of the book.

1. During the process of listening to sounds within the body, the physician heard abnormal crackling sounds when the patient breathed in.

   _____

   _____

2. It was unclear from the chest x-ray whether the patient had blood in the chest cavity or pus in the chest cavity.

   _____

   _____

3. The results of the lab test for the levels of oxygen and carbon dioxide present in the blood revealed an insufficient amount of oxygen in the body.

   _____

   _____

4. The patient underwent a surgical removal of a lung lobe after the discovery of a malignant lung tumor originating in the bronchi.

   _____

   _____

5. Mr. Scott's slow breathing was so severe that he had a blue color to his skin.

   _____

   _____

6. Carlyn went to the one who studies the lung when she noticed spitting up of blood several mornings is a row.

   _____

   _____

7. The physician ordered a test to grow and observe bacteria from sputum because Lars was coughing up phlegm with pus in it.

_____

_____

8. The patient underwent diagnostic procedures to assess respiratory function using an instrument to measure breathing and an instrument to measure oxygen.

_____

_____

9. The patient had long-term irreversible condition in which air flow to and from the lungs is decreased and as a result had developed hypertrophy of the right ventricle of the heart.

_____

_____

10. An x-ray with dye injected into the blood vessels of the lungs was ordered to determine whether a blood clot was in a pulmonary artery.

_____

_____

Spelling

Some of the following terms are misspelled. Identify the incorrect terms and spell them correctly in the blank provided.

1. pneumoconeosis _____

2. pneumonia _____

3. phlegm _____

4. ventilater _____

5. prurulent _____

6. influenza _____

7. asphyxia _____

8. hyperopnea _____

9. mediastinal _____

10. alveololar _____

Labeling Exercise

Write the name of each structure on the numbered line. Also use this space to write the combining form where appropriate.

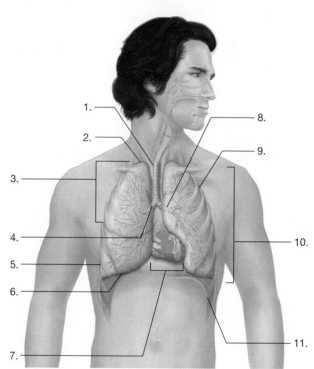

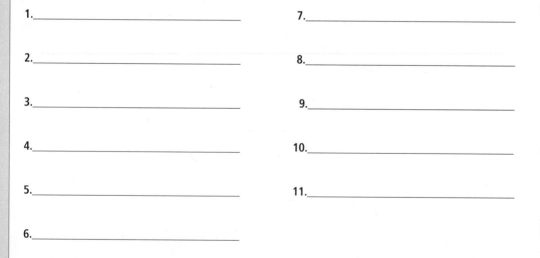

1._____

2._____

3._____

4._____

5._____

6._____

7._____

8._____

9._____

10._____

11._____

Build Medical Terms

Use each of the following word parts to build the indicated medical terms.

The combining form bronch/o means bronchus.

1. bronchus record _____

2. bronchus visual exam _____

3. bronchus involuntary muscle contraction _____

The combining form pneumon/o means lung.

4. lung puncture to withdraw fluid _____

5. lung surgical removal _____

6. lung surgical removal _____

7. lung cutting into _____

The suffix -ectasis means dilated or expanded.

8. incomplete expansion _____

9. bronchus expansion _____

The combining form trache/o means trachea.

10. trachea create new opening _____

11. trachea surgical repair _____

12. trachea inflammation _____

The suffix -pnea means breathing.

13. no breathing _____

14. fast breathing _____

15. difficult breathing _____

Fill in the Blank

Fill in the blank to complete each of the following sentences.

1. Jenny's _____ attacks were brought on by her allergies and always involved bronchospasms and coughing.

2. Mr. Wu had a _____ to examine the inside of his bronchial tubes for possible cancer.

3. Mr. Michael's many years of smoking destroyed his alveolar walls; he had developed _____.

4. A sweat test confirmed that the new infant had _____.

5. The _____ is commonly called the *windpipe*.

6. The respiratory therapist used a _____ to conduct a pulmonary function test.

7. Breathing too fast and too deep results in _____.

8. Hyaline membrane disease is also known as _____.

9. When air collects in the pleural cavity, causing the lung to collapse, it is referred to as a _____.

10. The patient had a pulmonary angiography to determine whether she had a(n) _____.

Abbreviation Matching

Match each abbreviation with its definition.

_____ 1. CXR   **A.** pulmonary embolism

_____ 2. SOB   **B.** temperature, pulse, respiration

_____ 3. TB   **C.** adult respiratory distress syndrome

_____ 4. PE   **D.** chest x-ray

_____ 5. LLL   **E.** arterial blood gases

_____ 6. TPR   **F.** tuberculosis

_____ 7. ET   **G.** chronic obstructive pulmonary disease

_____ 8. ABGs   **H.** shortness of breath

_____ 9. COPD   **I.** endotracheal

_____ 10. ARDS   **J.** left lower lobe

Medical Term Analysis

Examine each of the following terms. Begin by dividing it into its word parts and writing them in the indicated blanks (P = prefix, WR = word root; CF = combining form; S = suffix). Follow with the definition of each word part and then finally the meaning of the full term.

1. **thoracocentesis**

    CF _____

    means _____

    S _____

    means _____

    Term Meaning: _____

    _____

2. **cyanosis**

    WR _____

    means _____

    S _____

    means _____

    Term Meaning: _____

    _____

3. **pneumothorax**

    CF _____

    means _____

    S _____

    means _____

    Term Meaning: _____

    _____

4. **endotracheal**

    P _____

    means _____

    WR _____

    means _____

    S _____

    means _____

    Term Meaning: _____

    _____

5. **pneumoconiosis**

    CF _____

    means _____

    WR _____

    means _____

    S _____

    means _____

    Term Meaning: _____

    _____

6. **oximeter**

    CF _____

    means _____

    S _____

    means _____

    Term Meaning: _____

    _____

7. **orthopnea**

CF _____

means _____

S _____

means _____

Term Meaning: _____

_____

8. **pleurodynia**

CF _____

means _____

S _____

means _____

Term Meaning: _____

_____

9. **bronchiectasis**

WR _____

means _____

S _____

means _____

Term Meaning: _____

_____

10. **lobectomy**

WR _____

means _____

S _____

means _____

Term Meaning: _____

_____

Photomatch Challenge

Match each pulmonary condition with its name in the Word Bank.

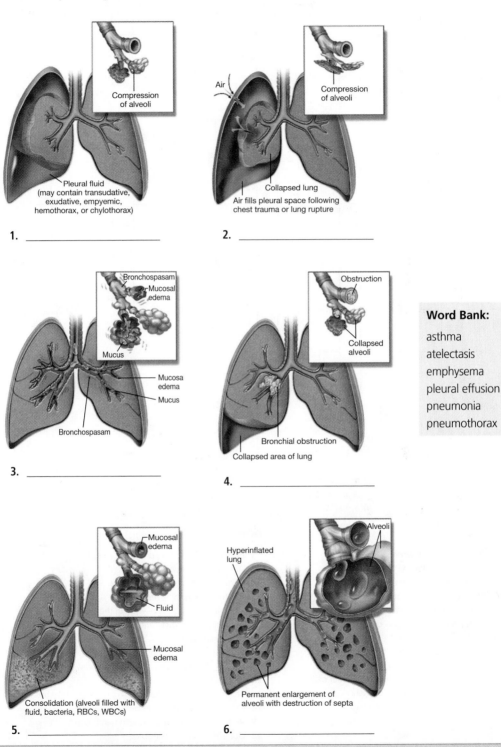

Compression of alveoli

Pleural fluid
(may contain transudative,
exudative, empyemic,
hemothorax, or chylothorax)

1. _____

Air

Compression of alveoli

Collapsed lung
Air fills pleural space following
chest trauma or lung rupture

2. _____

Bronchospasam
Mucosal edema

Mucus

Mucosa edema

Mucus

Bronchospasam

3. _____

Obstruction

Collapsed alveoli

Bronchial obstruction

Collapsed area of lung

4. _____

Word Bank:

asthma

atelectasis

emphysema

pleural effusion

pneumonia

pneumothorax

Mucosal edema

Fluid

Mucosal edema

Consolidation (alveoli filled with
fluid, bacteria, RBCs, WBCs)

5. _____

Alveoli

Hyperinflated lung

Permanent enlargement of
alveoli with destruction of septa

6. _____

Crossword Puzzle

Use the definitions given to complete the crossword puzzle.

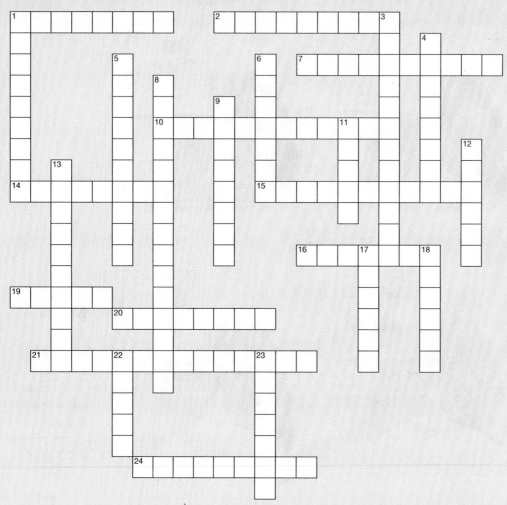

ACROSS

1. Inflammation of pleura
2. Highly contagious viral infection
7. Term meaning spitting up blood
10. Results in collapse of lung
14. Inhaling fluid into airways
15. Condition with collapse of lung tissue
16. Difficulty breathing
19. _____ test, a diagnostic test for cystic fibrosis
20. Sputum _____, test for cancer cells
21. Medication that widens bronchi
24. Condition that destroys alveolar walls

DOWN

1. Infection in which fluid fills the alveoli
3. Also called suffocation
4. Term describing blue skin color
5. Another name for a respirator
6. Term for insufficient oxygen in the body
8. Breathing too slowly and too shallowly
9. Containing pus
11. Crackling breath sounds
12. _____ fibrosis, genetic condition with thick mucus
13. Instrument to measure breathing
17. Thick mucus secreted by lining of respiratory tract
18. Condition that results in bronchospasms
22. Viral infection in children with harsh cough
23. Commonly called windpipe

11

Gastroenterology
Digestive System

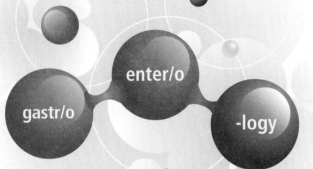

enter/o

gastr/o

-logy

A Brief Introduction to Gastroenterology

 UNDERSTAND the functions of the digestive system.

The **gastrointestinal,** or **digestive system,** is responsible for digesting the food we eat and absorbing the nutrient molecules. These processes occur as food passes through the organs of the gastrointestinal tract: the **mouth, pharynx, esophagus, stomach, intestine, colon, rectum,** and **anus.** Digestion also requires the assistance of accessory organs, the **liver, gallbladder,** and **pancreas.**

+ TERMINOLOGY TIDBIT

The gastrointestinal tract is also referred to as the *alimentary canal*. This name comes from the Latin word *alimentum* meaning "nourishment."

DESCRIBE the medical specialty of gastroenterology.

Gastroenterology is the branch of medicine specializing in the diagnosis and treatment of diseases and conditions affecting the lower gastrointestinal (GI) tract, which includes the organs between the esophagus and rectum. Conditions often treated by a **gastroenterologist** include bleeding, cancer, infections, nutritional disorders, inflammatory disorders, diverticulosis, gallbladder disease, liver disease, gastroesophageal reflux, and ulcers.

Gastroenterology Combining Forms

The following list presents new combining forms important for building and defining gastroenterology terms.

an/o	anus	esophag/o	esophagus
appendic/o	appendix	gastr/o	stomach
append/o	appendix	hepat/o	liver
chol/e	bile	ile/o	ileum
cholangi/o	bile duct	jejun/o	jejunum
cholecyst/o	gallbladder	lapar/o	abdomen
choledoch/o	common bile duct	pancreat/o	pancreas
col/o	colon	polyp/o	polyps
colon/o	colon	proct/o	rectum and anus
diverticul/o	diverticulum	rect/o	rectum
duoden/o	duodenum	sigmoid/o	sigmoid colon
enter/o	intestine		

The following list presents combining forms that are not specific to the digestive system but are also used for building and defining gastroenterology terms.

hemat/o	blood
lith/o	stone

Suffix Review

These suffixes and prefixes were introduced in Chapters 2 and 3. They are being reviewed in this chapter because they are especially important for building gastroenterology terms.

-al	pertaining to	-logy	study of
-algia	pain	-oma	tumor
-cele	protrusion	-osis	abnormal condition
-dynia	pain	-ostomy	surgically create an opening
-eal	pertaining to	-otomy	cutting into
-ectomy	surgical removal	-pepsia	digestion
-emesis	vomit	-phagia	eat, swallow
-gram	record	-plasty	surgical repair
-graphy	process of recording	-ptosis	dropping
-iasis	abnormal condition	-scope	instrument for viewing
-ic	pertaining to	-scopy	process of viewing
-itis	inflammation	-tripsy	surgical crushing
-logist	one who studies		

Prefix Review

a-	without		hyper-	excessive
brady-	slow		poly-	many
dys-	painful, difficult			

 IDENTIFY the organs treated in gastroenterology.

Organs Commonly Treated in Gastroenterology

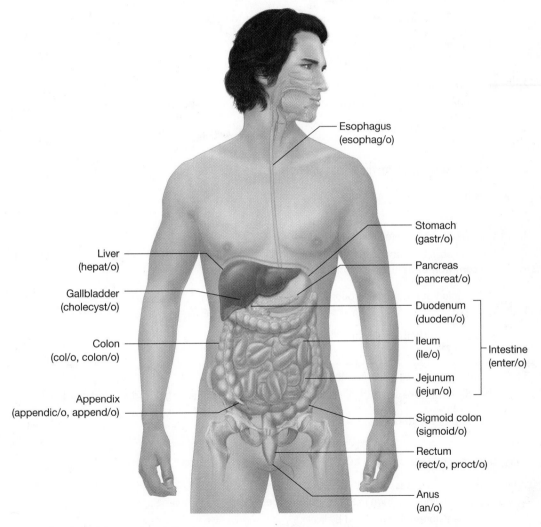

Esophagus
(esophag/o)

Stomach
(gastr/o)

Liver
(hepat/o)

Pancreas
(pancreat/o)

Gallbladder
(cholecyst/o)

Duodenum
(duoden/o)

Colon
(col/o, colon/o)

Ileum
(ile/o)

Intestine
(enter/o)

Jejunum
(jejun/o)

Appendix
(appendic/o, append/o)

Sigmoid colon
(sigmoid/o)

Rectum
(rect/o, proct/o)

Anus
(an/o)

>11.1 The organs of the gastrointestinal system

Building Gastroenterology Terms

This section presents word parts most often used to build gastroenterology terms. Following the explanation of the term, you have the opportunity to begin building your own vocabulary. Read the meaning for each term and then fill in the blanks to build a single medical term. Use the slashes to divide prefixes, word roots, combining vowels, and suffixes. To help you out you will find a key to the word parts underneath the blanks: r for word roots, p for prefix, cv for combining vowel, and s for suffix. Remember that not every term will contain all these word parts; it's up to you to decide which to use. As you gain experience, this process becomes easier. Answers can be found at the back of the book.

1. **an/o**–combining form meaning **anus**

   The anus is the distal opening of the digestive tract to outside of the body

   a. pertaining to anus   _____/_____
                                                  r   s

2. **appendic/o**–combining form meaning **appendix**

   The appendix is a small pouch attached to the cecum; serves no known purpose

   a. appendix inflammation   _____/_____
                                                  r   s

3. **append/o**–combining form meaning **appendix**

   a. surgical removal of appendix   _____/_____
                                                  r   s

4. **chol/e**–combining form meaning **bile**

   Bile is a substance produced by the liver and stored in the gallbladder; transported to duodenum by the **common bile duct;** aids in fat digestion; also called *gall*

   a. condition of having gall stones   _____/_____/_____/_____
                                                  r   cv   r   s

   b. surgical crushing of gall stones   _____/_____/_____/_____/_____
                                                  r   cv   r   cv   s

5. **cholangi/o**–combining form meaning **bile ducts**

   The bile ducts are a series of ducts to transport bile between liver, gallbladder, and duodenum

   a. record of bile duct   _____/_____/_____
                                                  r   cv   s

   b. process of recording bile duct   _____/_____/_____
                                                  r   cv   s

6. **cholecyst/o**–combining form meaning **gallbladder**

   This organ stores bile produced by liver

   a. gallbladder inflammation   _____/_____
                                                  r   s

   b. surgical removal of gallbladder   _____/_____
                                                  r   s

c. record of gallbladder

_____/_____/_____
r   cv   s

d. process of recording gallbladder

_____/_____/_____
r   cv   s

---

7. **choledoch/o**–combining form meaning **common bile duct**
   The common bile duct is the main duct that transports bile from liver or gallbladder to duodenum

   a. condition of stone in common bile duct

   _____/_____/_____/____
   r   cv   r   s

   b. surgical crushing of stone in common bile duct

   _____/___/_____/___/____
   r   cv   r   cv   s

---

8. **col/o**–combining form meaning **colon**
   The colon receives undigested food from intestine; allows for water to be reabsorbed into body; what remains are called *feces;* colon is divided into **ascending colon, transverse colon, descending colon,** and **sigmoid colon;** term *large intestine* includes **cecum,** appendix, colon, rectum, and anus

   >11.2 Colon

   a. Surgically create an opening in colon

   _____/_____
   r   s

   b. colon inflammation

   _____/_____
   r   s

   c. pertaining to colon and rectum

   _____/_____/_____/____
   r   cv   r   s

---

9. **colon/o**–combining form meaning **colon**

   a. instrument to visually examine colon

   _____/_____/_____
   r   cv   s

   b. process of visually examining colon

   _____/_____/_____
   r   cv   s

   c. pertaining to colon

   _____/_____
   r   s

---

10. **diverticul/o**–combining form meaning **diverticulum**
    Diverticula are small abnormal pouch that forms off intestinal or colon wall; can become inflamed and infected

    a. diverticulum inflammation

    _____/_____
    r   s

    b. abnormal condition of having diverticula

    _____/_____
    r   s

    c. surgical removal of diverticulum

    _____/_____
    r   s

---

11. duoden/o–combining form meaning **duodenum**

The duodenum is the first section of intestine; receives food from the stomach, digestive enzymes from the pancreas, and bile from the liver; final digestion of food and absorption of nutrients begins in duodenum

a. pertaining to duodenum

_____/_____
r   s

b. surgically create an opening in duodenum

_____/_____
r   s

12. -emesis–suffix meaning **to vomit**

a. vomiting blood

_____/_____
r   s

b. excessive vomiting

_____/_____
p   s

13. enter/o–combining form meaning **intestine**

The intestine receives food from the stomach, digestive enzymes from the pancreas, and bile from the liver; absorption of nutrients begins in intestine; consists of **duodenum, jejunum,** and **ileum**

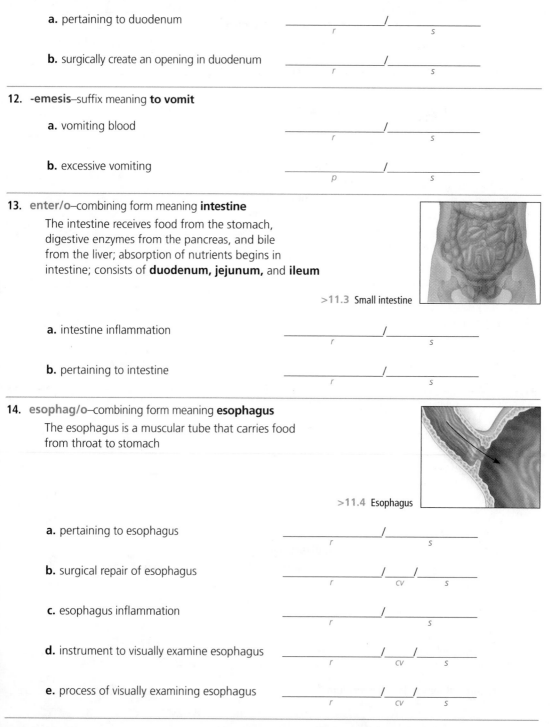

>11.3 Small intestine

a. intestine inflammation

_____/_____
r   s

b. pertaining to intestine

_____/_____
r   s

14. esophag/o–combining form meaning **esophagus**

The esophagus is a muscular tube that carries food from throat to stomach

>11.4 Esophagus

a. pertaining to esophagus

_____/_____
r   s

b. surgical repair of esophagus

_____/____/_____
r   cv   s

c. esophagus inflammation

_____/_____
r   s

d. instrument to visually examine esophagus

_____/____/_____
r   cv   s

e. process of visually examining esophagus

_____/____/_____
r   cv   s

15. gastr/o–combining form meaning **stomach**

The stomach is a muscular sac producing hydrochloric acid and digestive enzymes; begins digestive process by mixing food received from esophagus with acid; watery mixture, called **chyme,** leaves stomach and enters duodenum

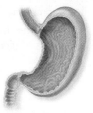

>11.5 Stomach

a. pertaining to stomach

_____/_____
          r   s

b. stomach inflammation

_____/_____
          r   s

c. stomach and intestine inflammation

_____/_____/_____/_____
      r   cv   r   s

d. surgical removal of stomach

_____/_____
          r   s

e. surgically create an opening in stomach

_____/_____
          r   s

f. instrument to visually exam stomach

_____/_____/_____
          r   cv   s

g. process of visually examining stomach

_____/_____/_____
          r   cv   s

h. stomach pain

_____/_____/_____
          r   cv   s

i. stomach pain

_____/_____
          r   s

j. one who studies stomach and intestine

_____/_____/_____/_____/_____
      r   cv   r   cv   s

k. study of stomach and intestine

_____/_____/_____/_____/_____
      r   cv   r   cv   s

16. hepat/o–combining form meaning **liver**

The liver is a complex abdominal organ; in gastroenterology, plays role in digestion by producing **bile** to aid in fat digestion

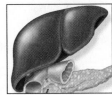

>11.6 Liver

a. liver inflammation

_____/_____
          r   s

b. pertaining to liver

_____/_____
          r   s

c. liver tumor

_____/_____
          r   s

17. ile/o–combining form meaning **ileum**

The ileum is the third section of intestine; receives digested food from jejunum and completes process of digestion and nutrient absorption

a. pertaining to ileum

_____/_____
r   s

b. surgically create a new opening in ileum

_____/_____
r   s

18. jejun/o–combining form meaning **jejunum**

The jejunum is the second portion of intestine; receives digested food from duodenum and continues process of digestion and nutrient absorption

a. pertaining to jejunum

_____/_____
r   s

b. surgically create a new opening in jejunum

_____/_____
r   s

19. lapar/o–combining form meaning **abdomen**

The abdomen is a body cavity that houses organs of digestion, reproduction, and excretion

a. cutting into abdomen

_____/_____
r   s

b. instrument to visually examine abdomen

_____/____/_____
r   CV   s

c. process of visually examining abdomen

_____/____/_____
r   CV   s

20. pancreat/o–combining form meaning **pancreas**

The pancreas is an organ that produces digestive enzymes; pancreatic duct carries these enzymes to duodenum where they aid in food digestion

>11.7 Pancreas

a. pertaining to pancreas

_____/_____
r   s

b. pancreas inflammation

_____/_____
r   s

21. -pepsia–suffix meaning **digestion**

a. without digestion

_____/_____
p   s

b. difficult digestion

_____/_____
p   s

c. slow digestion

_____/_____
p   s

22. **-phagia**–suffix meaning **eat** or **swallow**

 a. without swallowing

 _____/_____
 p   s

 b. difficult swallowing

 _____/_____
 p   s

 c. excessive eating

 _____/_____
 p   s

---

23. **polyp/o**–combining form meaning **polyp**

 Polyps are small mushroom-shaped tumors that grow on mucous membranes of colon and extend into lumen of colon; can become cancerous

 a. abnormal condition of having polyps

 _____/_____
 r   s

 b. surgical removal of polyp

 _____/_____
 r   s

---

24. **proct/o**–combining form meaning **rectum and anus**

 This combining form refers to both the rectum and anus

 a. drooping of rectum and anus

 _____/____/_____
 r   cv   s

 b. instrument to visually examine rectum and anus

 _____/____/_____
 r   cv   s

 c. process of visually examining rectum and anus

 _____/____/_____
 r   cv   s

 d. one who studies rectum and anus

 _____/____/_____
 r   cv   s

 e. study of rectum and anus

 _____/____/_____
 r   cv   s

---

25. **rect/o**–combining form meaning **rectum**

 The rectum is the final segment of colon; receives feces from the sigmoid colon and stores it prior to elimination

 a. protrusion of rectum

 _____/____/_____
 r   cv   s

 b. pertaining to rectum

 _____/_____
 r   s

---

26. **sigmoid/o**–combining form meaning **sigmoid colon**

 The sigmoid colon is an s-shaped region of colon; feces passes out of sigmoid colon and into rectum

 a. instrument to visually examine sigmoid colon

 _____/____/_____
 r   cv   s

 b. process of visually examining sigmoid colon

 _____/____/_____
 r   cv   s

Gastroenterology Vocabulary

The gastroenterology terms presented in this section include eponyms, modern English words, and those that contain Latin or Greek word parts but are not constructed solely from these word parts. When you recognize word parts within a term they will give you a hint about the word's meaning. In these instances, look for the word parts to follow the term.

Term	Explanation
ascites	Accumulation of fluid in abdominal cavity

+ TERMINOLOGY TIDBIT

The term *ascites* comes from the Latin word *askos* meaning "a bag." This describes the swollen appearance of the abdomen in a person with ascites.

Umbilicus may be protuberant

>11.8 Patient with swollen abdomen and protruding umbilicus characteristic of ascites

Bulging flank with fluid

barium enema (BE)	X-ray examination of intestine and colon using barium as contrast medium; also known as *lower GI series*
cirrhosis **-osis** = abnormal condition	Chronic liver disease

>11.9 Chronic destruction and scarring of liver due to cirrhosis

Crohn disease	Chronic inflammatory bowel disease (IBD) with mucous membrane ulcers; most often found in ileum
dysentery **dys-** = abnormal **enter/o** = intestine	Acute intestinal condition with pain, diarrhea, and blood and mucus in stools; usually caused by bacterial or parasitic infection
esophageal atresia **esophag/o** = esophagus **-eal** = pertaining to	Congenital lack of the connection between esophagus and stomach; food cannot enter stomach

+ TERMINOLOGY TIDBIT

The term *atresia* is formed by combining the Greek prefix *a-* meaning "without" and the word *tresis* meaning "a hole."

esophageal varices
  esophag/o =
  esophagus
  -eal = pertaining to

Varicose veins in esophagus; result in massive bleeding if rupture

>11.10 Blood clots forming from ruptured esophageal varices at point where esophagus meets the stomach

---

fecal occult blood test (FOBT)
  -al = pertaining to

Clinical lab test for presence of small amounts of blood in feces; also called *hemoccult test* or *stool guaiac test*

> **+ TERMINOLOGY TIDBIT**
>
> The term *occult* comes from the Latin word *occulere* meaning "hidden." This is a test for amounts of blood that are too small to see, even with a microscope.

---

gastric bypass
  gastr/o = stomach
  -ic = pertaining to

Surgical treatment for obesity; portion of stomach is stapled off and bypassed so that it holds less food; also called *stomach stapling*

> **+ TERMINOLOGY TIDBIT**
>
> The combining form for stomach, *gastr/o*, comes from the Greek word *gaster* meaning "stomach."

Flow of food
Esophagus
Small pouch of stomach that still receives food
Duodenum attached to small stomach pouch that receives food
Bypassed portion of stomach
Bypassed section of duodenum

>11.11 Gastric bypass surgery

---

gastroesophageal reflux disease (GERD)
  gastr/o = stomach
  esophag/o = esophagus
  -eal = pertaining to

Occurs when stomach acid backs up into esophagus

***Helicobacter pylori*
antibody test**

Clinical lab test for presence of bacteria known to cause gastric ulcers

---

hemorrhoids

Varicose veins in rectum

---

ileus

Obstruction of intestine that occurs when muscular movements stop moving food or blockage prevents food from moving through digestive tract

intussusception

Occurs when one section of intestine slips or telescopes into another section of intestine

>11.12 Intussusception. A short length of small intestine has telescoped into itself

irritable bowel syndrome (IBS)

Disturbance in normal functioning of bowel characterized by abdominal pain and diarrhea; often associated with stress; also called *spastic colon*

jaundice

Yellow-colored skin and whites of eyes associated with liver disease

>11.13 Yellow eyeballs of person with jaundice
Source: CDC, Dr. Thomas F. Sellers, Emory University

melena

Very dark, tarry stools due to presence of blood

nausea

Feeling of urge to vomit

+ TERMINOLOGY TIDBIT

The term *nausea* comes from the Latin word *nausia* meaning "seasickness."

ova and parasites (O&P)

Clinical lab test for presence lof parasites or their eggs in feces

>11.14 Hookworms attached to the intestinal lining. Eggs released by these parasites would be detected by an O&P
Source: Courtesy of the Centers for Disease Control & Prevention

peptic ulcer disease (PUD)

Craterlike erosion occurring on mucous membrane of lower esophagus, stomach, and/or duodenum; more dangerous if ulcer eats into blood vessel and becomes *bleeding ulcer,* or if ulcer eats through wall of stomach and becomes a *perforated ulcer* allowing stomach acids to escape into abdominal cavity

Gastric juices are released into the stomach

Duodenal ulcer

Gastric juices (acidic)

Acid secretions further break down the lining of the stomach, forming an ulcer

Gastric ulcer

>11.15 Figure illustrating the location and appearance of peptic ulcers in both the stomach and the duodenum

---

total parenteral nutrition (TPN)

Nutrient-complete solution given directly into bloodstream when person cannot eat by mouth

---

ulcerative colitis
col/o = colon
-itis = inflammation

Chronic inflammatory bowel disease (IBD) characterized by formation of ulcers on mucous membrane of colon

---

upper gastrointestinal series
gastr/o = stomach
-al = pertaining to

X-ray examination of esophagus and stomach using barium as contrast medium; also known as *barium swallow*

Barium

>11.16 Patient drinks liquid barium solution in order to outline her stomach for an upper GI series

---

volvulus

Length of bowel that becomes twisted around itself

Colon

Small intestine

Twisted portion of small intestine

>11.17 Volvulus. A length of small intestine has twisted around itself, cutting off blood circulation to the twisted loop

---

Vomit

Forceful return of stomach contents out of mouth

USE gastroenterology abbreviations.

Gastroenterology Abbreviations

The following list presents common gastroenterology abbreviations.

Ba	barium	**GERD**	gastroesophageal reflux disease
BE	barium enema	**GI**	gastrointestinal
BM	bowel movement	**IBD**	inflammatory bowel disease
BS	bowel sounds	**IBS**	irritable bowel syndrome
CBD	common bile duct	**N & V**	nausea and vomiting
CUC	chronic ulcerative colitis	**O & P**	ova and parasites
EGD	esophagogastroduodenoscopy	**PUD**	peptic ulcer disease
ERCP	endoscopic retrograde	**TPN**	total parenteral nutrition
	cholangiopancreatography	**UGI**	upper gastrointestinal series
GB	gallbladder		

CASE STUDY

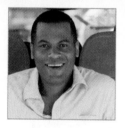

History of the Present Illness

The patient is a 35-year-old man who has had a gradual increase in upper abdominal pain for the past 8 months. He has no prior history of upper abdominal pain. He now reports a sharp pain in the epigastric area about 30 minutes after meals, which has been somewhat relieved by Tums or Rolaids or over-the-counter Zantac. Spicy foods make the pain more frequent and severe. Milk and ice cream relieve the pain sometimes. The pain is a deep aching feeling that does not radiate. The pain does not interfere with normal activities including work and sleep. On a scale from 1 (barely perceptible) to 10 (worst imaginable) he rates it a 3–4. It occurs almost daily and lasts about one hour. His appetite is good, and he has not lost weight. The patient denies dysphagia, substernal burning, N&V, lower abdominal pain, hematemesis, melena, and diarrhea. He has had intermittent constipation since his early 20s that he treats with Milk of Magnesia once every 2–3 months. Ten years ago he had some rectal bleeding from hemorrhoids. Other than that episode, he denies other GI problems.

Past Medical History

Hemorrhoids at age 25 requiring hemorrhoidectomy. He takes no regular prescriptions; does use over-the-counter antacids and Milk of Magnesia.

Family and Social History

Married with two children. College graduate. Works in accounting firm as a computer programmer. Smoked from ages 16 to 23. Social drinker. No illegal substance use. No travel or unusual exposures. Mother had colon cancer. Father had prostate cancer. Brother had hepatitis.

Physical Examination

No evidence of ascites, jaundice, hepatomegaly, abdominal mass.

Laboratory Findings

Test for *Helicobacter pylori* was positive.

Endoscopic Findings
EGD revealed gastritis without hemorrhage or ulcer.

Diagnosis
Dyspepsia without evidence of gastric or duodenal ulcer.

Plan of Treatment
1. Patient will be placed on medication to block release of acidic stomach secretions for the gastritis and an antibiotic to treat the *Helicobacter pylori* infection
2. Repeat GED in 3 months if symptoms do not resolved

Critical Thinking Questions
Answer the following questions regarding this case study. Do not just copy words out of the case study; translate all medical terms. To answer some of these questions, you may need to look up information from another chapter of this text, in a medical dictionary, or online. Answers are found at the back of the book.

1. What complaint brought this patient to the doctor?
   _____
   _____

2. What foods make the pain better? What foods make it worse? What is the main thing this patient has done to treat the problem on his own?
   _____
   _____

3. Two diagnostic tests/procedures were performed. Name them, describe them, and explain the findings.
   _____
   _____

4. The history states the pain is in the epigastric region and does not radiate. Where is the epigastric region? This chapter does not explain what *radiating pain* means. What do you think it means?
   _____
   _____

5. Describe the symptoms the patient denies having.
   _____
   _____

6. Why is this patient's family history important to this episode?
   _____
   _____

7. Which of the following is NOT one of the symptoms denied by the patient in the history?
   a. vomiting blood
   b. difficulty swallowing
   c. yellow colored skin
   d. dark tarry stools

8. Explain the physician's plan of treatment.
   _____
   _____

Sound It Out

The following are some of the key terms from this chapter written as their phonetic spelling. Sound out each term and write it in the blank. Pronunciations for all terms are included in the audio glossary at www.mymedicalterminologylab.com <http://www.mymedicalterminologylab.com/>.

1. sig-MOYD-oh-scope _____

2. ay-PEP-see-ah _____

3. RECK-toh-seal _____

4. gas-TRY-tis _____

5. ah-SIGH-teez _____

6. koh-LAN-jee-oh-gram _____

7. sih-ROH-sis _____

8. koh-LYE-tis _____

9. koh-lon-OSS-koh-pee _____

10. kohl-oh-REK-tall _____

11. dye-ver-TIK-yoo-lum _____

12. ay-NALL _____

13. do-ODD-in-OS-toh-me _____

14. pol-ee-POH-sis _____

15. koh-lee-sis-TEK-toh-mee _____

16. dis-PEP-see-ah _____

17. ah-FAY-jee-ah _____

18. en-TARE-ik _____

19. eh-soff-ah-go-PLAS-tee _____

20. VOM-it _____

21. eh-soff-ah-GOS-koh-pee _____

22. gas-troh-en-ter-EYE-tis _____

23. JAWN-diss _____

24. GAS-troh-scope _____

25. hee-mah-TEM-eh-sis _____

26. ah-pen-dih-SIGH-tis _____

27. HEM-oh-roydz _____

28. dis-in-TARE-ee _____

29. koh-LED-oh-koh-lith-ee-ay-sis _____

30. high-per-EM-eh-sis _____

31. brad-ee-PEP-see-ah _____

32. ill-ee-OSS-toh-mee _____

33. jih-JUNE-all _____

34. lap-ar-OSS-koh-pee _____

35. lap-ah-ROT-oh-mee _____

36. me-LEE-nah _____

37. NAW-see-ah _____

38. pan-kree-AT-ik _____

39. dis-FAY-jee-ah _____

40. pol-ee-PEK-toh-me _____

41. gas-TREK-toh-mee _____

42. pol-ee-FAY-jee-ah _____

43. hep-AT-ik _____

44. VOL-vyoo-lus _____

45. prok-top-TOH-sis _____

46. RECK-tall _____

47. REK-tum _____

48. sig-moid-OS-koh-pee _____

49. ah-PEN-diks _____

50. prok-TOL-oh-jist _____

Transcription Practice

Each of the following sentences is written in common English. Underline any words or phrases that can be replaced by a medical term. Then rewrite the entire sentence using medical terms. Answers can be found at the end of the book.

1. Mr. Mercado was noted to have yellow skin color, leading to a diagnosis of liver inflammation.

   _____

   _____

2. Mrs. Mendez underwent a visual examination of her esophagus, stomach, and duodenum that revealed a craterlike erosion in her stomach.

   _____

   _____

3. Mr. Brown's severe inflamed pouch extending off his colon resulted in his having the pouch surgically removed.

   _____

   _____

4. The patient presented in the emergency room with severe urge to vomit and vomiting blood.

   _____

   _____

5. The physician ordered an x-ray of the colon using barium as a contrast medium because of concern that the patient could have an abnormal condition of mushroom-shaped tumors.

   _____

   _____

6. Because of her abnormal condition of gall stones, Ms. Katopolis had an cutting into in her abdomen and gallbladder removal.

   _____

   _____

7. Common symptoms of stomach acid backing up into the esophagus include difficulty swallowing and stomach pain.

   _____

   _____

8. The patient was found to have an obstruction in the intestine due to the loss of muscular movements and required a surgical creation of a new opening into the second section of intestine.

   _____

   _____

9. The bowel movement was tested for the presence of small amounts of blood in the feces and the presence of parasites or their eggs in the feces.

   _____

   _____

10. To evaluate Mr. Habib's very dark, tarry stools, his stomach and intestine specialist performed a visual exam of the rectum and anus, a visual exam of the S-shaped region of colon, and a visual exam of the colon.

    _____

    _____

Labeling Exercise

Write the name of each organ on the numbered line. Also use this space to write the combining form where appropriate.

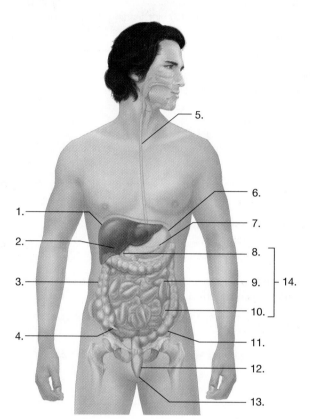

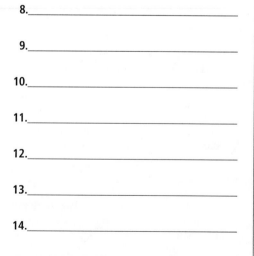

1. —

5.

6.

1. —
7.

2. —
8.

3. —
9. — 14.

10.

4. —
11.

12.

13.

1._____   8._____

2._____   9._____

3._____   10._____

4._____   11._____

5._____   12._____

6._____   13._____

7._____   14._____

Build Medical Terms

Use each of the following word parts to build the indicated medical terms.

The combining form *gastr/o* means stomach.

1. stomach inflammation _____

2. stomach surgical removal _____

3. instrument to visually examine the stomach _____

4. one term that means stomach pain _____

5. a different term that means stomach pain _____

The combining forms *proct/o* and *recto* both refer to the rectum.

6. Use *proct/o* to build rectum drooping. _____

7. Use *rect/o* to build rectum protrusion. _____

The combining form *cholecyst/o* means gallbladder.

8. gallbladder inflammation _____

9. gallbladder surgical removal _____

The suffix *-ostomy* means to create an artificial opening.

10. artificial opening in the duodenum _____

11. artificial opening in the colon _____

12. artificial opening in the stomach _____

The suffix *-pepsia* means digestion.

13. without digestion _____

14. difficult digestion _____

15. slow digestion _____

Abbreviation Matching

Match each abbreviation with its definition.

_____ 1. ERCP	**A.**	gastroesophageal reflux disease
_____ 2. GI	**B.**	barium
_____ 3. BE	**C.**	total parenteral nutrition
_____ 4. IBD	**D.**	gastrointestinal
_____ 5. TPN	**E.**	nausea and vomiting
_____ 6. GERD	**F.**	irritable bowel syndrome
_____ 7. Ba	**G.**	barium enema
_____ 8. IBS	**H.**	endoscopic retrograde cholangiopancreatography
_____ 9. EGD	**I.**	inflammatory bowel disease
_____ 10. N & V	**J.**	esophagogastroduodenoscopy

Fill in the Blank

Fill in the blank to complete each of the following sentences.

1. The patient had a nutrient-complete solution given directly into her bloodstream. The medical term for this is called _____.

2. In peptic ulcer disease, the ulcers may be found in the _____, _____, or _____.

3. The forceful return of stomach contents out of the mouth is to _____.

4. Another term for an upper GI series is _____.

5. Bile is produced by the _____ and stored in the _____.

6. The nurse's notes indicated that the patient's abdomen was swollen by fluid accumulating in the abdominal cavity. This accumulation is called _____.

7. The term that describes an intestinal blockage that occurs when the colon muscles stop pushing food through the colon is _____.

8. After finding ulcers on the mucous membrane of Mr. Fong's colon during a colonoscopy, the physician was able to tell him that he had a chronic condition called _____.

9. Miss Matthews did not recognize what condition she had when her doctor told her she had irritable bowel syndrome. She was more familiar with the name _____.

10. _____ is a surgical treatment for obesity.

Spelling

Some of the following terms are misspelled. Identify the incorrect terms and spell them correctly in the blank provided.

1. cholecystogram _____

2. esophogal _____

3. pancreasitis _____

4. duodenum _____

5. gastroitis _____

6. intussusception _____

7. *Helicobacter pylori* _____

8. cirhosis _____

9. volvolus _____

10. jaundice _____

Medical Term Analysis

*Examine each of the following terms. Begin by dividing it into its word parts and writing them in the indicated blanks (**P = prefix**, **WR = word root**; **CF = combining form**; **S = suffix**). Follow with the definition of each word part and then finally the meaning of the full term.*

1. **esophagoplasty**

   CF _____

   means _____

   S _____

   means _____

   Term Meaning: _____

   _____

2. **appendectomy**

   WR _____

   means _____

   S _____

   means _____

   Term Meaning: _____

   _____

3. **choledocholithotripsy**

   CF _____

   means _____

   CF _____

   means _____

   S _____

   means _____

   Term Meaning: _____

   _____

4. **hyperemesis**

   P _____

   means _____

   S _____

   means _____

   Term Meaning: _____

   _____

5. **gastroenteritis**

   CF _____

   means _____

   WR _____

   means _____

   S _____

   means _____

   Term Meaning: _____

   _____

6. **hepatoma**

   WR _____

   means _____

   S _____

   means _____

   Term Meaning: _____

   _____

7. **diverticulosis**

WR _____

means _____

S _____

means _____

Term Meaning: _____

_____

8. **ileostomy**

WR _____

means _____

S _____

means _____

Term Meaning: _____

_____

9. **laparoscope**

CF _____

means _____

S _____

means _____

Term Meaning: _____

_____

10. **polyphagia**

P _____

means _____

S _____

means _____

Term Meaning: _____

_____

mymedicalterminologylab

PEARSON

MyMedicalTerminologyLab is a premium online homework management system that includes a host of features to help you study. Registered users will find:

- Fun games and activities built within a virtual hospital
- Powerful tools that track and analyze your results—allowing you to create a personalized learning experience
- Videos, flashcards, and audio pronunciations to help enrich your progress
- Streaming lesson presentations and self-paced learning modules
- A space where you and your instructors can view and manage your assignments

Photomatch Challenge

Use the Word Bank below to build a term for each figure.

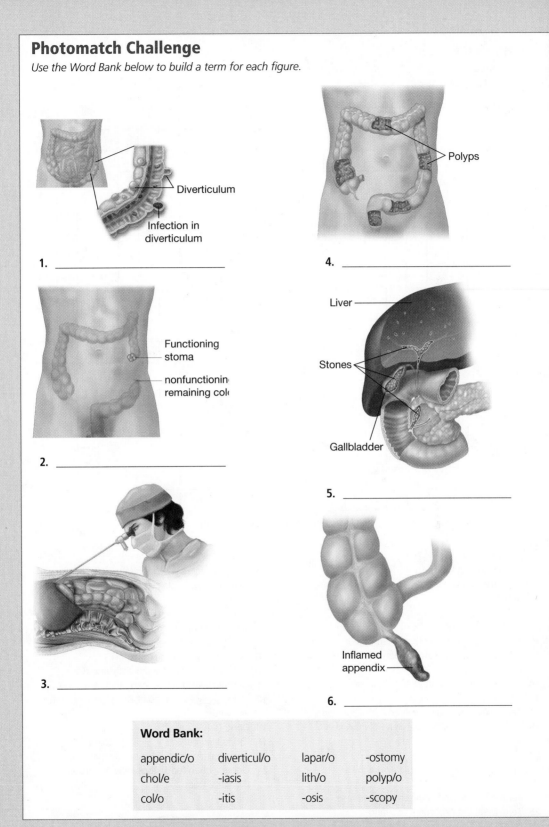

Diverticulum

Infection in diverticulum

1. _____

Polyps

4. _____

Functioning stoma

nonfunctioning remaining col[...]

2. _____

Liver

Stones

Gallbladder

5. _____

3. _____

Inflamed appendix

6. _____

Word Bank:

appendic/o	diverticul/o	lapar/o	-ostomy
chol/e	-iasis	lith/o	polyp/o
col/o	-itis	-osis	-scopy

Crossword Puzzle

Use the definitions given to complete the crossword puzzle.

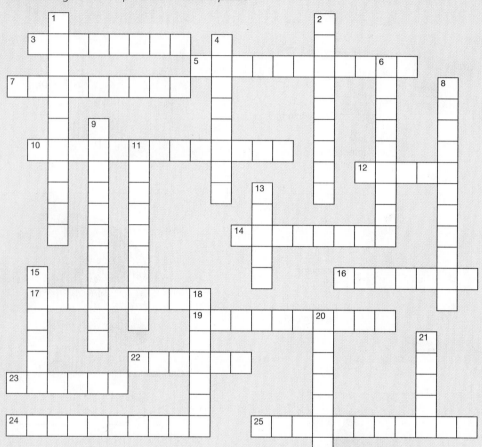

ACROSS

3 Term meaning liver tumor
5 Term meaning procedure to visually examine abdominal cavity
7 _____/o, the combining form for common bile duct
10 Term meaning gallbladder inflammation
12 Forceful return of stomach contents out of the mouth
14 Length of bowel twisted around itself
16 Term meaning not eating
17 Term meaning inflammation of small intestine
19 A(n) _____ ulcer has eaten a hole through the stomach wall
22 Urge to vomit
23 _____ enema is also called a lower GI series
24 Term meaning pertaining to the pancreas
25 Term meaning excessive vomiting

DOWN

1 Varicose veins in the rectum
2 Symptoms include pain, diarrhea, and blood in stools
4 Yellow-colored skin from liver disease
6 Term meaning abnormal condition of having polyps
8 Term meaning vomiting blood
9 TPN delivers nutrients directly into the _____
11 Chronic liver disease, can cause jaundice
13 _____/o, the combining form for rectum and anus
15 Dark, tarry stools
18 IBS is also called _____ colon
20 Accumulation of fluid in abdominal cavity
21 Occurs when food stops moving through digestive tract

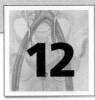

12

Urology and Nephrology
Urinary System and Male Reproductive System

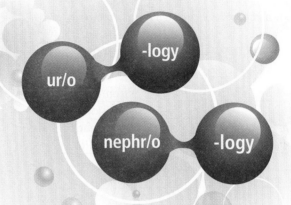

ur/o -logy

nephr/o -logy

A Brief Introduction to Urology and Nephrology

UNDERSTAND the functions of the urinary and male reproductive systems.

The urinary system is responsible for several very important processes necessary to maintain **homeostasis**, a stable internal environment. These processes include:

- Removing waste products
- Adjusting water and electrolyte levels in the body
- Maintaining normal pH

Beginning in the two **kidneys**, unneeded and unwanted substances are removed from the body along with excess water to produce **urine**. Urine then flows from each kidney through a **ureter** to the **urinary bladder** where it is stored. When urine is released from the body, it flows out through the **urethra**.

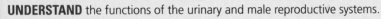

In males, the reproductive system is closely associated with the urinary system because both share the urethra. For this reason, these two systems are sometimes referred to as the **genitourinary system**. The testes are responsible for producing sperm and secreting testosterone, the male sex hormone. The remaining organs of this system include the **epididymis, vas deferens, seminal vesicles, prostate gland, bulbourethral gland, urethra**, and **penis**. These organs store and transport sperm or secrete seminal fluids to nourish the sperm.

DESCRIBE the medical specialties of urology and nephrology.

Two medical specialty areas are involved in the diagnosis and treatment of conditions affecting the urinary system: **urology** and **nephrology**. **Urologists** treat conditions of the female and male urinary tract. In addition, because of the overlap between organs of the urinary tract and male reproductive system, urologists also treat conditions affecting the testes, epididymis, vas deferens, prostate gland, seminal vesicles, bulbourethral glands, and penis. Nephrology is more specifically involved with treating kidney disease. Conditions commonly treated by **nephrologists** include renal failure, problems with fluid and electrolyte balance, kidney transplants, and kidney disease in dialysis patients.

DEFINE *urology* and nephrology-related combining forms, prefixes, and suffixes.

Urology and Nephrology Combining Forms

The following list presents new combining forms important for building and defining urology and nephrology terms.

balan/o	glans penis		**ren/o**	kidney
cyst/o	bladder		**semin/i**	semen
epididym/o	epididymis		**spermat/o**	sperm
glomerul/o	glomerulus		**sperm/o**	sperm
lith/o	stone		**testicul/o**	testicle
nephr/o	kidney		**ur/o**	urine
orchid/o	testes		**ureter/o**	ureter
orchi/o	testes		**urethr/o**	urethra
orch/o	testes		**urin/o**	urine
prostat/o	prostate gland		**vas/o**	vas deferens
pyel/o	renal pelvis		**vesicul/o**	seminal vesicle

The following list presents combining forms that are not specific to the urinary or male reproductive systems but are also used for building and defining urology and nephrology terms.

albumin/o	albumin		**hem/o**	blood
azot/o	nitrogen waste		**hydr/o**	water
bacteri/o	bacteria		**noct/i**	night
corpor/o	body		**olig/o**	scanty
crypt/o	hidden		**py/o**	pus
genit/o	genitals		**rect/o**	rectum
glycos/o	sugar, glucose		**ven/o**	vein
hemat/o	blood			

Suffix Review

These suffixes and prefixes were introduced in Chapters 2 and 3. They are being reviewed in this chapter because they are especially important for building urology and nephrology terms.

-al	pertaining to		**-megaly**	enlargement
-algia	pain		**-meter**	instrument for measuring
-ar	pertaining to		**-oma**	tumor, mass
-ary	pertaining to		**-osis**	abnormal condition
-cele	hernia, protrusion		**-ostomy**	surgically create an opening
-cyte	cell		**-otomy**	cutting into
-eal	pertaining to		**-ous**	pertaining to
-ectomy	surgical removal		**-pathy**	disease
-emia	blood condition		**-pexy**	surgical fixation
-genesis	produces, generates		**-plasty**	surgical repair
-gram	record, picture		**-ptosis**	drooping
-graphy	process of recording		**-rrhaphy**	suture
-ia	state		**-rrhea**	discharge, flow
-iasis	abnormal condition		**-sclerosis**	hardened condition
-ic	pertaining to		**-scope**	instrument for viewing
-ism	state of, condition		**-scopy**	process of visually examining
-itis	inflammation		**-stenosis**	narrowing
-lith	stone		**-tripsy**	crushing
-logist	one who studies		**-trophy**	development
-logy	study of		**-uria**	urine condition
-lysis	destruction			

Prefix Review

a-	without		**hyper-**	excessive
an-	without		**intra-**	within
dys-	abnormal		**poly-**	many
extra-	outside of		**trans-**	across

Organs Commonly Treated in Urology and Nephrology

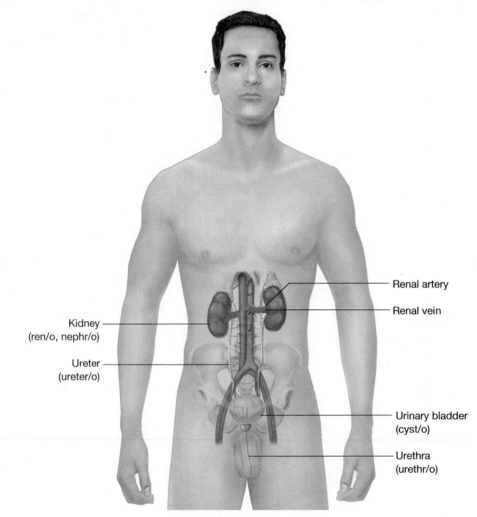

Renal artery

Renal vein

Kidney
(ren/o, nephr/o)

Ureter
(ureter/o)

Urinary bladder
(cyst/o)

Urethra
(urethr/o)

>12.1 The urinary system

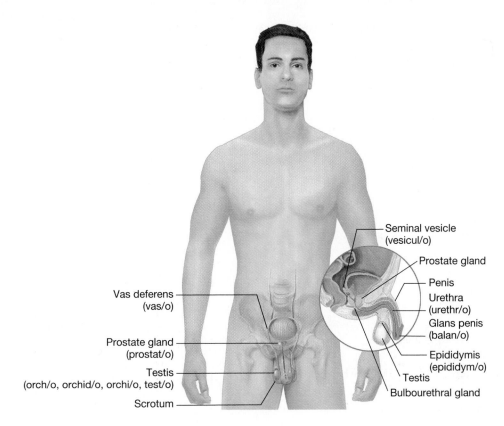

>12.2 The male reproductive system

 BUILD urology and nephrology medical terms from word parts.

Building Urology and Nephrology Terms

This section presents word parts most often used to build urology and nephrology terms. Following the explanation of the term, you have the opportunity to begin building your own vocabulary. Read the meaning for each term and then fill in the blanks to build a single medical term. Use the slashes to divide prefixes, word roots, combining vowels, and suffixes. To help you out you will find a key to the word parts underneath the blanks: r for word roots, p for prefix, cv for combining vowel, and s for suffix. Remember that not every term will contain all these word parts; it's up to you to decide which to use. As you gain experience, this process becomes easier. Answers can be found at the back of the book.

1. balan/o–combining form meaning **glans penis**

   The glans penis is the enlarged tip of the penis; glans is covered by the **prepuce** or **foreskin**

   a. glans penis inflammation

   _____/_____
                  r   s

   b. discharge from the glans penis

   _____/____/_____
                r   cv   s

2. cyst/o–combining form meaning **urinary bladder**

The urinary bladder is a muscular organ that stores urine produced by the kidneys; urine drains into bladder from ureters and exits bladder in urethra

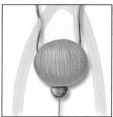

>12.3 Urinary bladder

a. bladder pain

_____/_____
　　　　　　　　　 r　　　　　s

b. protrusion of the bladder

_____/____/_____
　　　　 r　　 cv　　 s

c. surgical removal of the bladder

_____/_____
　　　　　　　 r　　　　　s

d. bladder inflammation

_____/_____
　　　　　　　 r　　　　　s

e. process of visually examining the bladder

_____/____/_____
　　　　 r　　 cv　　 s

f. record of the bladder

_____/____/_____
　　　　 r　　 cv　　 s

g. process of recording the bladder

_____/____/_____
　　　　 r　　 cv　　 s

h. instrument to visually examine the bladder

_____/____/_____
　　　　 r　　 cv　　 s

i. pertaining to the bladder

_____/_____
　　　　　　　 r　　　　　s

j. stone in the bladder

_____/____/_____
　　　　 r　　 cv　　 s

3. epididym/o–combining form meaning **epididymis**

The epididymis sits on surface of each testis; stores sperm as they are made by the testes

a. epididymis inflammation

_____/_____
　　　　　　　 r　　　　　s

b. pertaining to the epididymis

_____/_____
　　　　　　　 r　　　　　s

4. lith/o–combining form meaning **stone**

Stones form in many parts of body, usually formed from organic or inorganic salts

a. surgical crushing of a stone

_____/____/_____
　　　　 r　　 cv　　 s

b. abnormal condition of stone in ureter

_____/____/_____/____
　　　 r　　 cv　　　 r　　 s

c. abnormal condition of stone in kidney

_____/____/_____/____
　　　 r　　 cv　　　 r　　 s

d. abnormal condition of stone in bladder

_____/____/_____/____
　　　 r　　 cv　　　 r　　 s

5. nephr/o–combining form meaning **kidney**

One kidney is located on either side of spine at level of lower ribs; each consists of thousands of **nephrons**; **glomerulus** portion of each nephron filters waste products and excess water and electrolytes out of blood to produce urine; urine drains out of kidney into ureter and on to urinary bladder for storage

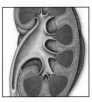

>12.4 Kidney

a. surgical removal of the kidney

_____/_____
r   s

b. kidney inflammation

_____/_____
r   s

c. enlarged kidney

_____/____/_____
r   cv   s

d. kidney tumor

_____/_____
r   s

e. drooping kidney

_____/____/_____
r   cv   s

f. cutting into the kidney

_____/_____
r   s

g. kidney disease

_____/____/_____
r   cv   s

h. surgical fixation of the kidney

_____/____/_____
r   cv   s

i. hardening of the kidney

_____/____/_____
r   cv   s

j. glomerulus and kidney inflammation

_____/____/_____/___
r   cv   r   s

k. kidney stone

_____/____/_____
r   cv   s

l. abnormal condition of the kidney

_____/_____
r   s

6. orchid/o–combining form meaning **testes**

The testes are the male reproductive organs that produce sperm and **testosterone**; the two testes are suspended outside body in the **scrotum**; as sperm are produced, they travel to epididymis for storage; singular form is testis; another term for testes is **testicles** (singular, testicle)

>12.5 Testes

a. surgical removal of testes

_____/_____
r   s

7. orchi/o–combining form meaning **testes**

a. surgical fixation of the testes

_____/____/_____
r   cv   s

b. testes pain

_____/_____
r   s

8. orch/o–combining form meaning **testes**

    a. condition of being without testes

                _____/_____/_____
                                  _p_   _r_   _s_

    b. testes inflammation

                _____/_____
                                _r_   _s_

    c. condition of hidden testes

                _____/_____/_____
                                _r_   _r_   _s_

---

9. -ostomy–suffix meaning **to create a surgical opening**

This suffix describes the creation of new opening between two organs or between organ and external surface of body; new opening on surface of body is called **stoma**

    a. surgically create an opening in the bladder

                _____/_____
                                _r_   _s_

    b. surgically create an opening in the kidney

                _____/_____
                                _r_   _s_

    c. surgically create an opening in the ureter

                _____/_____
                                _r_   _s_

    d. surgically create an opening in the renal pelvis

                _____/_____
                                _r_   _s_

    e. surgically create an opening in the urethra

                _____/_____
                                _r_   _s_

    f. surgically create an opening between (one section of) vas deferens and (another section of) vas deferens

                _____/_____/_____/_____
                            _r_   _cv_   _r_   _s_

---

10. prostat/o–combining form meaning **prostate gland**

The prostate gland is one of the male reproductive glands found surrounding urethra at base of bladder; secretes milky fluid that makes up much of liquid portion of semen and serves to nourish sperm

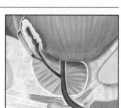

>**12.6** Prostate gland

    a. surgical removal of prostate gland

                _____/_____
                                _r_   _s_

    b. prostate gland inflammation

                _____/_____
                                _r_   _s_

    c. pertaining to prostate gland

                _____/_____
                                _r_   _s_

---

11. pyel/o–combining form meaning **renal pelvis**

The renal pelvis is an area inside each kidney where urine collects as it is being made; each renal pelvis then drains into one of the ureters

    a. renal pelvis and kidney inflammation

                _____/_____/_____/_____
                            _r_   _cv_   _r_   _s_

    b. record of the renal pelvis

                  _____/_____/_____
                              _r_   _cv_   _s_

    c. process of recording the renal pelvis

                  _____/_____/_____
                              _r_   _cv_   _s_

---

12. ren/o–combining form meaning **kidney**

    a. pertaining to kidney

                              _____/_____
                                             r   *s*

    b. record of kidney

            _____/_____/_____
                     r   *cv*   *s*

    c. process of recording kidney

        _____/_____/_____
                    r   *cv*   *s*

13. semin/i–combining form meaning **semen**

Semen is the fluid ejaculated from penis during intercourse; contains sperm and fluids secreted by reproductive glands: prostate gland, seminal vesicles, and bulbourethral gland

    a. pertaining to semen

        _____/_____
                    r   *s*

    b. condition of semen in urine

        _____/_____
                    r   *s*

14. spermat/o –combining form meaning **sperm**

Sperm are the male reproductive cells; produced in testes and ejaculated from body in semen; contain one-half of normal complement of chromosomes; when sperm fertilizes ovum (which also has one-half set of chromosomes from mother), new baby is created with full set of chromosomes

    a. generates sperm

        _____/_____/_____
                    r   *cv*   *s*

    b. destruction of sperm

        _____/_____/_____
                    r   *cv*   *s*

    c. pertaining to sperm

        _____/_____
                    r   *s*

    d. sperm cell

        _____/_____/_____
                    r   *cv*   *s*

15. sperm/o–combining form meaning **sperm**

    a. state of being without sperm

        _____/_____/_____
                  p   *r*   *s*

    b. state of having scanty sperm

        _____/_____/_____/____
                  r   *cv*   *r*   *s*

16. testicul/o–combining form meaning **testicle**

    a. pertaining to a testicle

        _____/_____
                    r   *s*

17. ureter/o–combining form meaning **ureter**

The ureter is a tube leading away from renal pelvis of each kidney, carries urine from kidney to urinary bladder

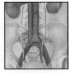

>12.7 **Ureters**

    a. ureter inflammation

        _____/_____
                    r   *s*

    b. narrowing of ureter

        _____/_____/_____
                    r   *cv*   *s*

    c. pertaining to ureter

        _____/_____
                    r   *s*

18. urethr/o–combining form meaning **urethra**

The single urethra leads out of bladder and carries urine to outside of body; external opening is **meatus**

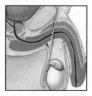

>12.8 **Male urethra**

a. surgical repair of urethra
_____/_____/_____
_r _{cv} _s

b. urethra pain
_____/_____
_r _s

c. urethra inflammation
_____/_____
_r _s

d. instrument for visually examining urethra
_____/_____/_____
_r _{cv} _s

e. process of visually examining urethra
_____/_____/_____
_r _{cv} _s

f. narrowing of urethra
_____/_____/_____
_r _{cv} _s

g. cutting into urethra
_____/_____
_r _s

h. pertaining to urethra
_____/_____
_r _s

19. -uria–suffix meaning **condition of the urine**

This suffix is used with a prefix or combining form to indicate something found in urine or associated with urination

a. sugar urine condition
_____/_____
_r _s

b. night urine condition
_____/_____
_r _s

c. scanty urine condition
_____/_____
_r _s

d. pus urine condition
_____/_____
_r _s

e. without urine condition
_____/_____
_p _s

f. abnormal urine condition
_____/_____
_p _s

g. blood urine condition
_____/_____
_r _s

h. much urine condition
_____/_____
_p _s

i. albumin (protein) urine condition
_____/_____
_r _s

j. nitrogen waste urine condition
_____/_____
_r _s

k. bacteria urine condition
_____/_____
_r _s

20. **urin/o**–combining form meaning **urine**

Urine is the fluid produced by nephrons of each kidney as they filter wastes, water, and dissolved substances from blood

    a. pertaining to urine

_____/_____
               r   s

    b. instrument to measure urine

_____/____/_____
            r   cv   s

21. **ur/o**–combining form meaning **urine**

    a. study of urine

_____/____/_____
            r   cv   s

    b. one who studies urine

_____/____/_____
            r   cv   s

    c. condition of urine in blood

_____/_____
               r   s

22. **vas/o**–combining form meaning **vas deferens**

The vas deferens is a long tube that carries sperm from epididymis to urethra; reproductive glands add fluids to sperm as they pass by, making semen

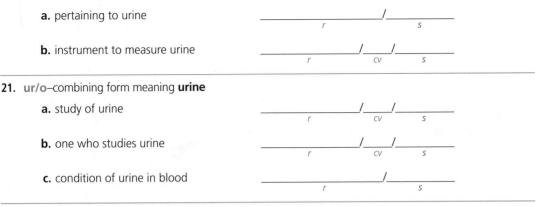

A   **B**   **C**   **D**

>12.9 Steps in performing a vasectomy: (A) vas deferens are located; (B) small skin incision is made; (C) vas deferens are cut and ends are cauterized; (D) vas deferens are returned to scrotum and skin is sutured

    a. surgical removal of vas deferens

_____/_____
               r   s

    b. suture vas deferens

_____/____/_____
            r   cv   s

23. **vesicul/o**–combining form meaning **seminal vesicles**

The seminal vesicles are the male reproductive glands found behind bladder; add fluids to sperm as they pass in vas deferens

    a. seminal vesicle inflammation

_____/_____
               r   s

    b. surgical removal of seminal vesicle

_____/_____
               r   s

    c. pertaining to seminal vesicle

_____/_____
               r   s

Urology and Nephrology Vocabulary

The urology and nephrology terms presented in this section include eponyms, modern English words, and those that contain Latin or Greek word parts but are not constructed solely from these word parts. When you recognize word parts within a term they will give you a hint about the word's meaning. In these instances, look for the word parts to follow the term.

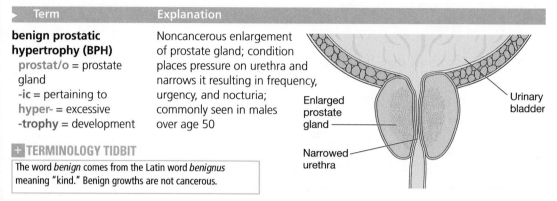

Term	Explanation
benign prostatic hypertrophy (BPH) prostat/o = prostate gland -ic = pertaining to hyper- = excessive -trophy = development	Noncancerous enlargement of prostate gland; condition places pressure on urethra and narrows it resulting in frequency, urgency, and nocturia; commonly seen in males over age 50

＋ TERMINOLOGY TIDBIT

The word *benign* comes from the Latin word *benignus* meaning "kind." Benign growths are not cancerous.

>12.10 Benign prostatic hypertrophy. The enlarged prostate gland pinches the urethra making urination difficult

Term	Explanation
blood urea nitrogen (BUN)	Blood test to determine kidney function by measuring level of nitrogenous waste, urea, in blood
calculus	Term for "stone formed within organ"; most are formed from mineral salts; commonly found in kidney, renal pelvis, ureters, bladder, or urethra; plural is *calculi*

＋ TERMINOLOGY TIDBIT

The word *calculus* comes from the Latin word *calculus* meaning "pebble."

>12.11 Common location for calculi in the urinary system: kidney, renal pelvis, ureter, and bladder

chlamydia

Bacterial sexually transmitted disease; causes inflammation of urethra of males or cervix of females with purulent discharge

circumcision

Surgical removal of prepuce or foreskin from glans penis; commonly performed on newborn male at request of parents; primary reason is for ease of hygiene; also a ritual practiced in some religions

> **+ TERMINOLOGY TIDBIT**
>
> The word *circumcision* comes from the Latin word *circumcido* meaning "to cut around." This describes the incision required to remove the prepuce.

clean catch specimen (CC)

Procedure for obtaining urine sample after cleaning off urethral meatus and catching urine in midstream (halfway through urination process) to minimize contamination from skin

digital rectal exam (DRE)
  rect/o = rectum
  -al = pertaining to

Direct examination for presence of enlarged prostate gland performed by palpating (feeling) prostate gland with fingers (digital) through wall of rectum

erectile dysfunction (ED)

Inability to achieve erection of penis for coitus; also called *impotence*

extracorporeal shockwave lithotripsy (ESWL)
  extra- = outside of
  corpor/o = body
  -eal = pertaining to
  lith/o = stone
  -tripsy = crushing

Treatment procedure for urinary system stones; utilizes ultrasound waves to break up stones; process is noninvasive, meaning it does not require surgery

Beam focused on kidney stones

Shockwave generator

Reflector

>12.12 Extracorporeal shockwave lithotripsy, a noninvasive procedure using high frequency sound waves to shatter kidney stones

frequency

Condition of feeling urge to urinate more often than normal but without increase in total daily volume of urine; can indicate inflammation of bladder or urethra or benign prostatic hypertrophy

genital herpes
  genit/o = genitals
  -al = pertaining to

Highly infectious viral sexually transmitted disease; causes blisterlike lesions on penis of males or cervix and vagina of females

gonorrhea
  -rrhea = discharge

Bacterial sexually transmitted disease; infects mucous membranes and can spread throughout entire genitourinary system; often does not cause many symptoms until widespread

Term	Explanation
hemodialysis (HD) **hem/o** = blood	Treatment for renal failure using artificial kidney machine to filter waste from blood >**12.13** Patient undergoing hemodialysis. Her blood passes through the hemodialysis machine for cleansing and is then returned to her body
hesitancy	State of difficulty initiating flow of urine; often symptom of blockage along urethra, such as caused by benign prostatic hypertrophy
hydrocele **hydr/o** = water **-cele** = protrusion	Accumulation of fluid within scrotum
intravenous pyelogram (IVP) **intra-** = within **ven/o** = vein **-ous** = pertaining to **pyel/o** = renal pelvis **-gram** = record	X-ray of kidney following injection of dye into vein to visualize renal pelvis as kidney filters dye out of bloodstream and puts it into urine
peritoneal dialysis **-al** = pertaining to	Artificial means to remove waste substances from body by placing warm, chemically balanced solutions into peritoneal cavity; treatment for renal failure >**12.14** In peritoneal dialysis, a chemically balanced solution is placed into the abdominal cavity to draw impurities out of the bloodstream. It is removed after several hours
phimosis	Narrowing of prepuce over glans penis; can cause difficulty with urination and infection; treatment is circumcision **TERMINOLOGY TIDBIT** The word *phimosis* comes from the Greek word *phimos* meaning "to muzzle." This describes how the prepuce constricts the glans penis.
polycystic kidney disease (PKD) **poly-** = many **cyst/o** = sacs **-ic** = pertaining to	Inherited kidney disease characterized by presence of multiple cysts throughout kidney tissue; eventually destroys kidneys and results in kidney failure

prostate-specific antigen (PSA)	Blood test to screen for prostate cancer

prostatic cancer
  prostat/o = prostate gland
  -ic = pertaining to
	Common and slow-growing cancer of prostate gland occurring in males over age 50; prostate-specific antigen (PSA) test is used to assist in early detection of this disease

renal failure
  ren/o = kidney
  -al = pertaining to
	Inability of kidneys to filter wastes from blood and/or produce urine; treatment of severe renal failure is dialysis or renal transplant

renal transplant
  ren/o = kidney
  -al = pertaining to
	Replacement of diseased kidney by donor kidney

>12.15 Figure illustrates the location of transplanted donor kidney

Transplanted kidney
Internal iliac artery and vein
Grafted ureter
External iliac artery and vein

retrograde pyelogram (RP)
  pyel/o = renal pelvis
  -gram = record
	X-ray of urinary bladder, ureters, and renal pelvis following insertion of dye through urethra

semen analysis	Evaluation of semen for fertility; sperm in semen analyzed for number, swimming strength, and shape; procedure would also be used to determine whether vasectomy has been successful
sexually transmitted disease (STD)	Contagious disease acquired through sexual contact; formerly referred to as *venereal disease (VD)*
sterility	Inability to produce children; in males, usually due to problem with sperm production, such as aspermia or oligospermia; also called *infertility*
syphilis	Bacterial sexually transmitted disease; begins as localized ulcer at point of infection; chronic disease that spreads through lymph nodes to nervous system after years, causing death

testicular cancer
  testicul/o = testes
  -ar = pertaining to
	Cancer of one or both testicles; commonly seen in young men or boys

transurethral resection (TUR)
trans- = across
urethr/o = urethra
-al = pertaining to

Surgical removal of prostate gland tissue by inserting device called *resectoscope* through urethra and removing prostate tissue

trichomoniasis
-iasis = abnormal condition

Protozoan sexually transmitted disease; causes inflammation of genitourinary tract in both men and women

undescended testicle

Congenital anomaly involving failure of one or both of testes to descend into scrotal sac before birth; surgical procedure called *orchiopexy* can be required to bring testes down into scrotum permanently; also called *cryptorchism*

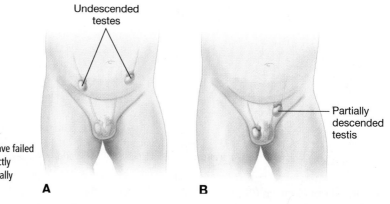

Undescended testes

Partially descended testis

>12.16 Undescended testicle or cryptorchism. In (A) both testes have failed to descend. In (B) one testis correctly descended while the other is partially descended

A   B

urgency

Force or impulse of needing need to urinate immediately

urinalysis (U/A, UA)
urin/o = urine

Laboratory test that consists of physical, chemical, and microscopic examination of urine

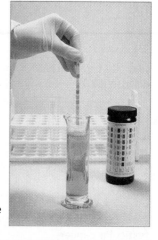

>12.17 A dipstick is used to conduct a chemical analysis of urine testing, for example, for the presence of sugar

urinary catheterization (cath)

urin/o = urine
-ary = pertaining to

Insertion of flexible tube, catheter, into urinary bladder through urethra; used to withdraw urine or insert dye

＋ TERMINOLOGY TIDBIT

The word *catheter* comes from the Greek word *katheter* meaning "to let down." This refers to the use of a catheter to remove fluid from the body.

A

B

>12.18 Urinary catheterization in both (A) female and (B) male patients

---

urinary incontinence

urin/o = urine
-ary = pertaining to

Involuntary urination; also called *enuresis*

＋ TERMINOLOGY TIDBIT

The word *incontinence* comes from the Latin word *incontinentia* meaning "unable to hold together."

---

urinary tract infection (UTI)

urin/o = urine
-ary = pertaining to

Infection of urethra and/or urinary bladder

Urine Exam

Bacteriuria (over 100,000/cu ml)

Leukocytes and white cell casts

>12.19 Urinary tract infection characterized by fever, low back or abdominal pain, and burning pain during urination. A urinalysis reveals the presence of bacteria and white blood cells

---

urine culture & sensitivity (C&S)

Diagnostic lab procedure that identifies bacterial infection of urinary system and determines best antibiotic to treat it; involves growing bacteria in culture medium and testing different antibiotics on it

---

varicocele

-cele = protrusion

Development of varicose veins of veins leading to testes in scrotum

---

voiding cystourethrography (VCUG)

cyst/o = bladder
urethr/o = urethra
-graphy = process of recording

X-ray made while patient voids dye that has been placed in urinary bladder through urethra

Urology and Nephrology Abbreviations

The following list presents common urology and nephrology abbreviations.

ARF	acute renal failure	**I & O**	intake and output
BPH	benign prostatic hypertrophy	**IVP**	intravenous pyelogram
BUN	blood urea nitrogen	**KUB**	kidney, ureter, bladder
cath	catheterization	**PKD**	polycystic kidney disease
CC	clean-catch urine specimen	**PSA**	prostate-specific antigen
CRF	chronic renal failure	**RP**	retrograde pyelogram
C & S	culture and sensitivity test	**STD**	sexually transmitted disease
cysto	cystoscopy	**TUR**	transurethral resection
DRE	digital rectal exam	**TURP**	transurethral resection and
ESRD	end-stage renal disease		prostatectomy
ESWL	extracorporeal shock-wave lithotripsy	**U/A, UA**	urinalysis
GU	genitourinary	**UC**	urine culture
HD	hemodialysis	**UTI**	urinary tract infection
HPV	human papilloma virus	**VCUG**	voiding cystourethrography

CASE STUDY

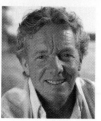

History of Present Illness

The patient is a 57-year-old male seen in the urologist's office to follow up an above normal prostate-specific antigen level found on his annual exam. His prostate-specific antigen values have been in the normal range but have gradually risen over the past three years. He reports nocturnal frequency and hesitancy but denies urinary incontinence or erectile dysfunction.

Past Medical History

Patient has a history of an acute myocardial infarction 2 years ago, which was treated by a percutaneous transluminal coronary angioplasty. He also had an inguinal herniorrhaphy 10 years ago. Patient has taken medication for hypertension for 4 years and for hyperlipidemia for 2 years.

Family and Social History

Patient is a professional golfer but has been unable to tolerate walking long distances for the past 3 years. He quit smoking following his myocardial infarction and denies using alcohol or illicit drugs. He is married and has three children. Family history is negative for cardiac problems. His father died of bone cancer and his mother is alive but in poor health with metastatic breast cancer.

Physical Examination

Patient is an average size male, alert and oriented x3, does not appear in any distress. His vital signs are normal, his abdomen is soft to palpation without organomegaly or lymphadenopathy. Digital rectal exam reveals a uniformly enlarged prostate gland but no nodules.

Diagnostic Tests

Urinalysis was positive for red blood cells but negative for bacteria, and a urine culture and sensitivity was negative. Multiple prostatic biopsies were taken. One biopsy revealed prostatic cancer. A bone scan and computed tomography scan of the abdomen and pelvis failed to demonstrate any evidence of metastases.

Diagnosis

Localized prostatic cancer without apparent metastases.

Plan of Treatment

1. Patient elected to undergo a prostatectomy
2. Because the tumor was well localized in the prostate gland and all lymph nodes were clear of metastatic disease, oncology did not recommend radiation or chemotherapy at this time
3. He is to have a repeat prostate-specific antigen level every 3 months

Critical Thinking Questions

Answer the following questions regarding this case study. Do not just copy words out of the case study; translate all medical terms. To answer some of these questions, you may need to look up information from another chapter of this text, in a medical dictionary, or online. Answers are found at the back of the book.

1. Describe the two urinary tract symptoms this patient does have and the two he does not complain of.

   _____

   _____

2. An elevated prostate-specific antigen level is often associated with:
   a. benign prostatic hypertrophy
   b. syphilis
   c. epispadias
   d. prostatic cancer

3. What are the vital signs?

   _____

   _____

4. Several terms in this case study can be replaced by an abbreviation. List five of them and their abbreviations.

   _____

   _____

5. What is a urinalysis? Describe the results of this patient's urinalysis.

   _____

   _____

6. What is an oncologist? Explain the oncologist's recommendations.

   _____

   _____

7. Two tests did not find any evidence of metastases. What were these tests, and what are *metastases*?

_____

_____

8. This patient has had a myocardial infarction that was treated with a percutaneous transluminal coronary angioplasty. Define these cardiology terms.

_____

_____

Sound It Out

The following are some of the key terms from this chapter written as their phonetic spelling. Sound out each term and write it in the blank. Pronunciations for all terms are included in the audio glossary at www.mymedicalterminologylab.com <http://www.mymedicalterminologylab.com/>.

1. yoo-ree-ter-oh-sten-OH-sis _____

2. bah-lah-noh-REE-ah _____

3. yoo-RAL-oh-jee _____

4. krip-TOR-kizm _____

5. yoo-rin-OH-meter _____

6. ah-SPER-mee-ah _____

7. SIS-toh-seel _____

8. tess-TOSS-ter-own _____

9. neh-FROH-ma _____

10. dis-YOO-ree-ah _____

11. en-yoo-REE-sis _____

12. ep-ih-did-ih-MYE-tis _____

13. glom-AIR-yoo-lus _____

14. veh-SIC-yoo-LYE-tis _____

15. hee-mah-TOO-ree-ah _____

16. klah-MID-ee-ah _____

17. hee-moh-dye-AL-ih-sis _____

18. gon-oh-REE-ah _____

19. pye-eh-loh-neh-FRYE-tis _____

20. SIS-toh-lith _____

21. neh-FROH-sis _____

22. LITH-oh-trip-see _____

23. mee-AY-tus _____

24. fih-MOH-sis _____

25. nef-roh-skleh-ROH-sis _____

26. glye-kohs-YOO-ree-ah _____

27. nok-TOO-ree-ah _____

28. ol-ih-goh-SPER-mee-ah _____

29. or-kid-EK-toh-mee _____

30. OR-kee-oh-PECK-see _____

31. pol-ee-YOO-ree-ah _____

32. sper-mah-TOL-ih-sis _____

33. pross-tah-TYE-tis _____

34. yoo-REE-ter _____

35. pye-YOO-ree-ah _____

36. ree-NOG-rah-fee _____

37. SIM-eh-nal _____

38. sper-mat-oh-JEN-eh-sis _____

39. tes-TIK-yoo-lar _____

40. yoo-REE-thral _____

41. KAL-kew-lus _____

42. trik-oh-moh-NYE-ah-sis _____

43. yoo-REE-mee-ah _____

44. sis-TEK-toh-me _____

45. yoo-REE-throh-scope _____

46. vas-EK-toh-mee _____

47. yoo-rih-NAL-ih-sis _____

48. VAIR-ih-koh-seel _____

49. nef-roh-MEG-ah-lee _____

50. NEF-roh-pek-see _____

Transcription Practice

Each of the following sentences is written in common English. Underline any words or phrases that can be replaced by a medical term. Then rewrite the entire sentence using medical terms. Answers can be found at the end of the book.

1. A procedure to visually examine the bladder revealed the presence of a bladder stone, and the patient underwent a surgical procedure to crush the stone.

   _____
   _____

2. When noting the discharge from the glans penis and the inflammation of the glans penis, the physician knew she needed to determine whether the patient had a developed a disease following sexually activity.

   _____
   _____

3. An x-ray record of the renal pelvis made after the insertion of a dye through the urethra confirmed the diagnosis of inflammation of the renal pelvis and kidney.

   _____
   _____

4. An evaluation of the semen for fertility performed 6 weeks after the surgical removal of the vas deferens confirmed the lack of sperm.

   _____
   _____

5. The patient's kidneys forming many small cysts resulted in the inability of his kidneys to filter waste from the blood, necessitating the use of a machine to filter the blood.

   _____
   _____

6. The results of the physical examination of the urine showed that there was pus in the urine, bacteria in the urine, and sugar in the urine.

_____

_____

7. After the patient developed an absence of urine, a kidney record revealed that the patient had developed hardening of the kidney.

_____

_____

8. The elderly gentleman required the surgical removal of the prepuce for narrowing of the prepuce.

_____

_____

9. The patient required a creation of a new opening to the ureter following the removal of the bladder for bladder cancer.

_____

_____

10. Bob developed the abnormal condition of stones in the kidneys and underwent a procedure utilizing ultrasound waves to break up the stones.

_____

_____

Abbreviation Matching

Match each abbreviation with its definition.

_____ **1.** ARF   **A.** blood urea nitrogen

_____ **2.** UTI   **B.** hemodialysis

_____ **3.** PSA   **C.** genitourinary

_____ **4.** HD   **D.** digital rectal exam

_____ **5.** BUN   **E.** intravenous pyelogram

_____ **6.** IVP   **F.** prostate-specific antigen

_____ **7.** TUR   **G.** urinary tract infection

_____ **8.** UA   **H.** urinalysis

_____ **9.** DRE   **I.** transurethral resection

_____ **10.** GU   **J.** acute renal failure

Labeling Exercise

Write the name of each structure on the numbered line. Also use this space to write the combining form where appropriate.

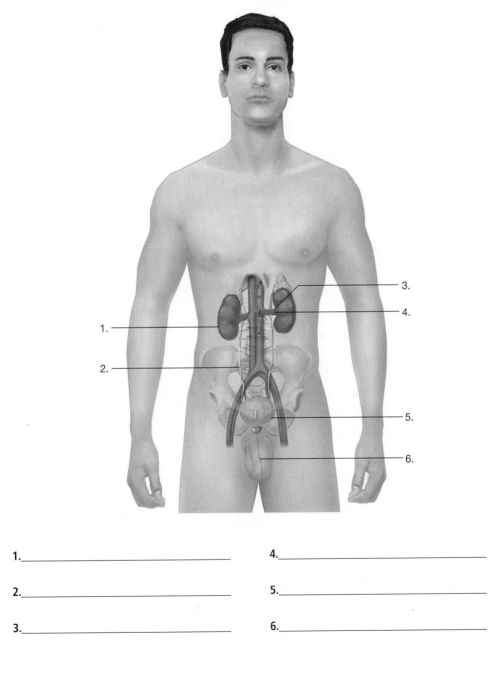

1._____

2._____

3._____

4._____

5._____

6._____

Build Medical Terms

Use each of the word parts below to build the indicated medical terms.

The combining form *nephr/o* means kidney.

1. kidney study of _____

2. kidney enlarged _____

3. kidney disease _____

4. kidney drooping _____

5. kidney surgical fixation _____

The combining form *spermat/o* means sperm.

6. sperm destruction _____

7. sperm pertaining to _____

The combining form *cyst/o* means bladder.

8. bladder record _____

9. bladder procedure to view _____

The combining form *prostate/o* means prostate gland.

10. prostate gland inflammation _____

11. prostate gland surgical removal _____

The suffix *-uria* means urine condition.

12. blood urine condition _____

13. night urine condition _____

14. abnormal urine condition _____

15. sugar urine condition _____

Fill in the Blank

Fill in the blank to complete each of the following sentences.

1. The development of varicose veins leading to the testes is called _____.

2. _____ is the noncancerous enlargement of the prostate gland.

3. The male sex hormone is _____.

4. In a semen analysis, the sperm are checked for _____, _____, and
_____.

5. An x-ray made while the persons voids dye that has been placed in the bladder is called a(n)
_____.

6. The treatment for phimosis is _____.

7. _____ is difficulty initiating the flow of urine.

8. _____ is a blood test used to screen for prostate cancer.

9. A _____ is a blood test to determine kidney function by
measuring the level of nitrogenous waste in the blood.

10. The term for a stone formed within an organ is a(n) _____.

Spelling

Some of the following terms are misspelled. Identify the incorrect terms and spell them correctly in the blank provided.

1. epidydimitis _____

2. nefrolithiasis _____

3. orchidectomy _____

4. pylography _____

5. ureterostenosis _____

6. catheterization _____

7. hidrocele _____

8. tricomoniasis _____

9. urinalysis _____

10. varicocele _____

Medical Term Analysis

*Examine each term of the following terms. Begin by dividing it into its word parts and writing them in the indicated blanks (**P = prefix**, **WR = word root**; **CF = combining form**, **S = suffix**). Follow with the definition of each word part and then finally the meaning of the full term.*

1. **balanitis**

   WR _____

   means _____

   S _____

   means _____

   Term Meaning: _____

   _____

2. **vasectomy**

   WR _____

   means _____

   S _____

   means _____

   Term Meaning: _____

   _____

3. **pyuria**

   WR _____

   means _____

   S _____

   means _____

   Term Meaning: _____

   _____

4. **ureterostomy**

   WR _____

   means _____

   S _____

   means _____

   Term Meaning: _____

   _____

5. **nephrolithiasis**

   CF _____

   means _____

   WR _____

   means _____

   S _____

   means _____

   Term Meaning: _____

   _____

6. **urology**

   CF _____

   means _____

   S _____

   means _____

   Term Meaning: _____

   _____

7. testicular

WR _____

means _____

S _____

means _____

Term Meaning: _____

8. cryptorchism

WR _____

means _____

WR _____

means _____

S _____

means _____

Term Meaning: _____
_____

9. prostatectomy

WR _____

means _____

S _____

means _____

Term Meaning: _____
_____

10. cystoscope

CF _____

means _____

S _____

means _____

Term Meaning: _____
_____

PEARSON
mymedicalterminologylab

MyMedicalTerminologyLab is a premium online homework management system that includes a host of features to help you study. Registered users will find:

- Fun games and activities built within a virtual hospital
- Powerful tools that track and analyze your results—allowing you to create a personalized learning experience
- Videos, flashcards, and audio pronunciations to help enrich your progress
- Streaming lesson presentations and self-paced learning modules
- A space where you and your instructors can view and manage your assignments

Photomatch Challenge

Match each scrotal condition with its name in the Word Bank.

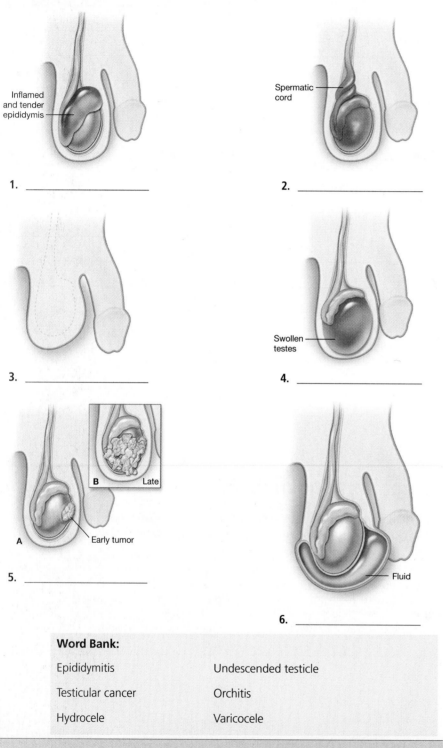

Inflamed and tender epididymis

1. _____

Spermatic cord

2. _____

3. _____

Swollen testes

4. _____

B   Late

A   Early tumor

5. _____

Fluid

6. _____

Word Bank:

Epididymitis   Undescended testicle

Testicular cancer   Orchitis

Hydrocele   Varicocele

Crossword Puzzle

Use the definitions given to complete the crossword puzzle.

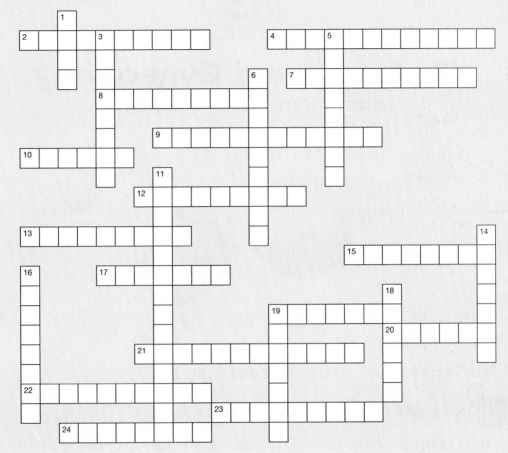

ACROSS

2 Varicose veins in scrotal veins
4 Another term for undescended testicle
7 Organ that stores sperm made by the testes
8 Accumulation of fluid within scrotum
9 Using artificial kidney machine to filter waste
10 Genital _____, highly infectious viral STD
12 Urge to urinate more often than normal
13 Another term for erectile dysfunction
15 Term meaning scanty amount of urine
17 Testes are suspended outside body in the _____
19 Need to urinate immediately
20 Transports urine between kidney and bladder
21 Surgical removal of prepuce
22 Laboratory test to examine urine
23 Inability to produce children
24 Another term for urinary incontinence

DOWN

1 A BUN tests for the level of _____ in the blood
3 Flexible tube inserted into the bladder
5 Narrowing of prepuce over glans penis
6 Difficulty initiating flow of urine
11 Protozoan sexually transmitted disease
14 Renal _____, inability of kidneys to filter wastes
16 Term for a stone formed within an organ
18 Term meaning pus in the urine
19 The U in UTI

13

Obstetrics and Gynecology
Female Reproductive System

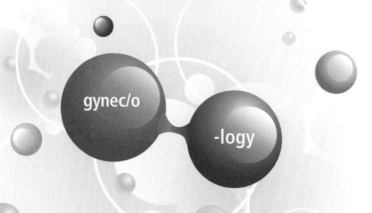

gynec/o

-logy

A Brief Introduction to Obstetrics and Gynecology

 UNDERSTAND the function of the female reproductive system.

The female reproductive system is vital to the continuation of the human race. **Ovaries** begin the process by producing egg cells called **ova** (singular is *ovum*). **Fertilization,** the joining of ovum and sperm, typically occurs in the **fallopian** (or **uterine**) **tubes.** The fertilized ovum then implants in the lining of the **uterus** where the new embryo develops. During birth, the baby passes through the **vagina** as it enters the world. The newborn is then nourished by milk made by the mother's **breasts.** In addition, the ovaries secrete the female sex hormones **estrogen** and **progesterone,** which regulate the reproductive cycle and produce the female secondary sexual characteristics.

 DESCRIBE the medical specialties of obstetrics and gynecology.

Gynecology is the branch of medicine that diagnoses and treats conditions of the female reproductive organs as well as provides general medical care for women. **Obstetrics** specializes in pregnancy and childbirth. Most physicians in this field train as both **gynecologists** and **obstetricians** at the same time. However, they can choose to further specialize in only one of the two areas.

Obstetrics and Gynecology Combining Forms

The following list presents new combining forms important for building and defining obstetrics and gynecology terms.

amni/o	amnion		mast/o	breast
cervic/o	neck, cervix		men/o	menses, menstruation
chori/o	chorion		metr/o	uterus
colp/o	vagina		nat/o	birth
embry/o	embryo		o/o	egg
episi/o	vulva		oophor/o	ovary
fet/o	fetus		ovari/o	ovary
gynec/o	woman, female		salping/o	fallopian tubes, uterine tubes
hyster/o	uterus		uter/o	uterus
lapar/o	abdomen		vagin/o	vagina
mamm/o	breast			

The following list presents combining forms that are not specific to the female reproductive system but are also used for building and defining obstetrics and gynecology terms.

carcin/o	cancer		olig/o	scanty
cyst/o	bladder		pelv/o	pelvis
fibr/o	fibrous		rect/o	rectum
hem/o	blood			

Suffix Review

These suffixes and prefixes were introduced in Chapters 2 and 3. They are being reviewed in this chapter because they are especially important for building obstetrics and gynecology terms.

-al	pertaining to		-lytic	destruction
-algia	pain		-metry	process of measuring
-an	pertaining to		-nic	pertaining to
-ary	pertaining to		-oid	resembling
-cele	protrusion		-oma	tumor
-centesis	puncture to withdraw fluid		-osis	abnormal condition
-cyesis	pregnancy		-otomy	cutting into
-cyte	cell		-para	to bear (offspring)
-ectomy	surgical removal		-partum	childbirth
-genesis	generates		-pexy	surgical fixation
-genic	producing		-plasty	surgical repair
-gram	record		-rrhagia	bursting forth
-graphy	process of recording		-rrhaphy	suture
-gravida	pregnancy		-rrhea	flow
-ic	pertaining to		-rrhexis	rupture
-ine	pertaining to		-scope	instrument for view
-itis	inflammation		-scopy	process of viewing
-logist	one who studies		-tic	pertaining to
-logy	study of			

Prefix Review

a-	without		multi-	many
ante-	before		neo-	new
dys-	painful		post-	after
endo-	inner		pre-	before
intra-	inside		primi-	first
nulli-	none		trans-	across

 IDENTIFY the organs treated in obstetrics and gynecology.

Organs Commonly Treated in Obstetrics and Gynecology

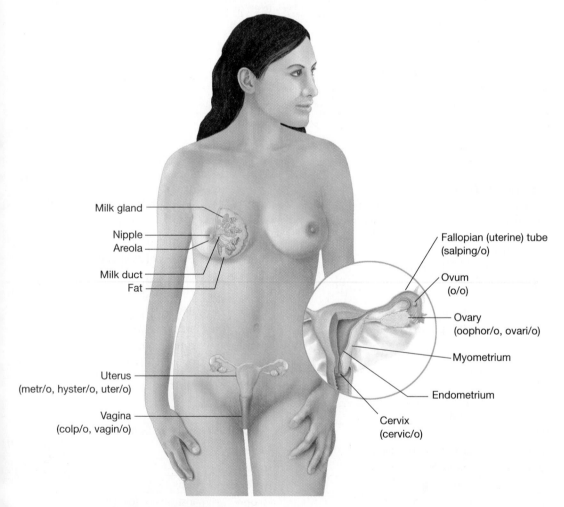

>13.1 Female reproductive system, anterior view

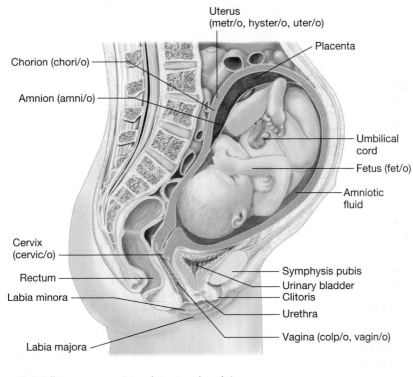

Uterus
(metr/o, hyster/o, uter/o)

Placenta

Chorion (chori/o)

Amnion (amni/o)

Umbilical cord

Fetus (fet/o)

Amniotic fluid

Cervix (cervic/o)

Rectum

Labia minora

Symphysis pubis

Urinary bladder

Clitoris

Urethra

Vagina (colp/o, vagin/o)

Labia majora

>13.2 Full-term pregnancy, internal structures, lateral view

 BUILD obstetrics and gynecology medical terms from word parts.

Building Obstetrics and Gynecology Terms

This section presents word parts most often used to build obstetrics and gynecology terms. Following the explanation of the term, you have the opportunity to begin building your own vocabulary. Read the meaning for each term and then fill in the blanks to build a single medical term. Use the slashes to divide prefixes, word roots, combining vowels, and suffixes. To help you out you will find a key to the word parts underneath the blanks: r for word roots, p for prefix, cv for combining vowel, and s for suffix. Remember that not every term will contain all these word parts; it's up to you to decide which to use. As you gain experience, this process becomes easier. Answers can be found at the back of the book.

1. **amni/o**–combining form meaning **amnion**

    The amnion is the inner sac surrounding fetus; contains **amniotic fluid** in which fetus floats

    a. pertaining to amnion

    _____/____/_____
    r   cv   s

    b. cutting into amnion

    _____/_____
    r   s

    c. flow of amniotic (fluid)

    _____/____/_____
    r   cv   s

    d. puncture of amnion to withdraw fluid

    _____/____/_____
    r   cv   s

    e. rupture of amnion

    _____/____/_____
    r   cv   s

2. **cervic/o**–combining form meaning **cervix**

   The cervix is the narrow, lower portion of uterus; opens into vagina; also called *neck of the uterus*

   a. pertaining to cervix   _____/_____
                                                r   *s*

   b. surgical removal of cervix   _____/_____
                                                r   *s*

   c. cervix inflammation   _____/_____
                                              r   *s*

   d. inflammation within cervix   _____/_____/_____
                                  p   *r*   *s*

   e. surgical repair of cervix   _____/____/_____
                                          r   *cv*   *s*

3. **chori/o**–combining form meaning **chorion**

   The chorion is the outer sac surrounding and protecting fetus; forms part of **placenta**

   a. pertaining to chorion   _____/____/_____
                                      r   *cv*   *s*

   b. cancerous tumor of chorion   _____/____/_____/_____
                                 r   *cv*   *r*   *s*

4. **colp/o**–combining form meaning **vagina**

   The vagina is the muscular tube extending from cervix to outside of body; receives penis and semen during intercourse; also called *birth canal*

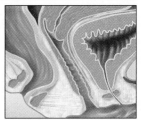

   >13.3 Vagina

   a. instrument to visually examine vagina   _____/____/_____
                                      r   *cv*   *s*

   b. process of visually examining vagina   _____/____/_____
                                      r   *cv*   *s*

   c. surgical removal of vagina   _____/_____
                                          r   *s*

   d. suture the vagina   _____/____/_____
                                      r   *cv*   *s*

5. **embry/o**–combining form meaning **embryo**

   The embryo is an early stage of human development from time of fertilization until approximately end of second month of pregnancy

   a. pertaining to embryo   _____/____/_____
                                      r   *cv*   *s*

   b. producing an embryo   _____/____/_____
                                      r   *cv*   *s*

   c. study of embryo   _____/____/_____
                                      r   *cv*   *s*

6. **episi/o**–combining form meaning **vulva**

   Vulva is a general term for all female external genitalia including **labia majora, labia minora, and clitoris**

   a. suture vulva

   _____/_____/_____
   r   cv   s

   b. surgical repair of vulva

   _____/_____/_____
   r   cv   s

   c. cutting into vulva

   _____/_____
   r   s

7. **fet/o**–combining form meaning **fetus**

   The fetus is a later stage of human development from approximately beginning of third month to birth

   >13.4 Photograph showing fetus in the uterus

   a. pertaining to fetus

   _____/_____
   r   s

   b. process of measuring fetus

   _____/_____/_____
   r   cv   s

   c. instrument for visually examining fetus

   _____/_____/_____
   r   cv   s

   d. process of visually examining fetus

   _____/_____/_____
   r   cv   s

8. **-gravida**–suffix meaning **pregnancy**

   Gestation is length of time of a pregnancy; normal gestation for humans is 40 weeks

   a. no pregnancies

   _____/_____
   p   s

   b. first pregnancy

   _____/_____
   p   s

   c. many pregnancies

   _____/_____
   p   s

9. **gynec/o**–combining form meaning **female**

   a. study of female

   _____/_____/_____
   r   cv   s

   b. one who studies female

   _____/_____/_____
   r   cv   s

10. **hyster/o**–combining form meaning **uterus**

The uterus is the hollow pear-shaped organ in lower pelvic cavity between urinary bladder and rectum; **fundus** is upper portion between where fallopian tubes enter; **body** of uterus is largest central region; **cervix** is narrow lowest region that opens into vagina; **endometrium** is inner lining that thickens during the month and is sloughed off during **menstrual period; myometrium** is thick muscular wall which contracts to push fetus through birth canal

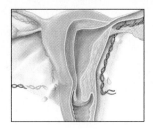

>13.5 **Uterus**

a. surgical fixation of uterus

_____/____/_____
　　　　r　　　　cv　　　s

b. ruptured uterus

_____/____/_____
　　　　r　　　　cv　　　s

c. surgical removal of uterus

_____/_____
　　　　r　　　　　　s

d. process of recording uterus

_____/____/_____
　　　　r　　　　cv　　　s

e. record of uterus

_____/____/_____
　　　　r　　　　cv　　　s

11. **lapar/o**–combining form meaning **abdomen**

a. cutting into abdomen

_____/_____
　　　　r　　　　　　s

b. instrument for visually examining abdomen

_____/____/_____
　　　　r　　　　cv　　　s

c. process of visually examining abdomen

_____/____/_____
　　　　r　　　　cv　　　s

12. **mamm/o**–combining form meaning **breast**

The breast is a collection of glands to produce milk to nourish infant

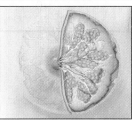

>13.6 **Breast**

a. pertaining to breast

_____/_____
　　　　r　　　　　　s

b. record of breast

_____/____/_____
　　　　r　　　　cv　　　s

c. process of recording breast

_____/____/_____
　　　　r　　　　cv　　　s

d. surgical repair of breast

_____/____/_____
　　　　r　　　　cv　　　s

13. mast/o–combining form meaning **breast**

    a. breast pain

                            _____/_____
                                  r   *s*

    b. breast inflammation

                            _____/_____
                                  r   *s*

    c. surgical removal of breast

                            _____/_____
                                  r   *s*

---

14. men/o–combining form meaning **menstruation**

Menstruation is the period of time during the monthly period when endometrial lining of uterus is shed; appears as bloody flow through cervix and vagina

    a. without menstrual flow

          _____/_____/____/_____
               p   *r*   *CV*   *s*

    b. painful menstrual flow

          _____/_____/____/_____
               p   *r*   *CV*   *s*

    c. scanty menstrual flow

          _____/____/_____/____/____
              r   *CV*   *r*   *CV*   *s*

    d. menstruation bursting forth

          _____/____/_____
                  r   *CV*   *s*

---

15. metr/o–combining form meaning **uterus**

    a. inner uterus inflammation

          _____/_____/_____
                   p   *r*   *s*

    b. flow from uterus

          _____/____/_____
                  r   *CV*   *s*

    c. bursting forth from uterus

          _____/____/_____
                  r   *CV*   *s*

---

16. nat/o–combining form meaning **birth**

    a. pertaining to birth

          _____/_____
                  r   *s*

    b. pertaining to a newborn

          _____/_____/_____
                   p   *r*   *s*

    c. study of newborn

          _____/_____/____/_____
                p   *r*   *CV*   *s*

    d. one who studies newborn

          _____/_____/____/_____
                p   *r*   *CV*   *s*

---

17. o/o–combining form meaning **egg**

The ovum is the egg cell that carries the mother's half of chromosomes; combines with sperm to form new human

    a. egg cell

          _____/____/_____
                  r   *CV*   *s*

    b. produces an egg

          _____/____/_____
                  r   *CV*   *s*

---

18. oophor/o–combining form meaning **ovary**

The ovaries are almond-shaped pair of organs located on each side of uterus; connected to uterus by fallopian (or uterine) tube; produce ova; release of ovum from ovary is called **ovulation;** secrete female hormones, estrogen, and progesterone

>13.7 Ovary

a. ovary inflammation

_____/_____
r   s

b. surgical removal of ovary

_____/_____
r   s

c. surgical fixation of ovary

_____/____/_____
r   CV   s

---

19. ovari/o–combining form meaning **ovary**

a. pertaining to ovary

_____/_____
r   s

b. ovary and fallopian tube inflammation

_____/____/_____/____
r   CV   r   s

---

20. -para–suffix meaning **to bear (birth)**

This suffix refers to the number of times a pregnancy has successfully ended with birth of infant

a. no births

_____/_____
p   s

b. first birth

_____/_____
p   s

c. many births

_____/_____
p   s

---

21. -partum–suffix meaning **childbirth**

a. before childbirth

_____/_____
p   s

b. after childbirth

_____/_____
p   s

---

22. salping/o–combining form meaning **fallopian (or uterine) tube**

The fallopian tubes are narrow tubes that run from the area around each ovary to upper uterus; ova travels from ovary to uterus through fallopian tube; normal location for **fertilization;** also called **uterine tube**

>13.8 Fallopian tube

a. surgical removal of fallopian tube

_____/_____
r   s

b. fallopian tube inflammation

_____/_____
r   s

c. process of recording fallopian tube

_____/____/_____
r   CV   s

d. record of fallopian tube

_____/____/_____
r   CV   s

e. pregnancy in fallopian tube

_____/____/_____
r   CV   s

23. uter/o–combining form meaning **uterus**

a. pertaining to uterus

_____/_____
r   s

b. surgical repair of uterus

_____/____/_____
r   cv   s

c. instrument for visually examining uterus

_____/____/_____
r   cv   s

d. process of visually examining uterus

_____/____/_____
r   cv   s

e. pertaining to inside uterus

_____/_____/_____
p   r   s

24. vagin/o–combining form meaning **vagina**

a. pertaining to vagina

_____/_____
r   s

b. vagina inflammation

_____/_____
r   s

c. pertaining to across vagina

_____/_____/_____
p   r   s

EXPLAIN obstetrics and gynecology medical terms.

Obstetrics and Gynecology Vocabulary

The obstetrics and gynecology terms presented in this section include eponyms, modern English words, and those that contain Latin or Greek word parts but are not constructed solely from these word parts. When you recognize word parts within a term they will give you a hint about the word's meaning. In these instances, look for the word parts to follow the term.

Term	Explanation
abortion (AB)	Discharge of embryo from uterus before about 20th week of gestation; *spontaneous abortion* (miscarriage) is unplanned and due to death of embryo; *elective abortion* is legal termination of pregnancy; *therapeutic abortion* is necessary for mother's health
abruptio placentae	Emergency condition occurring when placenta tears away from uterine wall prior to birth of fetus; requires baby's immediate birth

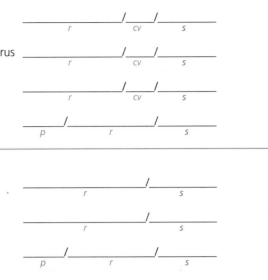

+ TERMINOLOGY TIDBIT

The term *abruptio* comes from the Latin word *abruptus* meaning "to break off." The term *placenta* comes from the Greek word *plakous* meaning "flat cake." This word was used to describe the appearance of the placenta.

>13.9 Illustration showing the premature separation of the placenta in abruptio placentae

Term	Explanation
atresia **a-** = without	Lack of normal body opening; for example, *hysteratresia* is closing of cervix, usually from scarring

Term	Explanation
breast cancer	Malignant tumor of breast; usually forms in milk glands or lining of milk ducts

Tumor

Lactiferous glands

>13.10 Breast with a malignant tumor growing in the milk gland and duct

Term	Explanation
cervical cancer **cervic/o** = cervix **-al** = pertaining to	Malignant tumor of cervix; some cases caused by *human papilloma virus* (HPV), sexually transmitted virus for which there is now vaccine; regular Pap smear used for early detection
cesarean section (CS, C-section)	Surgical birth of baby through incision into abdominal and uterine walls; named for Roman emperor, Julius Caesar, who is said to have been the first person born using this method

>13.11 The head of a fetus emerges from the uterus during a cesarean section

Term	Explanation
chorionic villus sampling (CVS) **chori/o** = chorion **-nic** = pertaining to	Removal of small piece of chorion for genetic analysis; can be done at earlier stage of pregnancy than amniocentesis
conization	Surgical removal of a core of cervical tissue for biopsy
cystocele **cyst/o** = bladder **-cele** = protrusion	Hernia or outpouching of bladder protrudes into vagina; can cause urinary frequency and urgency and block vagina

dilation and curettage (D&C)

Surgical procedure consisting of widening cervix and scraping or suctioning out endometrial lining of uterus; often performed after spontaneous abortion or to stop excessive bleeding from other causes

> **+ TERMINOLOGY TIDBIT**
>
> The term *curettage* comes from the French word *curer* meaning "to cleanse."

---

ectopic pregnancy
 -ic = pertaining to

Pregnancy occurring outside of uterus, usually in fallopian tubes; growing fetus will rupture fallopian tube requiring a salpingectomy

> **+ TERMINOLOGY TIDBIT**
>
> The term *ectopic* comes from the Greek word *ektopos* meaning "out of place."

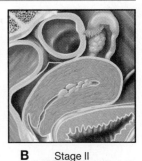

Interstitial
pregnancy

Ovarian
pregnancy

>13.12 Illustration of common sites for ectopic pregnancy

---

endometriosis
 endo- = inner
 metr/o = uterus
 -osis = abnormal condition

Occurs when endometrial tissue appears throughout pelvic or abdominal cavity; causes recurring pain and scarring

---

endometrial cancer
 endo- = inner
 metr/o = uterus
 -al = pertaining to

Cancerous tumor forms in lining of uterus

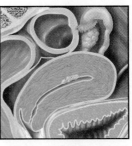

A   Stage I

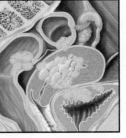

B   Stage II

>13.13 Illustration showing the stages of endometrial cancer
(A) Stage I-localized tumor forms in endometrial tissue. (B) Stage II-tumor grows larger within the uterus. (C) Stage III-tumor spreads to nearby organs. (D) Stage IV-cancerous tumors appear throughout the body

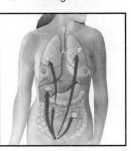

C   Stage III

D   Stage IV

Term	Explanation

fetal monitoring
fet/o = fetus
-al = pertaining to

Use of electronic equipment placed on mother's abdomen or fetus' scalp to check fetal heart rate (FHR) and fetal heart tone (FHT) during labor; normal FHR ranges from 120 to 160 beats per minute; drop in fetal heart rate indicates fetal distress

---

fibrocystic breast disease
fibr/o = fibrous
cyst/o = bladder
[not urinary in this case]
-ic = pertaining to

Benign cysts in breast tissue; not precancerous

Adipose
Cysts
Lactiferous glands

>13.14 Illustration showing the location of a fibrocystic lump in the adipose tissue of the breast

---

fibroid tumor
fibr/o = fibrous
-oid = resembling

Benign tumor of fiberlike tissue; the most common type of tumor in women

Under the perimetrium
Within the myometrium
Under the endometrium

>13.15 Common sites for the development of fibroid tumors

---

fistula

Abnormal passageway that develops between two structures; *vesicovaginal fistula* is between urinary bladder and vagina; *rectovaginal fistula* is between rectum and vagina

+ TERMINOLOGY TIDBIT

The term *fistula* comes directly from the Latin word *fistula* meaning "a pipe."

---

hemolytic disease of the newborn (HDN)
hem/o = blood
-lytic = destruction

Condition developing in fetus when mother's blood type is Rh-negative and baby's blood is Rh-positive; antibodies in mother's blood enter fetus' bloodstream through placenta and destroy fetus' red blood cells; causes anemia, jaundice, and enlargement of spleen; treated with intrauterine blood transfusion; also called *erythroblastosis fetalis*

---

in vitro **fertilization (IVF)**

Infertility treatment; ova are removed from woman and fertilized by sperm externally; resulting embryos are returned to uterus for development; commonly called *test tube baby*

---

infertility

Inability to produce children; generally defined as no pregnancy after properly timed intercourse for one year

---

ovarian cancer
ovari/o = ovary
-an = pertaining to

Cancerous tumor formed within ovary

Papanicolaou (Pap) smear

Test for early detection of cervical cancer; named after developer, George Papanicolaou, a Greek physician; cells are removed from cervix by simple scraping and examined under microscope

pelvic inflammatory disease (PID)
pelv/o = pelvis
-ic = pertaining to

Chronic or acute infection, usually bacterial, that ascends through female reproductive tract and out into pelvic cavity; can result in scarring that interferes with fertility

placenta previa

Placenta forms in lower portion of uterus and blocks birth canal; can require C-section for birth

Umbilical cord

Fetus

>13.16 Illustration of placenta previa showing the placenta growing over the opening of the cervix

Placenta
Severe bleeding

premature birth
pre- = before

Birth of fetus before 37 weeks of gestation

>13.17 A premature infant
Source: Courtesy of Lisa Smith-Pedersen, RN, MSN, NNP-BC./Pearson Education

premenstrual syndrome (PMS)
pre- = before

Symptoms that develop just prior to onset of menstrual period; can include irritability, headache, tender breasts, and anxiety

prolapsed uterus

Fallen uterus that can cause cervix to protrude through vaginal opening

+ TERMINOLOGY TIDBIT

The term *prolapse* comes from the Latin word *prolapsus* meaning "falling."

Prolapsed uterus

Severely prolapse uterusd

>13.18 Illustration of (A) mild and (B) severe prolapsed uterus **A**

B

Term	Explanation
rectocele rect/o = rectum -cele = protrusion	Protrusion or herniation of rectum into vagina
stillbirth (SB)	Birth in which viable-age fetus dies shortly before or at time of birth
tubal ligation -al = pertaining to	Surgical tying off of fallopian tubes to prevent pregnancy

Forceps

Operating laparoscope

Uterine cannula

Sterilization

>13.19 Ilustration show laparoscope being used to perform a tubal ligation

USE obstetrics and gynecology abbreviations.

Obstetrics and Gynecology Abbreviations

The following list presents common obstetrics and gynecology abbreviations.

AB	abortion	**HPV**	human papilloma virus
BSE	breast self-examination	**HRT**	hormone replacement therapy
CS, C-section	cesarean section	**HSG**	hysterosalpingography
CVS	chorionic villus sampling	**IUD**	intrauterine device
Cx	cervix	**IVF**	*in vitro* fertilization
D&C	dilation and curettage	**LMP**	last menstrual period
EMB	endometrial biopsy	**NB**	newborn
ERT	estrogen replacement therapy	**OB**	obstetrics
FHR	fetal heart rate	**OCPs**	oral contraceptive pills
FHT	fetal heart tone	**PAP**	Papanicolaou test
FTND	full-term normal delivery	**PI, para I**	first birth
GI, grav I	first pregnancy	**PID**	pelvic inflammatory disease
GYN, gyn	gynecology	**PMS**	premenstrual syndrome
HDN	hemolytic disease of the newborn	**SB**	stillbirth
		TAH-BSO	total abdominal hysterectomy–bilateral salpingo-oophorectomy

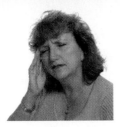

History of Present Illness
The patient is a 52-year-old female who reports postmenopausal vaginal bleeding for the past 2 months. She states that her last known menstrual period was 3 years ago. She also reports mild to moderate uterine cramps, lower abdominal pain, and painful intercourse.

Past Medical History
Patient reports having migraine headaches about once every 3 months, asthma since her mid-20s, and hyperlipemia. She is grav2 para2. Patient currently uses pain medication prn for headaches and a bronchodilator to relieve asthma symptoms. She is not treating hyperlipemia.

Family and Social History
Patient is divorced. Her two living children are well.

Physical Examination
Patient appears her stated age and is in no distress. She is obese. Pelvic examination revealed normal appearing cervix and vagina. A small amount of bright red blood was apparent, but no likely source of bleeding was identified.

Diagnostic Tests
An Hg and HCT revealed anemia. Pap smear was negative. Pelvic ultrasound revealed no uterine fibroids or pelvic masses. A D&C was conducted and pathologist reports no abnormal findings. Finally, hysteroscopy was performed. During course of this procedure, a single small area of active bleeding was identified within the uterine cavity and EMB was completed. Results indicated endometrial cancer.

Diagnosis
Endometrial cancer, stage unknown

Plan of Treatment
1. Schedule patient for total abdominal hysterectomy with lymphadenectomy to stage the cancer
2. Begin iron supplement for anemia, can require transfusion prior to surgery
3. MRI to look for metastases
4. Referral to oncologist for evaluation for possible radiation therapy, hormone therapy, or chemotherapy

Critical Thinking Questions
Answer the following questions regarding this case study. Do not just copy words out of the case study; translate all medical terms. In order to answer some of these questions, you may need to look up information from another chapter of this text, in a medical dictionary, or online. Answers are found at the back of the book.

1. From the patient's history of present illness, explain why it was surprising and troublesome that she was experiencing vaginal bleeding. What are her additional symptoms?

   _____

   _____

2. Interpret the following abbreviations used in this case study: prn, grav2, para2, D&C, EMB.

   _____

   _____

(continued)

(continued)

3. List this patient's three previous medical conditions and the treatment she is using for each.

4. What is a Pap smear used to diagnose? Why was it not surprising that it was negative?

5. What are an Hbg and HCT? What is a possible explanation for why this patient is anemic?

6. Go to the following website, www.oncologychannel.com, click on "Endometrial cancer" and then "Staging." Describe the four main stages, I-IV (ignore the substages such as IA and IB), for endometrial cancer. If cancer cells are found in this patient's lymph nodes, what stage will her cancer be?

7. Carefully read the results of the D&C and hysteroscopy. Suggest why it might be possible that the D&C missed the cancer cells but the hysteroscopy found them.

8. What does lymphadenectomy mean and why is it helpful for determining this patient's diagnosis and treatment?

Sound It Out

The following are some of the key terms from this chapter written as their phonetic spelling. Sound out each term and write it in the blank. Pronunciations for all terms are included in the audio glossary at www.mymedicalterminologylab.com <http://www.mymedicalterminologylab.com/>.

1. ah-men-oh-REE-ah _____

2. am-nee-oh-sen-TEE-sis _____

3. AM-nee-on _____

4. ah-TREE-she-ah _____

5. SER-vih-koh-plas-tee _____

6. SER-viks _____

7. KOH-ree-oh-car-sih-no-mah _____

8. KOR-ree-on _____

9. kol-poe-RAH-fee _____

10. kol-POSS-koh-pee _____

11. kon-ih-ZAY-shun _____

12. SIS-toh-seel _____

13. dis-men-oh-REE-ah _____

14. EM-bree-oh _____

15. en-doh-ser-vih-SIGH-tis _____

16. en-doh-mee-tree-OH-sis _____

17. eh-peez-ee-OT-oh-mee _____

18. fee-TOM-eh-tree _____

19. FEE-tus _____

20. FIS-tyoo-lah _____

21. gigh-neh-KOL-oh-jee _____

22. hiss-ter-EK-toh-me _____

23. hiss-ter-OG-rah-fee _____

24. IN-tra-YOU-ter-in _____

25. lap-ar-OSS-koh-pee _____

26. lap-ah-ROT-oh-mee _____

27. MAM-moh-gram _____

28. mass-TEK-toh-mee _____

29. mas-TYE-tis _____

30. men-oh-RAY-jee-ah _____

31. mull-TIP-ah-rah _____

32. NEE-oh-NAY-tall _____

33. null-ih-GRAV-ih-dah _____

34. ob-STET-riks _____

35. ol-lih-goh-men-oh-REE-ah _____

36. oh-off-oh-REK-toh-mee _____

37. OH-vah-reez _____

38. oh-VAIR-ee-oh-sal-pin-JIH-tis _____

39. OH-vum _____

40. plah-SEN-tah _____

41. post-PAR-tum _____

42. prem-ih-GRAV-ih-dah _____

43. RECK-toh-seal _____

44. sal-ping-go-sigh-EE-sis _____

45. tranz-VAJ-ih-nal _____

46. YOU-ter-oh-plas-tee _____

47. YOU-ter-us _____

48. vah-JIGH-nah _____

49. vaj-ih-NIGH-tis _____

50. VULL-vah _____

Transcription Practice

Each of the following sentences is written in common English. Underline any words or phrases that can be replaced by a medical term. Then rewrite the entire sentence using medical terms. Answers are found at the end of the book.

1. Mrs. Scott's painful menstrual flow was treated with a surgical procedure to widen the cervix and scrape the endometrial lining.

   _____

   _____

2. Over time Mrs. Martinez had developed an abnormal passageway between her bladder and vagina.

   _____

   _____

3. The one who studies newborns assisted with the birth through an incision in the abdominal and uterine walls.

   _____

   _____

4. Jean's inability to produce children after properly timed intercourse for one year was the result of scarring caused by chronic bacterial infections ascending through the female reproductive tract.

   _____

   _____

5. A surgical removal of the uterus became necessary due to extensive endometrial tissue appearing outside the uterus in the pelvic cavity.

   _____

   _____

6. The new patient at the gynecologist's office was in her first pregnancy and had no births.

   _____

   _____

7. Maria was happy to find out she had a benign breast tumor of fiberlike tissue, not a malignant tumor of the milk glands of the breast.

   _____

   _____

8. A surgical removal of a fallopian tube was necessary following the discovery of a pregnancy occurring outside of the uterus in the fallopian tubes.

   _____

   _____

9. Following abnormal test results in which cells were removed from the cervix by scraping, Tawanda's malignant tumor of the cervix was diagnosed by removal of a core of cervical tissue for biopsy.

_____

_____

10. A process of viewing the abdomen was conducted to examine the patient for a cancerous tumor forming within the ovary.

_____

_____

Build Medical Terms

Use each of the following word parts to build the indicated medical terms.

The combining form *hyster/o* means uterus.

1. uterus surgical fixation _____

2. uterus surgical removal _____

3. uterus ruptured _____

4. uterus record _____

The combining form *fet/o* means fetus.

5. pertaining to fetus _____

6. fetus process of measuring _____

The suffix *-partum* means childbirth.

7. before childbirth _____

8. after childbirth _____

The combining form *men/o* means menstruation.

9. without menstrual flow _____

10. painful menstrual flow _____

11. scanty menstrual flow _____

12. menstruation bursting forth _____

The combining form *mast/o* means breast.

13. breast pain _____

14. breast inflammation _____

15. breast surgical removal _____

Spelling

Some of the following terms are misspelled. Identify the incorrect terms and spell them correctly in the blank provided.

1. histerectomy _____

2. laparoscopy _____

3. mammary _____

4. oogenesis _____

5. premenstral _____

6. antipartum _____

7. menorhagia _____

8. ovariosalpingitis _____

9. anmiotomy _____

10. endometriosis _____

Fill in the Blank

Fill in the blank to complete each of the following sentences.

1. Fertilization typically occurs in the _____ (or _____) tubes.

2. _____ is the branch of medicine that treats conditions of the female reproductive

    tract, and _____ is the branch that specializes in pregnancy.

3. The inner lining of the uterus is called the _____, and the muscular
    layer of the uterus is called the _____.

4. _____ is the removal of a small piece of chorion for genetic analysis.

5. Fetal monitoring uses equipment to check the _____ and
    _____.

6. Erythroblastosis fetalis is another name for _____.

7. An abnormal passageway that develops between two structures is called a(n) _____.

8. Tying off the fallopian tubes to prevent pregnancy is called _____.

9. A prolapsed uterus can cause the _____ to protrude through the vaginal opening.

10. A(n) _____ occurs when the fetus dies shortly before time of birth.

Labeling Exercise

Write the name of each structure on the numbered line. Also use this space to write the combining form where appropriate.

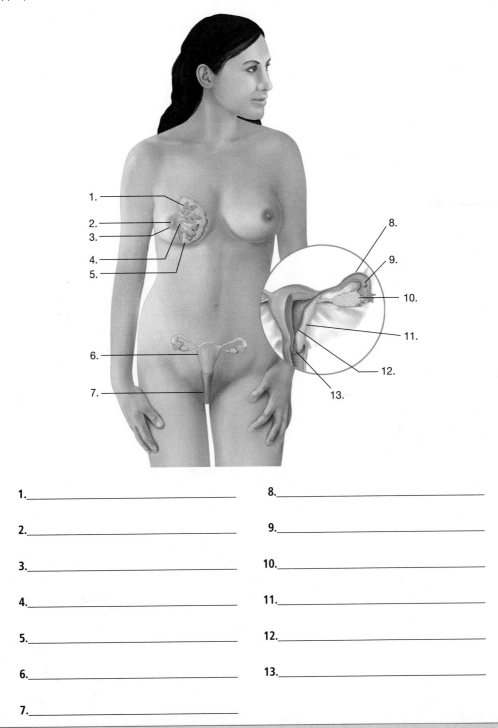

1._____

2._____

3._____

4._____

5._____

6._____

7._____

8._____

9._____

10._____

11._____

12._____

13._____

Medical Term Analysis

*Examine each of the following terms. Begin by dividing it into its word parts and writing them in the indicated blanks (**P = prefix, WR = word root; CF = combining form; S = suffix**). Follow with the definition of each word part and then finally the meaning of the full term.*

1. **oophoropexy**

   CF _____

   means _____

   S _____

   means _____

   Term Meaning: _____

   _____

2. **colposcope**

   CF _____

   means _____

   S _____

   means _____

   Term Meaning: _____

   _____

3. **choriocarcinoma**

   CF _____

   means _____

   WR _____

   means _____

   S _____

   means _____

   Term Meaning: _____

   _____

4. **intrauterine**

   P _____

   means _____

   WR _____

   means _____

   S _____

   means _____

   Term Meaning: _____

   _____

5. **transvaginal**

   P _____

   means _____

   WR _____

   means _____

   S _____

   means _____

   Term Meaning: _____

   _____

6. **embryonic**

   CF _____

   means _____

   S _____

   means _____

   Term Meaning: _____

   _____

7. oocyte

CF _____

means _____

S _____

means _____

Term Meaning: _____

_____

8. cervicoplasty

CF _____

means _____

S _____

means _____

Term Meaning: _____

_____

9. ovariosalpingitis

CF _____

means _____

WR _____

means _____

S _____

means _____

Term Meaning: _____

_____

10. episiotomy

WR _____

means _____

S _____

means _____

Term Meaning: _____

_____

Abbreviation Matching

Match each abbreviation with its definition.

_____	**1.** NB	**A.**	hysterosalpingography
_____	**2.** Cx	**B.**	*in vitro* fertilization
_____	**3.** FHR	**C.**	cervix
_____	**4.** HSG	**D.**	estrogen replacement therapy
_____	**5.** HPV	**E.**	premenstrual syndrome
_____	**6.** IVF	**F.**	newborn
_____	**7.** grav I	**G.**	abortion
_____	**8.** ERT	**H.**	human papilloma virus
_____	**9.** AB	**I.**	fetal heart rate
_____	**10.** PMS	**J.**	first pregnancy

Photomatch Challenge

Match each procedure with its name in the Word Bank.

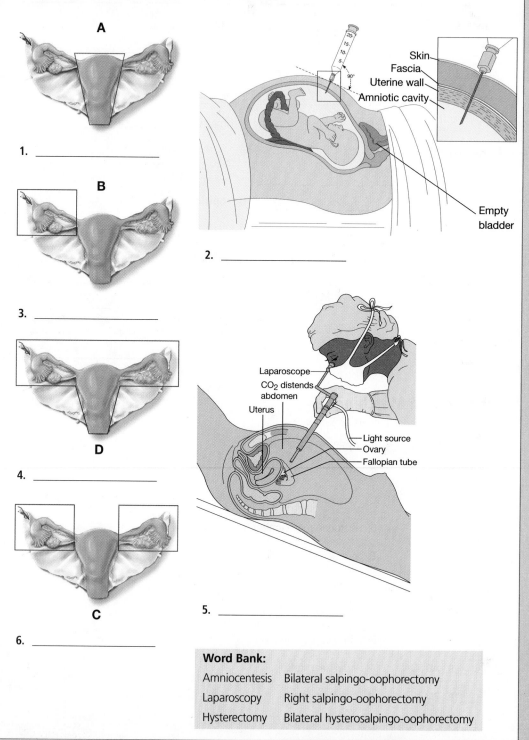

A

1. _____

B

Skin
Fascia
Uterine wall
Amniotic cavity

Empty bladder

2. _____

3. _____

Laparoscope
CO$_2$ distends abdomen
Uterus

Light source
Ovary
Fallopian tube

D

4. _____

C

5. _____

6. _____

Word Bank:

Amniocentesis	Bilateral salpingo-oophorectomy
Laparoscopy	Right salpingo-oophorectomy
Hysterectomy	Bilateral hysterosalpingo-oophorectomy

Crossword Puzzle

Use the definitions given to complete the crossword puzzle.

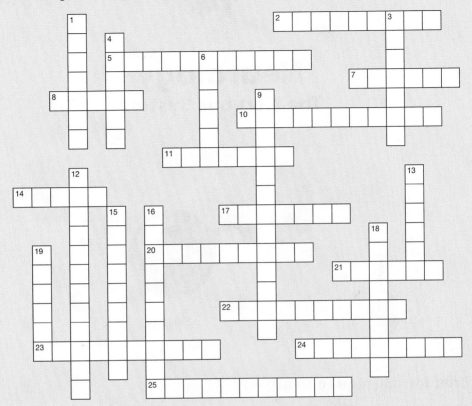

ACROSS

2 Term meaning first birth
5 Inner lining of the uterus
7 Glands to produce milk are found in the

    _____

8 Term meaning external genitalia
10 Inability to produce children
11 Outer sac around the fetus
14 Later stage of human development, beginning at third month
17 Pregnancy occurring outside of uterus
20 Release of ovum from ovary
21 Organ also called birth canal
22 The suffix -partum means _____
23 Fetus dies shortly before or at time of birth
24 Herniation of rectum into vagina
25 Another term for spontaneous abortion

DOWN

1 Abnormal passageway
3 Lack of a normal body opening
4 Narrow region of uterus, opens into vagina
6 Early stage of human development, ends at second month
9 Endometrial tissue appears throughout pelvic cavity
12 Term meaning no pregnancies
13 Inner sac around the fetus
15 Hernia of bladder into vagina
16 Muscular wall of uterus
18 Surgical tying off of fallopian tube
19 Upper portion of the uterus

14

Neurology
The Nervous System

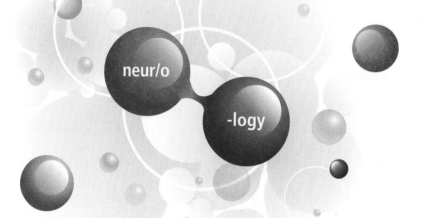

neur/o

-logy

A Brief Introduction to Neurology

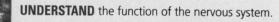

 UNDERSTAND the function of the nervous system.

The nervous system consists of the **brain, spinal cord,** and **nerves** and is responsible for coordinating all of the body's activity. This task involves receiving information from **sensory receptors** and then using that information to adjust the activity of **muscles** and **glands** to match the body's needs. The nervous system is divided into the **central nervous system (CNS)** and the **peripheral nervous system (PNS).** The CNS consists of the brain and spinal cord; the PNS comprises all of the nerves carrying electrical impulses between the CNS and all of the body's organs.

The structures of the nervous system are composed of **neurons.** These cells conduct the electrical impulses necessary to carry information between the CNS and body. The point at which one neuron meets another is called a **synapse.** Electrical impulses cannot pass directly across the gap between two neurons, called the **synaptic cleft.** They instead require the help of a chemical messenger, called a **neurotransmitter.** Many neurons are covered by **myelin,** an insulating substance that helps neurons conduct their electrical impulses faster.

DESCRIBE the medical specialty of neurology.

Neurology is the branch of medicine that specializes in the diagnosis and treatment of conditions affecting the nervous system including the brain, spinal cord, and nerves. A **neurologist** can also treat muscle conditions that are caused by nervous system problems. Another specialty, **neurosurgery,** includes surgical procedures in treating nervous system conditions.

Neurology Combining Forms

The following list presents new combining forms important for building and defining neurology terms.

cerebell/o	cerebellum		myel/o	spinal cord
cerebr/o	cerebrum		neur/o	nerve
encephal/o	brain		pont/o	pons
medull/o	medulla oblongata		thalam/o	thalamus
mening/o	meninges			

The following list presents combining forms that are not specific to the nervous system but are also used for building and defining neurology terms.

cephal/o	head		my/o	muscle
electr/o	electricity		scler/o	hardening
hemat/o	blood		spin/o	spine
hydr/o	water		vascul/o	blood vessels
lumb/o	low back			

Suffix Review

These suffixes and prefixes were introduced in Chapters 2 and 3. They are being reviewed in this chapter because they are especially important for building neurology terms.

-al	pertaining to		-logist	one who studies
-algia	pain		-logy	study of
-ar	pertaining to		-malacia	softening
-ary	pertaining to		-oma	tumor
-asthenia	weakness		-osis	abnormal condition
-cele	hernia, protrusion		-otomy	cutting into
-eal	pertaining to		-pathy	disease
-ectomy	surgical removal		-phasia	speech
-esthesia	feeling, sensation		-plasty	surgical repair
-gram	record		-plegia	paralysis
-graphy	process of recording		-rrhaphy	suture
-ic	pertaining to		-sclerosis	hardening
-ine	pertaining to		-trophic	development
-itis	inflammation			

Prefix Review

a-	without		hyper-	excessive
an-	without		mono-	one
anti-	against		poly-	many
di-	two		quadri-	four
dys-	painful, difficult		sub-	under
hemi-	half			

 IDENTIFY the organs treated in neurology.

Organs Commonly Treated in Neurology

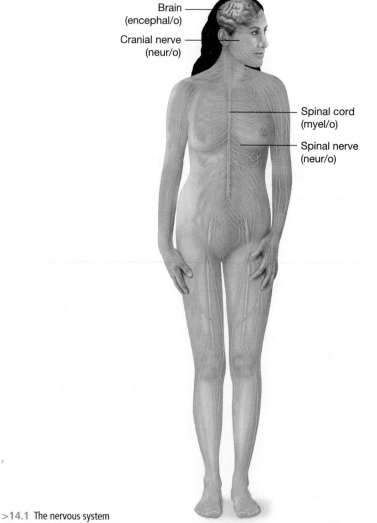

Brain
(encephal/o)

Cranial nerve
(neur/o)

Spinal cord
(myel/o)

Spinal nerve
(neur/o)

>14.1 The nervous system

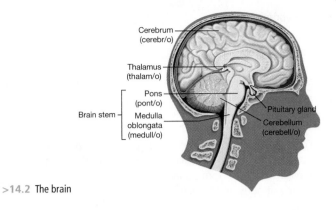

Cerebrum
(cerebr/o)

Thalamus
(thalam/o)

Pons
(pont/o)

Brain stem

Medulla
oblongata
(medull/o)

Pituitary gland

Cerebellum
(cerebell/o)

>14.2 The brain

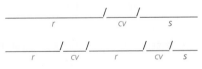

BUILD neurology medical terms from word parts.

Building Neurology Terms

This section presents word parts most often used to build neurology terms. Following the explanation of the term, you have the opportunity to begin building your own vocabulary. Read the meaning for each term and then fill in the blanks to build a single medical term. To help you out you will find a key to the word parts underneath the blanks: r for word roots, p for prefix, cv for combining vowel, and s for suffix. Remember that not every term will contain all these word parts; it's up to you to decide which to use. As you gain experience, this process becomes easier. Answers can be found at the back of the book

1. **cerebell/o**–combining form meaning **cerebellum**

   The cerebellum is the second largest part of brain; coordinates body movement and maintains balance

   a. pertaining to cerebellum

   _____/_____
               r   s

   b. cerebellum inflammation

   _____/_____
               r   s

2. **-cele**–suffix meaning **hernia** or **protrusion**

   In neurology this suffix refers to a birth defect in which portion of nervous system protrudes through opening in vertebral column

   a. protrusion of meninges

   _____/____/_____
               r   cv   s

   b. protrusion of meninges and spinal cord protrusion

   _____/____/_____/____/____
     r   cv   r   cv   s

3. **cerebr/o**–combining form meaning **cerebrum**

   The cerebrum is the largest part of brain; receives sensory information and sends motor commands; also responsible for memory, problem solving, and language; divided into **frontal, parietal, temporal,** and **occipital lobes**

   a. pertaining to cerebrum

   _____/_____
               r   s

   b. pertaining to cerebrum and spine

   _____/____/_____/_____
     r   cv   r   s

   c. cerebrum inflammation

   _____/_____
               r   s

   d. softening of cerebrum

   _____/____/_____
               r   cv   s

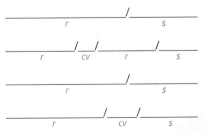

e. hardening of cerebrum

_____ / _____ / _____
r   CV   s

f. pertaining to cerebral blood vessels

_____ / _ / _____ / _____
r   CV   r   s

g. cutting into cerebrum

_____ / _____
r   s

---

4. **encephal/o**–combining form meaning **brain**

The brain is one of largest organs in body; coordinates most body activities; four sections of brain are **cerebrum, cerebellum, thalamus, and brain stem;** each section performs specific duties; right side of brain controls left side of body and left side of brain controls right side of body

>14.3 The brain

a. pertaining to brain

_____ / _____
r   s

b. record of electricity of brain

_____ / _ / _____ / _ / ___
r   CV   r   CV   s

c. process of recording electricity of brain

_____ / _ / _____ / _ / ___
r   CV   r   CV   s

d. brain pain

_____ / _____
r   s

e. brain inflammation

_____ / _____
r   s

f. brain disease

_____ / _ / _____
r   CV   s

g. brain tumor

_____ / _____
r   s

h. softening of brain

_____ / _ / _____
r   CV   s

i. hardening of brain

_____ / _ / _____
r   CV   s

---

5. **-esthesia**–suffix meaning **feeling, sensation**

a. without sensation

_____ / _____
p   s

b. excessive sensations

_____ / _____
p   s

---

6. **medull/o**–combining form meaning **medulla oblongata**

The medulla oblongata is part of the brain stem; connects rest of brain to spinal cord; contains control centers for respiration, heart rate, temperature, and blood pressure

a. pertaining to medulla oblongata

_____ / _____
r   s

---

7. **mening/o**–combining form meaning **meninges**

The meninges for a three-layer protective sac around brain and spinal cord; outer layer is **dura mater,** middle layer is **arachnoid layer,** inner layer is **pia mater**

   a. pertaining to meninges   _____/_____
                                                       r   s

   b. meninges inflammation   _____/_____
                                                       r   s

   c. meninges and spinal cord inflammation   _____/__/_____/_____
                                               r   cv   r   s

---

8. **myel/o**–combining form meaning **spinal cord**

The spinal cord is a column of nervous tissue providing path for messages traveling to and from brain

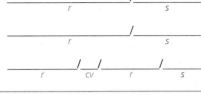

   >14.4 The spinal cord

   a. record of spinal cord   _____/____/_____
                                               r   cv   s

   b. process of recording spinal cord   _____/____/_____
                                               r   cv   s

   c. spinal cord inflammation   _____/_____
                                               r   s

   d. softening of spinal cord   _____/____/_____
                                               r   cv   s

   e. spinal cord and nerve inflammation   _____/__/_____/_____
                                              r   cv   r   s

   f. spinal cord disease   _____/____/_____
                                               r   cv   s

   g. hardening of spinal cord   _____/____/_____
                                               r   cv   s

   h. cutting into spinal cord   _____/_____
                                               r   s

---

9. **neur/o**–combining form meaning **nerve**

A nerve is a cordlike bundle of neurons carrying messages between CNS and muscles and organs of body; **sensory nerves** carry information to CNS; **motor nerves** carry messages from CNS to muscles and organs

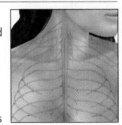

   >14.5 Nerves

   a. pertaining to nerves   _____/_____
                                               r   s

   b. nerve pain   _____/_____
                                               r   s

   c. surgical removal of a nerve   _____/_____
                                               r   s

   d. study of nerves   _____/____/_____
                                               r   cv   s

e. one who studies nerves

_____/____/_____
       r   CV   s

f. nerve tumor

_____/_____
       r   s

g. nerve disease

_____/____/_____
       r   CV   s

h. surgical repair of nerve

_____/____/_____
       r   CV   s

i. inflammation of many nerves

_____/_____/_____
   p   r   s

j. suture a nerve

_____/____/_____
       r   CV   s

---

10. -phasia–suffix meaning **speech**

a. without speech

_____/_____
       p   s

b. difficult speech

_____/_____
       p   s

---

11. -plegia–suffix meaning **paralysis**

a. paralysis of one (limb)

_____/_____
       p   s

b. paralysis of two (limbs)

_____/_____
       p   s

c. paralysis of four (limbs)

_____/_____
       p   s

d. half paralysis

_____/_____
       p   s

e. nerve paralysis

_____/____/_____
       r   CV   s

---

12. pont/o–combining form meaning **pons**

The pons is another part of the brain stem; connects cerebellum to rest of brain

a. pertaining to pons

_____/_____
       r   s

b. pertaining to pons and cerebellum

_____/___/_____/_____
   r   CV   r   s

c. pertaining to pons and medulla oblongata _____/___/_____/_____
   r   CV   r   s

---

13. thalam/o–combining form meaning **thalamus**

The thalamus is the part of the brain that relays incoming sensory information to correct part of cerebrum

a. pertaining to thalamus

_____/_____
       r   s

b. cutting into thalamus

_____/_____
       r   s

Neurology Vocabulary

The neurology terms presented in this section include eponyms, modern English words, and those that contain Latin or Greek word parts but are not constructed solely from these word parts. When you recognize word parts within a term they will give you a hint about the word's meaning. In these instances, look for the word parts to follow the term.

Term	Explanation
Alzheimer disease	Chronic brain condition involving progressive disorientation, speech and gait disturbances, and loss of memory
amyotrophic lateral sclerosis (ALS) a- = without my/o = muscle -trophic = development scler/o = hardening -osis = abnormal condition	Disease with muscular weakness and atrophy due to degeneration of motor neurons of spinal cord; commonly called *Lou Gehrig disease*
anticonvulsant anti- = against	Medication to reduce excitability of neurons and to prevent uncontrolled neuron activity associated with seizures
brain tumor	Intracranial mass, either benign or malignant; benign tumor of brain can still be fatal because it will grow and cause pressure on normal brain tissue

Glioma

>14.6 (A) Illustration of a large brain tumor and (B) PET scan image revealing brain tumor in the frontal lobe of the brain
Source: (B) Courtesy of Dr. Giovanni DiChiro and Dr. Ramesh Raman of the Neuroimaging Branch, National Institute of Neurological Disorders and Stroke, National Institutes of Health.

A   **B**

cerebral contusion cerebr/o = cerebrum -al = pertaining to	Bruising of brain from impact; symptoms last longer than 24 hours and include unconsciousness, dizziness, vomiting, unequal pupil size, and shock

＋ TERMINOLOGY TIDBIT

The term *contusion* comes from the Latin word *contundere* meaning "to bruise or crush."

Term	Explanation

cerebral palsy (CP)
cerebr/o = cerebrum
-al = pertaining to

Nonprogressive brain damage resulting from defect in fetal development or trauma or oxygen deprivation at time of birth

+ TERMINOLOGY TIDBIT

The term *palsy* comes from the Old French word *paralisie* meaning "paralysis."

---

cerebrospinal fluid analysis
cerebr/o = cerebrum
spin/o = spine
-al = pertaining to

Laboratory examination of clear, watery, colorless fluid from within brain and spinal cord; detects infections or bleeding of brain

---

cerebrovascular accident (CVA)
cerebr/o = cerebrum
vascul/o = blood vessels
-ar = pertaining to

Development of brain infarct due to loss in blood supply to brain; can be caused by ruptured blood vessel (hemorrhage), floating clot (embolus), stationary clot (thrombosis), or compression; extent of damage depends on size and location of infarct and can include dysphasia and hemiplegia; commonly called *stroke*

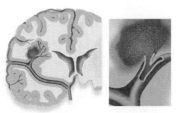

Cerebral hemorrhage: Cerebral artery ruptures and bleeds into brain tissue.

Cerebral embolism: Embolus from another area lodges in cerebral artery and blocks blood flow.

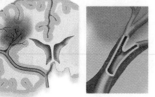

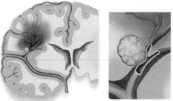

>14.7 The four common causes of cerebrovascular accidents: hemorrhage, embolism, thrombosis, and compression

Cerebral thrombosis: Blood clot forms in cerebral artery and blocks blood flow.

Compression: Pressure from tumor squeezes adjacent blood vessel and blocks blood flow.

---

coma

Profound unconsciousness or stupor resulting from illness or injury

+ TERMINOLOGY TIDBIT

The term *coma* comes from the Greek word *koma* meaning "deep sleep or trance."

---

concussion

Injury to brain when brain is shaken inside skull because of impact; symptoms last 24 hours or less and can include dizziness, vomiting, unequal pupil size, and shock

+ TERMINOLOGY TIDBIT

The term *concussion* comes from the Latin word *concutere* meaning "to shake violently."

dementia	Progressive impairment of intellectual function that interferes with performing activities of daily living

epilepsy	Recurrent disorder of brain; seizures and loss of consciousness occur as result of uncontrolled neuron electrical activity

+ TERMINOLOGY TIDBIT

The term *epilepsy* comes from the Greek word *epilepsia* meaning "seizure or attack."

hydrocephalus hydr/o = water cephal/o = head	Buildup of cerebrospinal fluid within brain, causing head to be enlarged; treated by creating shunt from brain to abdomen to drain excess fluid

Bulging fontanel

A Enlarged ventricles

B Catheter tip in ventricle

Valve

Blocked aqueduct

Shunt

>14.8 (A) A child with the enlarged ventricles of hydrocephalus. (B) the same child with a shunt to send the excess cerebrospinal fluid to the abdominal cavity

lumbar puncture (LP) lumb/o = low back -ar = pertaining to	Puncture with needle into lumbar vertebral area (usually space between fourth and fifth lumbar vertebrae) to withdraw fluid for examination or for injection of medication; also called *spinal puncture* or *spinal tap*

Skin
Fat
Interspinous ligament
L4
L5
Extradural "space"

Tip end of spinal cord
CSF in lumbar cistern
Dura mater
Sacrum

L1 vertebra
Lumbar puncture needle
Coccyx

>14.9 A lumbar puncture. The needle is inserted between the lumbar vertebrae and into the spinal canal

Term	Explanation
migraine	Specific type of headache characterized by severe head pain, sensitivity to light, dizziness, and nausea
multiple sclerosis (MS) scler/o = hardening -osis = abnormal condition	Inflammatory autoimmune disease of central nervous system; immune system damages myelin around neurons and results in extreme weakness and numbness
myasthenia gravis my/o = muscle -asthenia = weakness	Autoimmune disease with severe muscular weakness and fatigue due to difficulty of electrical impulse passing across synapse from one nerve to the next
paralysis	Temporary or permanent loss of muscle function and movement
Parkinson disease	Chronic disorder of the nervous system with fine tremors, muscular weakness, rigidity, and shuffling gait
positron emission tomography (PET)	Use of positive radionuclides to reconstruct brain sections; measurement of oxygen and glucose uptake, cerebral blood flow, and blood volume can be taken; amount of glucose brain uses indicates its metabolic activity
seizure	Sudden, uncontrollable onset of symptoms; such as in epileptic seizure; *absence seizure* (petit mal seizure) appears as loss of awareness and absence of activity; *tonic-clonic seizure* (grand mal seizure) is characterized by muscle convulsions
shingles	Eruption of painful blisters on the body along nerve path; thought to be caused by a *Herpes zoster* virus infection of nerve root

+ TERMINOLOGY TIDBIT

The term *shingles* comes from the Latin word *cingulum* meaning "girdle." This word describes how the blisters form in a line that encircles the body.

Term	Explanation
spina bifida	Congenital defect in walls of spinal canal in which two sides of vertebra do not meet or close; can result in *meningocele* or *myelomeningocele*

Nerve fibers — Meninges — Tuft of hair — Dimpling of skin —

A. Spina bifida

Skin — Spinal cord — Cerebrospinal fluid — Meninges — Meninges sac

B. Meningocele

Skin — Spinal cord — Cerebrospinal fluid — Spinal cord and spinal nerves in meningeal sac

C. Myelomeningocele

>14.10 Spina bifida. (A) Spina bifida occulta, the vertebra is not complete, but there is no protrusion of nervous system structures, (B) meningocele, the meninges protrude through the opening in the vertebra, and (C) myelomeningocele, the meninges and spinal cord protrude through the opening in the vertebra

Term	Explanation
spinal cord injury (SCI) spin/o = spine -al = pertaining to	Damage to spinal cord as result of trauma; spinal cord can be bruised or completely severed

Term	Explanation
subdural hematoma sub- = under -al = pertaining to hemat/o = blood -oma = tumor	Mass of blood forming underneath dura mater when meninges are torn by trauma; can exert fatal pressure on brain if hematoma is not drained by surgery

>14.11 A subdural hematoma. A meningeal vein has ruptured and blood has accumulated in the subdural space producing pressure on the brain

- Torn cerebral vein
- Subdural hematoma
- Compressed brain tissue
- Dura mater
- Arachnoid layer

Term	Explanation
syncope	Fainting

+ TERMINOLOGY TIDBIT

The term *syncope* comes form the Greek word *sunkope* meaning "to cut short or swoon."

Term	Explanation
transient ischemic attack (TIA) -ic = pertaining to	Temporary reduction of blood supply to brain; causes symptoms such as syncope, numbness, and hemiplegia; can eventually lead to cerebrovascular accident

 USE neurology abbreviations.

Neurology Abbreviations

The following list presents common neurology abbreviations.

ALS	amyotrophic lateral sclerosis	**HA**	headache
ANS	autonomic nervous system	**ICP**	intracranial pressure
CNS	central nervous system	**LP**	lumbar puncture
CP	cerebral palsy	**MS**	multiple sclerosis
CSF	cerebrospinal fluid	**PET**	positron emission tomography
CVA	cerebrovascular accident	**PNS**	peripheral nervous system
CVD	cerebrovascular disease	**SCI**	spinal cord injury
EEG	electroencephalogram, electroen-cephalography	**TIA**	transient ischemic attack

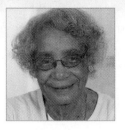

History of Present Illness

A 73-year-old African American female is brought to the ER via ambulance. She was found lying on the floor of her kitchen by her daughter. Patient is awake but unable to speak or move her left extremities. Daughter reports she has witnessed her mother have two short spells of numbness and clumsiness with her left hand over the past 3 months. She urged her mother to see her family physician but does not believe she has followed through. Medication for hypertension and NSAIDs for arthritis were brought to ER by the daughter, who states she believes her mother is hoarding her medication and not taking it as often as prescribed.

Past Medical History

Hypertension; arthritis in right hip requiring occasional use of quad cane for walking long distances; had hysterectomy at age 46 for endometriosis

Family and Social History

Patient is widowed and lives alone. She is a retired school bus driver. Daughter reports she is active in her church and tends a large vegetable garden each year. Multiple family members are hypertensive, but history is negative for neurological diseases.

Physical Examination

Patient is awake and calm. She is unable to answer any questions and does not follow any commands for moving left extremities and does not spontaneously move left extremities. Follows all commands with right extremities, and muscle strength appears normal for her age. Her blood pressure was 168/108.

Diagnostic Imaging

MRI of head shows area of cerebral hemorrhage on right side of brain. X-rays of head, spine, and hips were negative for fractures.

Diagnosis

Right CVA with left hemiplegia

Plan of Treatment

1. Admit to ICU and monitor for additional bleeding and worsening of symptoms
2. Aggressive medical treatment to reduce blood pressure
3. Begin rehabilitation with PT, OT, and speech therapy
4. Referral to medical social worker to begin discussions with patient, family, and rehabilitation therapists to determine alternate living arrangements

Critical Thinking Questions

Answer the following questions regarding this case study. Do not just copy words out of the case study; translate all medical terms. To answer some of these questions, you may need to look up information from another chapter of this text, in a medical dictionary, or online. Answers are found at the back of the book

1. In ER the patient was unable to speak or move the left extremities. What are the medical terms for these symptoms?

    _____

    _____

2. The patient's daughter reported that her mother has had short spells of numbness and clumsiness with the left hand. Review the conditions described in the Neurology Vocabulary and suggest a possible name for these episodes.

    _____

    _____

3. Which of the following is NOT one of the patient's previous medical diagnoses and operations?

    a. Endometrial tissue found throughout pelvic cavity
    b. High blood pressure
    c. Stomach protruding through hole in diaphragm
    d. Joint pain

4. What are NSAIDs, and why was this patient taking them? (*Hint:* Check the orthopedics chapter.)

    _____

    _____

5. Define the following abbreviations used in this medical record: ER, MRI, ICU, PT, OT.

    _____

    _____

6. Why do you think taking skeletal x-rays was a necessary part of this patient's evaluation?

    _____

    _____

7. Explain why the bleeding was found on the right side of the brain, but the paralysis was of the left extremities.

    _____

    _____

Sound It Out

The following are some of the key terms from this chapter written as their phonetic spelling. Sound out each term and write it in the blank. Pronunciations for all terms are included in the audio glossary at www.mymedicalterminologylab.com <http://www.mymedicalterminologylab.com/>.

1. men-in-JYE-tis _____

2. an-tye-kon-VULL-sant _____

3. noo-ROH-mah _____

4. ah-FAY-zee-ah _____

5. SER-eh-broh-mah-LAY-she-ah _____

6. ser-eh-BELL-ar _____

7. en SEFF-ah-low-skle-ROH-sis _____

8. ser-eh-BELL-um _____

9. seh-REE-bral _____

10. kon-KUSH-un _____

11. en-seff-ah-LYE-tis _____

12. dee-MEN-she-ah _____

13. an-es-THEE-zee-ah _____

14. SER-eh-broh-SPY-nal _____

15. dis-FAY-zee-ah _____

16. ee-lek-troh-en-SEFF-ah-loh-gram _____

17. MY-eh-LOP-ah-thee _____

18. EN-seh-FAL-ik _____

19. noo-REK-toh-mee _____

20. EP-ih-lep-see _____

21. hem-ee-PLEE-jee-ah _____

22. THAL-ah-mus _____

23. high-droh-SEFF-ah-lus _____

24. MED-you-lair-ee _____

25. meh-NIN-jee-all _____

26. kwod-rih-PLEE-jee-ah _____

27. tha-LAM-ik _____

28. meh-NING-goh-seel _____

29. noo-ROR-ah-fee _____

30. MY-grain _____

31. seh-REE-brum _____

32. MY-eh-lin _____

33. noo-rol-oh-jee _____

34. my-eh-LOG-rah-fee _____

35. ser-eh-BROT-oh-me _____

36. MY-eh-LOT-oh-me _____

37. NOO-rall _____

38. noo-RAL-jee-ah _____

39. NOO-ron _____

40. meh-NIN-jeez _____

41. pon-TEEN _____

42. NOOR-oh-plas-tee _____

43. pah-RAL-ih-sis _____

44. en-seff-ah-LOW-mah _____

45. pol-ee-noo-RYE-tis _____

46. my-eh-LYE-tis _____

47. PONZ _____

48. SEE-zyoor _____

49. SER-eh-broh-VASS-kyoo-lar _____

50. SIN-koh-pee _____

Transcription Practice

Each of the following sentences is written in common English. Underline any words or phrases that can be replaced by a medical term. Then rewrite the entire sentence using medical terms. Answers are found at the end of the book.

1. Jon took medication to reduce neuron excitability to control his epileptic sudden, uncontrolled onset of symptoms.

   _____

   _____

2. As a result of the development of a brain infarct due to loss in blood supply, Mr. van Pelt was in a profound state of unconsciousness.

   _____

   _____

3. The auto accident victim developed paralysis of all four limbs following a severing of the spinal cord as a result of trauma.

   _____

   _____

4. During the temporary reduction of blood supply to the brain, Mr. Edelstein had the inability to speak.

   _____

   _____

5. Ilina's paralysis of one limb was caused by an inflammatory autoimmune disease of the central nervous system.

   _____

   _____

6. Antonio went to the physician who studies nerves because he was having severe headaches with sensitivity to light, dizziness, and nausea.

   _____

   _____

7. An image made using positive radionuclides was completed to see whether the tumor was in the largest part of the brain or the second largest part of the brain.

   _____

   _____

8. A puncture with a needle into the lumbar vertebral area was performed to analyze cerebrospinal fluid for signs of brain inflammation.

   _____

   _____

9. Mr. Larsen's severe leg pain was caused by inflammation of many nerves.

   _____

   _____

10. The elderly gentleman with chronic brain condition involving progressive speech and gait disturbances and loss of memory eventually developed impaired intellectual function that interfered with activities of daily living.

    _____

    _____

▶Labeling Exercise

Write the name of each structure on the numbered line. Also use this space to write the combining form where appropriate.

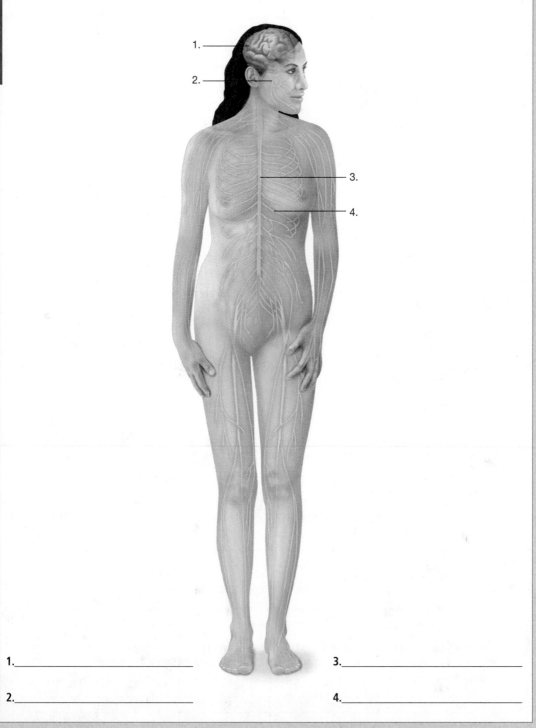

1.

2.

3.

4.

1._____

2._____

3._____

4._____

Build Medical Terms

Use each of the following word parts to build the indicated medical terms.

The combining form *neur/o* means nerve

1. nerve pain _____

2. nerve tumor _____

3. study of nerves _____

4. surgical repair of nerves _____

5. nerve disease _____

The combining form *thalam/o* means thalamus.

6. pertaining to thalamus _____

7. cutting into thalamus _____

The suffix *-plegia* means paralysis.

8. paralysis of two (limbs) _____

9. paralysis of half _____

The combining form *mening/o* means meninges.

10. pertaining to meninges _____

11. meninges inflammation _____

The combining form *myel/o* means spinal cord.

12. record of spinal cord _____

13. spinal cord softening _____

14. spinal cord hardening _____

15. spinal cord inflammation _____

PEARSON mymedicalterminologylab™

***MyMedicalTerminologyLab* is a premium online homework management system that includes a host of features to help you study. Registered users will find:**

- Fun games and activities built within a virtual hospital
- Powerful tools that track and analyze your results—allowing you to create a personalized learning experience
- Videos, flashcards, and audio pronunciations to help enrich your progress
- Streaming lesson presentations and self-paced learning modules
- A space where you and your instructors can view and manage your assignments

Fill in the Blank

Fill in the blank to complete each of the following sentences.

1. Amyotrophic lateral sclerosis causes degeneration of the _____ of the spinal cord.

2. Because his dizziness and vomiting lasted less than 24 hours, Ali had a _____ rather than a cerebral _____.

3. The medical term for fainting is _____.

4. The four sections of the brain are the _____, _____, _____, and _____.

5. The protective sac around the brain and spinal cord is called the _____.

6. _____ is brain damage caused by trauma or oxygen deprivation at the time of birth.

7. A tonic-clonic seizure used to be called a _____ seizure.

8. _____ is because of the difficulty of electrical impulse passing across synapse from one nerve to the next.

9. _____ disease is recognized by fine tremors, muscular weakness, rigidity, and a shuffling gait.

10. _____ is caused by a *Herpes zoster* virus of a nerve root.

Abbreviation Matching

Match each abbreviation with its definition.

_____ **1.** LP	**A.** electroencephalogram
_____ **2.** MS	**B.** transient ischemic attack
_____ **3.** PNS	**C.** multiple sclerosis
_____ **4.** EEG	**D.** cerebral palsy
_____ **5.** SCI	**E.** amyotrophic lateral sclerosis
_____ **6.** TIA	**F.** spinal cord injury
_____ **7.** CSF	**G.** intracranial pressure
_____ **8.** CP	**H.** lumbar puncture
_____ **9.** ICP	**I.** cerebrospinal fluid
_____ **10.** ALS	**J.** peripheral nervous system

Medical Term Analysis

Examine each of the following terms. Begin by dividing it into its word parts and writing them in the indicated blanks (P = prefix, WR = word root; CF = combining form; S = suffix). Follow with the definition of each word part and then finally the meaning of the full term.

1. **cerebellar**

   WR _____

   means _____

   S _____

   means _____

   Term Meaning: _____

   _____

2. **meningocele**

   CF _____

   means _____

   S _____

   means _____

   Term Meaning: _____

   _____

3. **cerebrospinal**

   CF _____

   means _____

   WR _____

   means _____

   S _____

   means _____

   Term Meaning: _____

   _____

4. **anesthesia**

   P _____

   means _____

   S _____

   means _____

   Term Meaning: _____

   _____

5. **meningomyelitis**

   CF _____

   means _____

   WR _____

   means _____

   S _____

   means _____

   Term Meaning: _____

   _____

6. **encephaloma**

   WR _____

   means _____

   S _____

   means _____

   Term Meaning: _____

   _____

7. dysphasia

P _____

means _____

S _____

means _____

Term Meaning: _____

_____

8. neurology

CF _____

means _____

S _____

means _____

Term Meaning: _____

_____

9. pontomedullary

CF _____

means _____

WR _____

means _____

S _____

means _____

Term Meaning: _____

_____

10. cerebrotomy

WR_____

means _____

S _____

means _____

Term Meaning: _____

_____

Spelling

Some of the following terms are misspelled. Identify the incorrect terms and spell them correctly in the blank provided.

1. neurorhaphy _____

2. encephalalgia _____

3. cerebromalacia _____

4. meningoitis _____

5. quadraplegia _____

6. pontine _____

7. electroencepalography _____

8. hydrocephalus _____

9. myesthenia gravis _____

10. syncope _____

Photomatch Challenge

Each combining form below stands for an area of the central nervous system. Write the name of the area in the blank following the combining form. Then translate the medical term on the second line.

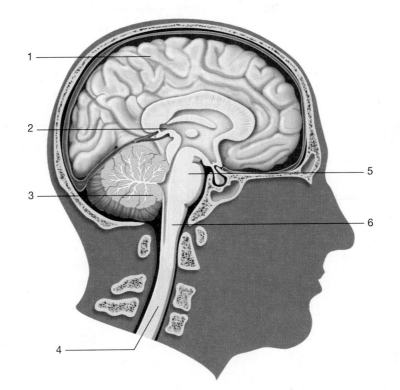

Word Bank:

1. cerebr/o _____

cerebromalacia _____

2. thalam/o _____

thalamotomy _____

3. cerebell/o _____

cerebellitis _____

4. myel/o _____

myelogram _____

5. pont/o _____

pontine _____

6. medull/o _____

medullary _____

Crossword Puzzle

Use the definitions given to complete the crossword puzzle.

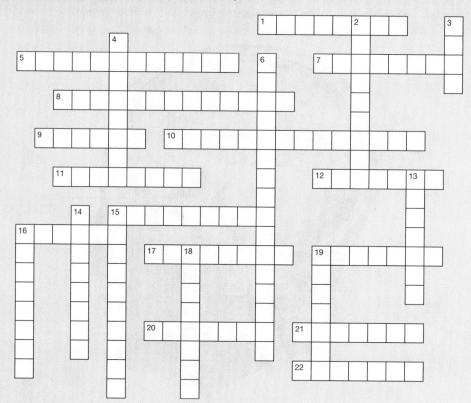

ACROSS

1 Seizures caused by uncontrolled neuron electrical activity
5 Term meaning paralysis of four (limbs)
7 Largest part of brain
8 Buildup of cerebrospinal fluid within brain
9 In multiple sclerosis, the immune system destroys _____
10 Medication that reduces neuron excitability
11 Progressive impairment of intellectual function
12 Petit mal is also called a(n) _____ seizure
15 Cerebral _____, bruising of the brain
16 Common name for cerebrovascular accident
17 Term meaning blood tumor
19 _____ nerves carry information to CNS
20 Fainting
21 Term meaning without speech
22 A sudden, uncontrollable onset of symptoms

DOWN

2 The temporary or permanent loss of muscle function
3 Profound unconsciousness
4 Headache with severe pain, dizziness, and nausea
6 Myasthenia gravis happens because of insufficient _____
13 Brain and spinal cord form the _____ nervous system
14 A PET scan uses _____ radionuclides
15 Coordinates body movement and maintains balance
16 Condition caused by Herpes zoster virus
18 Protective covering around brain and spinal cord
19 Point where one neuron meets another

15

Endocrinology
Endocrine System

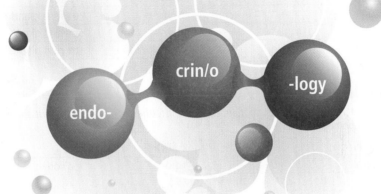

endo- crin/o -logy

A Brief Introduction to Endocrinology

UNDERSTAND the function of the endocrine system.

The **endocrine system** plays a vital role in maintaining **homeostasis,** a stable internal body environment. This system consists of a group of **glands** that secrete chemical messengers called **hormones** directly into the bloodstream. Hormones travel through the blood to **target organs** to adjust their activity to regulate factors such as growth, reproduction, metabolic rate, bone growth, and sugar levels. The endocrine system is made up of the following: two **adrenal glands,** two **ovaries** in the female, four **parathyroid glands,** the **pancreas,** the **pineal gland,** the **pituitary gland,** two **testes** in the male, the **thymus gland,** and the **thyroid gland.**

> **➕ TERMINOLOGY TIDBIT**
>
> The term *endocrine* literally means "to secrete within." This describes how these glands release their chemicals into the inside of the body by secreting directly into the bloodstream. On the other hand, exocrine glands, such as sweat glands, release their secretions the outside the body.

DESCRIBE the medical specialty of endocrinology.

Endocrinology is a subspecialty of internal medicine. **Endocrinologists** diagnose and treat diseases and conditions that develop as a result of a hormone imbalance. If a gland releases too much hormone, **hypersecretion,** or too little hormone, **hyposecretion,** the target organ functions improperly because it did not receive the correct message.

Endocrinology Combining Forms

The following list presents new combining forms important for building and defining endocrinology terms.

aden/o	gland		pancreat/o	pancreas
adren/o	adrenal glands		parathyroid/o	parathyroid gland
adrenal/o	adrenal glands		pineal/o	pineal gland
crin/o	secrete		pituitar/o	pituitary gland
glyc/o	sugar		testicul/o	testes
glycos/o	sugar		thym/o	thymus gland
oophor/o	ovary		thyr/o	thyroid gland
orchi/o	testes		thyroid/o	thyroid gland
ovari/o	ovary			

The following list presents combining forms that are not specific to the endocrine system but are also used for building and defining endocrinology terms.

acr/o	extremities		ophthalm/o	eye
carcin/o	cancer		toxic/o	poison
cyt/o	cell			

Suffix Review

These suffixes and prefixes were introduced in Chapters 2 and 3. They are being reviewed in this chapter because they are especially important for building endocrinology terms.

-al	pertaining to		-logy	study of
-an	pertaining to		-malacia	softening
-ar	pertaining to		-megaly	enlarged
-centesis	puncture to withdraw fluid		-oid	resembling
-cyte	cell		-oma	tumor
-dipsia	thirst		-osis	abnormal condition
-ectomy	surgical removal		-otomy	cutting into
-edema	swelling		-pathy	disease
-emia	blood condition		-pexy	surgical fixation
-ic	pertaining to		-plasty	surgical repair
-ism	state of, condition		-rrhexis	rupture
-itis	inflammation		-uria	urine condition
-logist	one who studies			

Prefix Review

endo-	within		hypo-	insufficient
ex-	outward		poly-	many, much
hyper-	excessive			

Organs Commonly Treated in Endocrinology

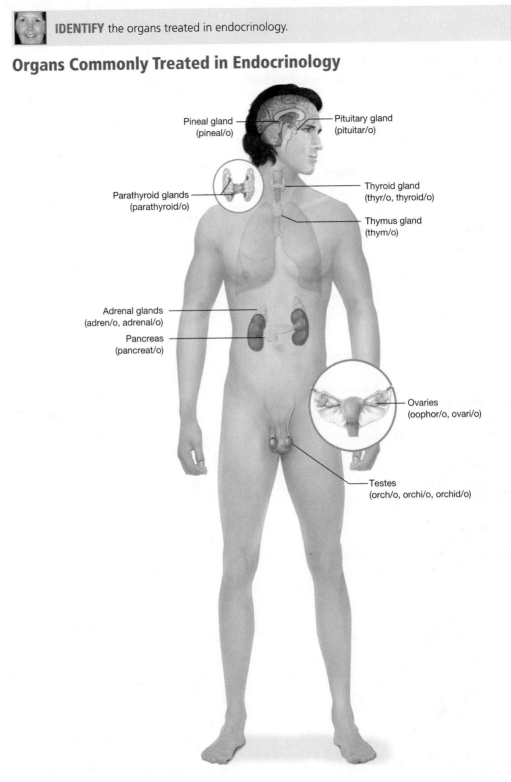

Pineal gland
(pineal/o)

Pituitary gland
(pituitar/o)

Parathyroid glands
(parathyroid/o)

Thyroid gland
(thyr/o, thyroid/o)

Thymus gland
(thym/o)

Adrenal glands
(adren/o, adrenal/o)

Pancreas
(pancreat/o)

Ovaries
(oophor/o, ovari/o)

Testes
(orch/o, orchi/o, orchid/o)

>15.1 The endocrine system

Building Endocrinology Terms

This section presents word parts most often used to build endocrinology terms. Following the explanation of the term, you have the opportunity to begin building your own vocabulary. Read the meaning for each term and then fill in the blanks to build a single medical term. Use the slashes to divide prefixes, word roots, combining vowels, and suffixes. To help you out you will find a key to the word parts underneath the blanks: r for word roots, p for prefix, cv for combining vowel, and s for suffix. Remember that not every term will contain all these word parts; it's up to you to decide which to use. As you gain experience, this process becomes easier. Answers can be found at the back of the book.

1. **aden/o**–combining form meaning **gland**

    A gland is a group of cells that work together to produce and secrete substances such as hormones

    a. cancerous tumor in gland

    _____/___/_____/_____
           r   *cv*   *r*   *s*

    b. gland cell

    _____/_____/_____
          r   *cv*   *s*

    c. resembling gland

    _____/_____
          r   *s*

    d. softening of gland

    _____/____/_____
          r   *cv*   *s*

2. **adren/o**–combining form meaning **adrenal gland**

    Each of two adrenal glands sits on top of a kidney; divided into outer **adrenal cortex** and inner **adrenal medulla;** adrenal cortex secretes **aldosterone** to regulate sodium levels in the body, **cortisol** to regulate carbohydrate metabolism, and sex hormones such as **estrogen** and **testosterone;** adrenal medulla secretes **epinephrine** (also called *adrenaline*) to help body respond to emergency situations

    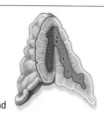

    >15.2 The adrenal gland

    ### TERMINOLOGY TIDBIT

    The term *cortex* is frequently used in anatomy to indicate the outer portion of an organ such as the adrenal gland or the kidney. The word *cortex* is Latin and means "bark" as in the bark of a tree. The word *medulla* means "marrow." Because marrow is found in the inner cavity of bones, the term came to stand for the middle of an organ.

    a. pertaining to the adrenal gland

    _____/_____
          r   *s*

    b. enlarged adrenal gland

    _____/____/_____
          r   *cv*   *s*

3. **adrenal/o**–combining form meaning **adrenal gland**

    a. surgical removal of adrenal gland

    _____/_____
          r   *s*

    b. adrenal gland inflammation

    _____/_____
          r   *s*

    c. adrenal gland disease

    _____/____/_____
          r   *cv*   *s*

4. **crin/o**–combining form meaning **to secrete**

    This combining form refers to glands releasing substances such as hormones

    a. study of (the glands that) secrete within   _____/_____/___/_____
                                                                            p   *r*   cv   *s*

    b. one who studies (the glands that) secrete within   _____/_____/___/_____
                                                                        p   *r*   cv   *s*

    c. tumor that secretes within   _____/_____/_____
                                        p   *r*   *s*

    d. disease that secretes within   _____/_____/___/_____
                                      p   *r*   cv   *s*

5. **glyc/o**–combining form meaning **sugar**

    Even though this combining form means sugar it usually refers to **glucose,** primary sugar used by body for energy production

    a. blood condition of excessive sugar   _____/_____/_____
                                        p   *r*   *s*

    b. blood condition of insufficient sugar   _____/_____/_____
                                        p   *r*   *s*

6. **glycos/o**–combining form meaning **sugar**

    a. condition of sugar in urine   _____/_____
                               r   *s*

7. **oophor/o**–combining form meaning **ovary**

    The ovaries are a pair of almond-shaped organs in female pelvic cavity; release ova for reproduction and female sex hormones such as **estrogen** to regulate menstrual cycle

    a. ovary inflammation   _____/_____
                               r   *s*

    b. surgical repair of ovary   _____/___/_____
                               r   cv   *s*

    c. cutting into ovary   _____/_____
                               r   *s*

    d. surgical removal of ovary   _____/_____
                               r   *s*

8. **orchi/o**–combining form meaning **testes**

    The testes are a pair of oval-shaped glands located in scrotum of males; releases sperm for reproduction and male sex hormone **testosterone**

    a. surgical removal of testes   _____/_____
                               r   *s*

    b. surgical fixation of testes   _____/___/_____
                               r   cv   *s*

    c. cutting into testes   _____/_____
                               r   *s*

9. **ovari/o**–combining form meaning **ovary**

   Another combining form meaning ovary

   a. pertaining to ovary

   _____/_____
                r   s

   b. puncture of ovary to remove fluid

   _____/_____/_____
                r   cv   s

   c. ruptured ovary

   _____/_____/_____
                r   cv   s

10. **pancreat/o**–combining form meaning **pancreas**

    The pancreas is located in the abdominal cavity along lower curvature of stomach; secretes **insulin** and **glucagon** to regulate blood sugar levels; insulin lowers blood sugar levels by allowing sugar to enter individual cells; glucagon raises blood sugar by stimulating liver to release stored sugar back into the bloodstream

    a. pertaining to pancreas

    _____/_____
                 r   s

    b. surgical removal of pancreas

    _____/_____
                 r   s

    c. pancreas inflammation

    _____/_____
                 r   s

    d. cutting into pancreas

    _____/_____
                 r   s

11. **parathyroid/o**–combining form meaning **parathyroid gland**

    The parathyroid glands are four small glands located on posterior surface of thyroid gland; secretes **parathyroid hormone** to raise blood levels of calcium

    a. pertaining to parathyroid gland

    _____/_____
                 r   s

    b. surgical removal of parathyroid gland

    _____/_____
                 r   s

    c. condition of excessive parathyroid gland (secretion)

    _____/_____/_____
                 p   r   s

    d. condition of insufficient parathyroid gland (secretion)

    _____/_____/_____
                 p   r   s

12. **pineal/o**–combining form meaning **pineal gland**

    The pineal gland is a small pine cone-shaped gland in thalamus region of brain; secretes **melatonin,** which plays a role in regulating body's circadian rhythm (24-hour clock)

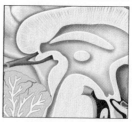

    >15.3 The pineal gland

    a. surgical removal of pineal gland

    _____/_____
                 r   s

13. **pituitar/o**–combining form meaning **pituitary gland**

The pituitary gland is a small marble-shaped gland that hangs down from underside of brain; often referred to as *master gland* because some of its hormones regulate other endocrine glands; divided into **anterior lobe** and **posterior lobe;** anterior lobe secretes **growth hormone** (stimulates body to grow larger), **thyroid-stimulating hormone** (regulates activity of thyroid gland), **adrenocorticotropin hormone** (regulates activity of adrenal cortex), **prolactin** (stimulates milk production by breast), **melanocyte-stimulating hormone** (stimulates melanocytes to produce more melanin), and **follicle-stimulating hormone** and **luteinizing hormone** (work together to regulate activity of ovary or testes); posterior lobe secretes **antidiuretic hormone** (regulates volume of water in body) and **oxytocin** (stimulates uterine contractions during labor and birth)

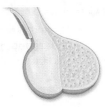

>15.4 The pituitary gland

a. condition of insufficient pituitary gland (secretion)   _____ / _____ / _____
p   r   s

b. condition of excessive pituitary gland (secretion)   _____ / _____ / _____
p   r   s

---

14. **poly**–prefix meaning **many or much**

This prefix meaning many or much; often used to indicate "too much" of a substance

a. too much thirst   _____ / _____
p   s

b. condition of (producing) too much urine   _____ / _____
p   s

---

15. **testicul/o**–combining form meaning **testes**

a. pertaining to testes   _____ / _____
r   s

---

16. **thym/o**–combining form meaning **thymus gland**

The thymus gland is located in mediastinum of chest behind sternum and above heart; secretes **thymosin,** which is important for immune system's development

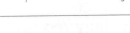

>15.5 The thymus gland

a. pertaining to thymus gland   _____ / _____
r   s

b. surgical removal of thymus gland   _____ / _____
r   s

c. thymus gland inflammation   _____ / _____
r   s

d. thymus gland tumor   _____ / _____
r   s

17. **thyr/o**–combining form meaning **thyroid gland**

Located in neck; has two lobes on either side of trachea; secretes **thyroxine** and **triiodothyronine,** which regulate body's metabolic rate; also secretes calcitonin to lower blood calcium levels

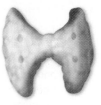

>15.6 The thyroid gland

a. enlarged thyroid gland

_____/_____/_____
          r   cv   s

b. cutting into thyroid gland

_____/_____
          r   s

18. **thyroid/o**–combining form meaning **thyroid gland**

Another combining form meaning thyroid gland

a. pertaining to thyroid gland

_____/_____
          r   s

b. thyroid gland inflammation

_____/_____
          r   s

c. surgical removal of thyroid gland

_____/_____
          r   s

d. condition of excessive thyroid gland (secretion)

_____/_____/_____
        p   r   s

e. condition of insufficient thyroid gland (secretion)

_____/_____/_____
        p   r   s

EXPLAIN endocrinology medical terms.

Endocrinology Vocabulary

The endocrinology terms presented in this section include eponyms, modern English words, and those that contain Latin or Greek word parts but are not constructed solely from these word parts. When you recognize word parts within a term they will give you a hint about the word's meaning. In these instances, look for the word parts to follow the term.

> Term	Explanation

acromegaly
  acr/o = extremities
  -megaly = enlarged
	Chronic condition developing in adults with excessive growth hormone; results in elongation and enlargement of bones of head and extremities

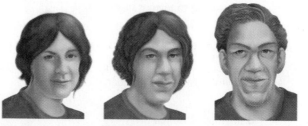

>15.7 Series of pictures of a woman with acromegaly. As she ages, the bones of her hands and face grow larger, but she will not grow taller

adrenal feminization
  adren/o = adrenal gland
  -al = pertaining to
	Development of female secondary sexual characteristics (such as breasts) in male as result of increased estrogen secretion by adrenal cortex

Term	Explanation
adrenal virilism adren/o = adrenal gland -al = pertaining to	Development of male secondary sexual characteristics (such as deeper voice and facial hair) in female as result of increased androgen secretion by adrenal cortex
blood serum test	Blood test to measure level of substances such as hormones in bloodstream; used to study function of endocrine glands
corticosteroids	In addition to its normal function, these hormones secreted by adrenal cortex also have strong anti-inflammatory action; can be used to treat severe chronic inflammatory diseases such as rheumatoid arthritis
cretinism -ism = state of	Congenital condition causing lack of thyroid hormones; results in poor physical and mental development
Cushing syndrome	Condition resulting from hypersecretion of adrenal cortex; can be product of adrenal gland tumor; symptoms include weakness, edema, excess hair growth, skin discoloration, and osteoporosis
diabetes insipidus (DI)	Condition caused by insufficient antidiuretic hormone secreted by posterior lobe of pituitary gland; symptoms include polyuria and polydipsia
diabetes mellitus (DM)	Chronic disorder of sugar metabolism; symptoms include hyperglycemia and glycosuria; two different forms of diabetes mellitus: *insulin-dependent diabetes mellitus* (IDDM) or *type 1*, and *noninsulin-dependent diabetes mellitus* (NIDDM) or *type 2*.
dwarfism -ism = state of	Being excessively short in height; can result from lack of growth hormone
exophthalmos ex- = out ophthalm/o = eye	Condition in which eyeballs protrude, such as in Graves disease; commonly caused by hypersecretion of thyroid hormones

+ TERMINOLOGY TIDBIT

The term *cretinism* comes from the French word *crestin*, which means "Christian." The intent of using this term was to remind people that persons with poor mental development were still people.

+ TERMINOLOGY TIDBIT

The term *diabetes* comes from the Greek word meaning "siphon" and was chosen to describe conditions in which large amounts of urine were excreted. The term *mellitus* comes from the Latin term meaning "sweet." Urine from persons with diabetes mellitus is sweet due to the large amount of glucose being released.

>15.8 Exophthalmos, a common symptom of hyperthyroidism

Term	Explanation
fasting blood sugar (FBS)	Blood test to measure amount of sugar in bloodstream after a 12-hour fast
gigantism **-ism** = state of	Excessive growth of body due to hypersecretion of growth hormone in a child or teenager
glucose tolerance test (GTT)	Test for initial diagnosis of diabetes mellitus; patient is given dose of glucose; then blood samples are taken at regular intervals to determine patient's ability to use glucose properly
goiter	Enlargement of the thyroid gland

＋ TERMINOLOGY TIDBIT

The term *goiter* comes from the Latin word *guttur* meaning "throat." This word was used to describe the greatly enlarged throat region seen in persons with a goiter.

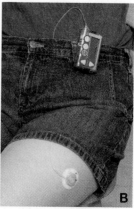

>15.9 A male with a very large goiter

Graves disease	Condition resulting from hypersecretion of thyroid hormones; symptoms include exophthalmos and goiter
Hashimoto disease	Chronic autoimmune form of thyroiditis, results in hyposecretion of thyroid hormones
hormone replacement therapy	Artificial replacement of hormones in patients with hyposecretion disorders; available in pill, injection, or adhesive skin patch forms
insulin-dependent diabetes mellitus (IDDM)	Also called *type 1 diabetes* mellitus; tends to develop early in life; pancreas stops producing insulin; can be autoimmune disease; patient must take insulin injections

>15.10 (A) Female checking her blood sugar level with a glucometer before using an insulin pen (an insulin injection system). (B) A person wearing an insulin pump, which delivers small amounts of insulin throughout the day

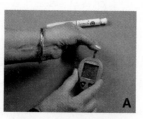

Term	Explanation
myxedema **-edema** = swelling	Condition resulting from hyposecretion of thyroid hormones in adult; symptoms include anemia, slow speech, swollen facial features, puffy and dry skin, drowsiness, and mental sluggishness
noninsulin-dependent diabetes mellitus (NIDDM)	Also called *type 2 diabetes mellitus;* typically develops later in life; pancreas produces normal to high levels of insulin but cells fail to respond; patients can take medication to improve insulin function
pheochromocytoma **cyt/o** = cell **-oma** = tumor	Usually benign tumor of adrenal medulla; secretes excessive amount of epinephrine; symptoms include anxiety, heart palpitations, dyspnea, hypertension, profuse sweating, headache, and nausea
radioactive iodine uptake (RAIU)	Test of thyroid function that measures how much radioactively tagged iodine is removed from the bloodstream by thyroid gland
radioimmunoassay (RIA)	Test used to measure levels of hormones in plasma of blood
tetany	Nerve irritability and painful muscle cramps resulting from hypocalcemia; hypoparathyroidism is one cause
thyroid function test (TFT)	Blood test to measure levels of thyroxine, triiodothyronine, and thyroid-stimulating hormone in the bloodstream to evaluate thyroid function
thyroid scan	Test in which radioactive iodine is administered and localizes in the thyroid gland; gland is visualized with scanning device; able to detect thyroid gland tumors

+ TERMINOLOGY TIDBIT

The term *tetany* comes from the Greek word *tetanos* meaning "muscular spasm."

>15.11 Radioactive iodine concentrates in the neck of a patient with a goiter. The actual scan is superimposed on a line drawing of the neck region

Goiter

Term	Explanation
thyrotoxicosis **thyr/o** = thyroid gland **toxic/o** = poison **-osis** = abnormal condition	Condition resulting from extreme hypersecretion of thyroid hormones; symptoms include rapid heart action, tremors, enlarged thyroid gland, exophthalmos, and weight loss

Endocrinology Abbreviations

The following list presents common endocrinology abbreviations.

ACTH	adrenocorticotropic hormone	Na^+	sodium
ADH	antidiuretic hormone	NIDDM	noninsulin-dependent diabetes mellitus
DI	diabetes insipidus	NPH	neutral protamine Hagedorn (insulin)
DM	diabetes mellitus	PRL	prolactin
FBS	fasting blood sugar	PTH	parathyroid hormone
FSH	follicle-stimulating hormone	RAI	radioactive iodine
GH	growth hormone	RIA	radioimmunoassay
GTT	glucose tolerance test	T_3	triiodothyronine
IDDM	insulin-dependent diabetes mellitus	T_4	thyroxine
K^+	potassium	TFT	thyroid function test
LH	luteinizing hormone	TSH	thyroid-stimulating hormone
MSH	melanocyte-stimulating hormone		

CASE STUDY

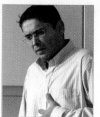

History of Present Illness

A 32-year-old male presented to ER thinking he was having a heart attack. States he monitors his blood pressure at home because he has hypertension and it has been higher than normal today. Also reports elevated heart rate, heart palpitations, diaphoresis, hand tremors, and extreme anxiety. States his father died of heart attack in his 50s, and he is quite concerned he is having a heart attack.

Past Medical History

Tonsillectomy at age 7. Fractured right femur at age 12 in bicycle accident. Appendectomy at age 19. Currently taking blood pressure medication for mild hypertension.

Social and Family History

Patient has a sedentary job at an accounting firm. Works out three times a week for weight control. He does not smoke and reports drinking about three beers per week. He is married with no children. Father died at age 52 from myocardial infarction. Mother is alive and well.

Physical Examination

Male patient who appears stated age. He is alert and answers all questions appropriately. BP is 184/98, pulse is 110 bpm, RR is 22 breaths/min. Height is 5'11", and weight is 220 lb. He is sweating profusely. He denies any dyspnea; however, patient appears very anxious and unable to sit or lie still on examination table.

Diagnostic Procedures

EKG, cardiac enzymes, and CXR were normal.
Blood tests show increased epinephrine.
Abdominal MRI reveals tumor in right adrenal medulla.

Diagnosis

Probable pheochromocytoma, right adrenal medulla

Plan of Treatment

1. Additional medication to control hypertension and slow down heart rate was started
2. Scheduled appointment with endocrinologist for follow-up care consisting of biopsy to verify diagnosis and determine whether tumor is malignant or benign, continued medical control of symptoms, and surgical removal of tumor

Critical Thinking Questions

Answer the following questions regarding this case study. Do not just copy words out of the case study; translate all medical terms. To answer some of these questions, you may need to look up information from another chapter of this text, in a medical dictionary, or online. Answers are found at the back of the book.

1. List and briefly describe each of the patient's presenting symptoms in the ER.

_____

_____

2. Which of the following is NOT part of this patient's medical history?

   a. Broken arm bone   c. Removal of appendix

   b. Removal of tonsils   d. High blood pressure

3. Read the information found at the following National Institute of Health website, http://www.nlm .nih.gov/medlineplus/ency/article/002341.htm, and look up the normal range for blood pressure, respiratory rate, and heart rate.

_____

_____

4. Define the following abbreviations: ER, EKG, CXR, BP, and bpm.

_____

_____

5. The patient's denial of dyspnea was noted; define the term.

_____

_____

6. What is the difference between malignant and benign?

_____

_____

7. What are the two purposes for performing a biopsy?

_____

_____

8. What is the term to describe the surgical removal of the adrenal gland?

_____

_____

Sound It Out

The following are some of the key terms from this chapter written as their phonetic spelling. Sound out each term and write it in the blank. Pronunciations for all terms are included in the audio glossary at www.mymedicalterminologylab.com <http://www.mymedicalterminologylab.com/>.

1. thigh-roh-MEG-ah-lee _____

2. AD-eh-no-mah-LAY-she-ah _____

3. ad-ree-noh-MEG-ah-lee _____

4. an-tye-dye-yoo-RET-ik _____

5. al-DOSS-ter-ohn _____

6. kor-tih-koh-STAIR-oydz _____

7. PAN-kree-ah-TYE-tis _____

8. KREE-tin-izm _____

9. pair-ah-thigh-royd-EK-toh-mee _____

10. DWARF-izm _____

11. ak-roh-MEG-ah-lee _____

12. en-doh-krin-ALL-oh-jee _____

13. ep-ih-NEF-rin _____

14. eks-off-THAL-mohs _____

15. GLOO-koh-gon _____

16. ad-ree-nal-EK-toh-mee _____

17. glye-kohs-YOO-ree-ah _____

18. GOY-ter _____

19. or-kee-EK-toh-mee _____

20. HIGH-per-pih-TOO-ih-tuh-rizm _____

21. IN-suh-lin _____

22. mel-ah-TOH-nin _____

23. miks-eh-DEE-mah _____

24. HIGH-poh-pair-ah-THIGH-royd-izm _____

25. JYE-gan-tizm _____

26. oh-OFF-or-oh-PLAS-tee _____

27. high-poh-THIGH-royd-izm _____

28. pol-ee-YOO-ree-ah _____

29. OR-kee-oh-PECK-see _____

30. oh-VAIR-ee-an _____

31. ox-see-TOH-sin _____

32. PAN-kree-ass _____

33. PAN-kree-ah-TEK-toh-mee _____

34. HIGH-per-gli-SEE-mee-ah _____

35. pan-kree-AT-ik _____

36. en-doh-krin-OP-ah-thee _____

37. fee-oh-kroh-moh-sigh-TOH-ma _____

38. PIN-ee-ah-LEK-toh-mee _____

39. try-eye-oh-doh-THIGH-roh-neen _____

40. pol-ee-DIP-see-ah _____

41. proh-LAK-tin _____

42. tes-TIK-yoo-lar _____

43. TET-ah-nee _____

44. thigh-MY-tis _____

45. thigh-MOH-sin _____

46. ah-DREE-nall _____

47. thigh-royd-EK-toh-mee _____

48. thigh-roh-toks-ih-KOH-sis _____

49. oh-off-oh-REK-toh-mee _____

50. thigh-ROKS-in _____

Transcription Practice

Each of the following sentences is written in common English. Underline any words or phrases that can be replaced by a medical term. Then rewrite the entire sentence using medical terms. Answers are found at the end of the book.

1. Gladys' blood test taken after she was given a dose of glucose confirmed the diagnosis of chronic disorder of sugar metabolism.

   _____

   _____

2. When Dr. Nguyen noted protruding eyeballs, she suspected a condition resulting from hypersecretion of thyroid hormones.

   _____

   _____

3. A surgical removal of the adrenal gland was necessary to treat the benign tumor of the adrenal medulla secreting excessive amounts of epinephrine.

   _____

   _____

4. Insufficient parathyroid gland (secretion) condition is one cause of nerve irritability resulting from hypocalcemia.

   _____

   _____

5. Two diagnostic tests were ordered: a scanned image of the thyroid gland after administering radioactive iodine and a blood test to measure levels of thyroxine, triiodothyronine, and thyroid-stimulating hormone.

   _____

   _____

6. Hypersecretion of growth hormone produces excessive body growth in a child or teenager, and lack of growth hormone can produce excessive shortness in height.

   _____

   _____

7. A person with a condition caused by insufficient antidiuretic hormone often has excessive thirst and frequent urination.

   _____

   _____

8. When Mrs. Ruiz developed facial hair and a deeper voice, a condition in which male secondary sexual characteristics appear in a female was suspected.

   _____

   _____

9. Adrenal cortex hormones with strong anti-inflammatory action were prescribed for the patient with rheumatoid arthritis.

   _____

   _____

10. Mr. McDonald's enlarged adrenal gland was caused by a cancerous glandular tumor.

    _____

    _____

Build Medical Terms

Use each of the following word parts to build the indicated medical terms.

The combining form *thyroid/o* means thyroid gland.

1. thyroid gland pertaining to _____

2. thyroid gland inflammation _____

3. thyroid gland surgical removal _____

4. excessive thyroid gland condition _____

5. insufficient thyroid gland condition _____

The combining form *glyc/o* means sugar.

6. excessive sugar blood condition _____

7. insufficient sugar condition _____

The prefix *poly-* means too much.

8. too much thirst _____

9. too much urine condition _____

The combining form *aden/o* means gland.

10. gland cancer tumor _____

11. gland resembling _____

12. gland softening _____

The combining form *pancreat/o* means pancreas.

13. pancreas pertaining to _____

14. pancreas inflammation _____

15. pancreas cutting into _____

PEARSON
mymedicalterminologylab

MyMedicalTerminologyLab is a premium online homework management system that includes a host of features to help you study. Registered users will find:

- Fun games and activities built within a virtual hospital
- Powerful tools that track and analyze your results—allowing you to create a personalized learning experience
- Videos, flashcards, and audio pronunciations to help enrich your progress
- Streaming lesson presentations and self-paced learning modules
- A space where you and your instructors can view and manage your assignments

Labeling Exercise

Write the name of each structure on the numbered line. Also use this space to write the combining form where appropriate.

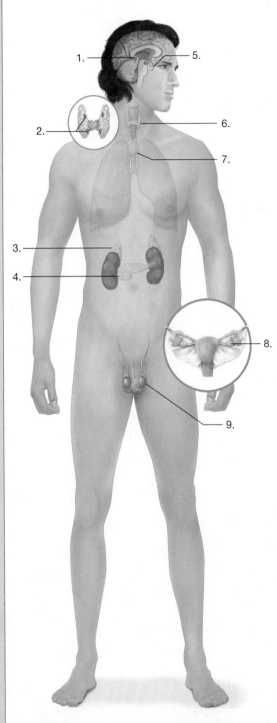

1._____

2._____

3._____

4._____

5._____

6._____

7._____

8._____

9._____

Spelling

Some of the following terms are misspelled. Identify the incorrect terms and spell them correctly in the blank provided.

1. hyperthyroidism _____

2. ovariocentesus _____

3. myxadema _____

4. pheochromocytoma _____

5. radioimmunoassay _____

6. teteny _____

7. exopthalmos _____

8. dwarfism _____

9. corticosteroids _____

10. virilizm _____

Fill in the Blank

Fill in the blank to complete each of the following sentences.

1. The endocrine system plays a vital role in maintaining a stable internal body environment referred to as _____.

2. Endocrine glands secrete chemical messengers called _____, which travel through the bloodstream to reach their _____.

3. Having too much of a hormone is called _____; having too little is called

   _____.

4. The adrenal glands sit on top of each _____ and are divided into the outer adrenal _____ and the inner adrenal _____.

5. _____ is secreted by the ovary and regulates the _____ cycle.

6. The two hormones secreted by the pancreas are _____ and _____.

7. Parathyroid hormone works to raise blood levels of _____.

8. The pineal gland secretes _____ that works to regulate the body's

   _____ rhythm.

9. The _____ gland is often referred to as the *master gland.*

10. The _____ gland is important for normal development of the immune system.

Abbreviation Matching

Match each abbreviation with its definition.

_____ **1.** PRL   **A.** noninsulin-dependent diabetes mellitus

_____ **2.** RAI   **B.** radioimmunoassay

_____ **3.** Na$^+$ **C.** radioactive iodine

_____ **4.** TFT   **D.** thyroxine

_____ **5.** RIA   **E.** prolactin

_____ **6.** LH   **F.** antidiuretic hormone

_____ **7.** T$_4$ **G.** fasting blood sugar

_____ **8.** NIDDM   **H.** sodium

_____ **9.** FBS   **I.** luteinizing hormone

_____ **10.** ADH   **J.** thyroid function test

Medical Term Analysis

Examine each of the following terms. Begin by dividing it into its word parts and writing them in the indicated blanks (**P = prefix, WR = word root; CF = combining form; S = suffix**). Follow with the definition of each word part and then finally the meaning of the full term.

1. orchiopexy

CF _____

means _____

S _____

means _____

Term Meaning: _____

_____

2. thyromegaly

CF _____

means _____

S _____

means _____

Term Meaning: _____

_____

3. adenocarcinoma

CF _____

means _____

WR _____

means _____

S _____

means _____

Term Meaning: _____

_____

4. **hypoparathyroidism**

P _____

means _____

WR _____

means _____

S _____

means _____

Term Meaning: _____

_____

5. **thyrotoxicosis**

CF _____

means _____

WR _____

means _____

S _____

means _____

Term Meaning: _____

_____

6. **pinealectomy**

WR _____

means _____

S _____

means _____

Term Meaning: _____

_____

7. **ovariorrhexis**

CF _____

means _____

S _____

means _____

Term Meaning: _____

_____

8. **thymitis**

WR _____

means _____

S _____

means _____

Term Meaning: _____

_____

9. **hyperglycemia**

P _____

means _____

WR _____

means _____

S _____

means _____

Term Meaning: _____

_____

10. **oophoroplasty**

CF _____

means _____

S _____

means _____

Term Meaning: _____

_____

Photomatch Challenge

This illustration shows the pituitary gland and its target organs. For each target, give its combining form. On the second line build the medical term.

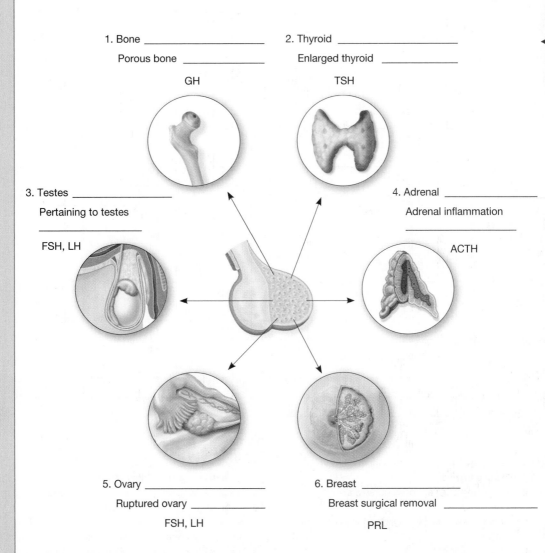

1. Bone _____

   Porous bone _____

   GH

2. Thyroid _____

   Enlarged thyroid _____

   TSH

3. Testes _____

   Pertaining to testes

   _____

   FSH, LH

4. Adrenal _____

   Adrenal inflammation

   _____

   ACTH

5. Ovary _____

   Ruptured ovary _____

   FSH, LH

6. Breast _____

   Breast surgical removal _____

   PRL

Crossword Puzzle

Use the definitions given to complete the crossword puzzle.

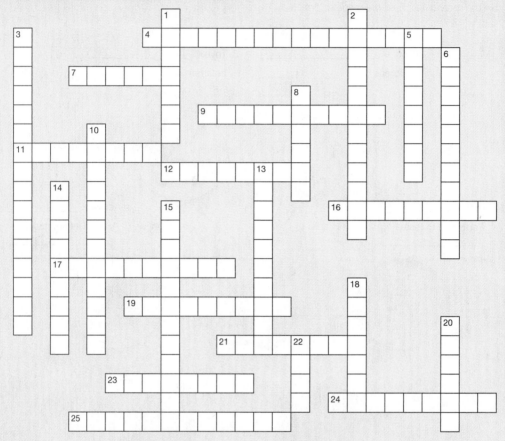

ACROSS

4 Usually benign tumor of adrenal medulla
7 Enlarged thyroid gland
9 Excessive growth of bones of head and extremities
11 Condition with swollen facial features and puffy, dry skin
12 Pancreas secretes insulin and _____
16 Excessive growth of entire body
17 Term meaning excessive thirst
19 _____ gland, also called master gland
21 Short body due to lack of growth hormone
23 Hormone secreted by thymus gland
24 Hormone secreted by pineal gland
25 Male sex hormone

DOWN

1 Hashimoto disease affects the _____ gland
2 Term meaning insufficient blood sugar level
3 Test measures levels of hormones in blood
5 Diabetes _____, one cause in insufficient insulin
6 Hormone secreted by adrenal medulla
8 Nerve irritability and painful muscle cramps
10 Term meaning softening of a gland
13 Term meaning sugar in the urine
14 Diabetes _____, caused by insufficient antidiuretic hormone
15 Protruding eyeballs
18 Chemical messenger secreted by endocrine glands
20 A thyroid scan uses radioactive _____
22 Number of parathyroid glands

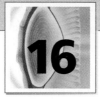

Ophthalmology
The Eye

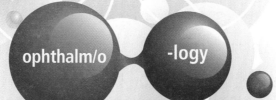

ophthalm/o   -logy

A Brief Introduction to Ophthalmology

 UNDERSTAND the function of the eye.

The **eyeball** is one of our special sense organs and is responsible for **vision.** Light rays entering the eyeball travel through the **cornea, pupil, iris, lens,** and land on the **retina** to produce an image. The image is then carried to the brain by the **optic nerve.** Accessory organs provide protection for the eye and include the **conjunctiva, eyelids,** and **lacrimal glands.** The two medical specialties providing eye care are ophthalmology and optometry. There is some degree of confusion regarding the difference in these two professions.

DESCRIBE the medical specialty of ophthalmology.

Ophthalmology is the diagnosis and treatment of diseases and conditions of the eye and vision. **Ophthalmologists** are medical doctors (MD or DO) who have completed at least four years of specialized training after completing medical school. They are involved in all aspects of eye care including vision examinations, corrective lens prescription, diagnosis and treatment of eye diseases and conditions, and eye surgery.

An **optometrist** obtains a doctor of optometry (OD) degree after completing four years at a school of optometry. **Optometry** specializes in assessing vision and prescribing corrective lens, treating glaucoma, corneal damage, and visual skill problems, providing pre and post-surgical care, as well as screening for other eye diseases.

Ophthalmology Combining Forms

The following list presents new combining forms important for building and defining ophthalmology terms.

aque/o	water		lacrim/o	tears
blephar/o	eyelid		ocul/o	eye
choroid/o	choroid layer		ophthalm/o	eye
conjunctiv/o	conjunctiva		opt/o	eye, vision
core/o	pupil		phac/o	lens
corne/o	cornea		pupill/o	pupil
cycl/o	ciliary body		retin/o	retina
dacry/o	tears		scler/o	sclera
ir/o	iris		ton/o	tension, pressure
irid/o	iris		vitre/o	glassy
kerat/o	cornea			

The following list presents combining forms that are not specific to the eye but are also used for building and defining ophthalmology terms.

aden/o	gland		dipl/o	double
ambly/o	dull or dim		myc/o	fungus
angi/o	vessel		nas/o	nose
chrom/o	color		phot/o	light
cry/o	cold		xer/o	dry
cyst/o	sac			

Suffix Review

These suffixes and prefixes were introduced in Chapters 2 and 3. They are being reviewed in this chapter because they are especially important for building ophthalmology terms.

-al	pertaining to		-logist	one who studies
-ar	pertaining to		-logy	study of
-ary	pertaining to		-lysis	destruction
-ectomy	surgical removal		-malacia	softening
-graphy	process of recording		-meter	instrument to measure
-ia	state, condition		-metry	process of measuring
-ic	pertaining to		-opia	vision
-ician	specialist		-osis	abnormal condition
-itis	inflammation		-otomy	cutting into
-lith	stone		-ous	pertaining to

-pathy	disease		**-ptosis**	drooping
-pexy	surgical fixation		**-rrhea**	flow
-phobia	fear		**-sclerosis**	hardening
-plasty	surgical repair		**-scope**	instrument to view
-plegia	paralysis		**-scopy**	process of viewing

Prefix Review

a–	without		**hyper–**	excessive
an–	without		**intra–**	within
hemi–	half		**micro–**	small

 IDENTIFY the structures treated in ophthalmology.

Structures of the Eye and Orbit

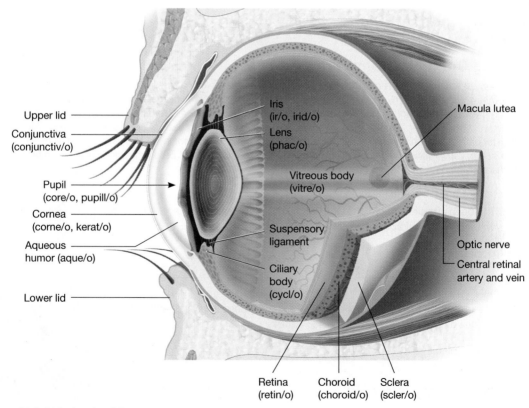

Upper lid

Conjunctiva
(conjunctiv/o)

Pupil
(core/o, pupill/o)

Cornea
(corne/o, kerat/o)

Aqueous
humor (aque/o)

Lower lid

Iris
(ir/o, irid/o)

Lens
(phac/o)

Vitreous body
(vitre/o)

Suspensory
ligament

Ciliary
body
(cycl/o)

Macula lutea

Optic nerve

Central retinal
artery and vein

Retina
(retin/o)

Choroid
(choroid/o)

Sclera
(scler/o)

>16.1 Sagittal section of the eye

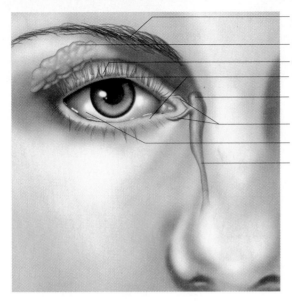

Eyebrow

Lacrimal (tear) gland (lacrim/o)

Cilia

Eyelid (blephar/o)

Lacrimal sac

Lacrimal canals

Eyeball (ocul/o, ophthalm/o)

Nasolacrimal duct
(drains into the nasal cavity)

>16.2 Anterior view of the eye orbit

BUILD ophthalmology medical terms from word parts.

Building Ophthalmology Terms

This section presents word parts most often used to build ophthalmology terms. Following the explanation of the term you have the opportunity to begin the process of building your own vocabulary. Read the meaning for each term and then fill in the blanks to build a single medical term. Use the slashes to divide prefixes, word roots, combining vowels, and suffixes. To help you out you will find a key to the word parts underneath the blanks: r for word roots, p for prefix, cv for combining vowel, and s for suffix. Remember that not every term will contain all these word parts; it's up to you to decide which to use. As you gain experience this process becomes easier. Answers can be found at the back of the book.

1. **aque/o**—combining form meaning **water**

    The open areas of the eye anterior to the lens are filled areas of eye anterior to the lens is filled with watery fluid called **aqueous humor**

    a. pertaining to water

    _____/_____
                  r   s

2. **blephar/o**—combining form meaning **eyelid**

    The upper and lower eyelids are folds of skin that close to protect anterior surface of eyeball; eyelashes are called **cilia**

    a. drooping eyelid

    _____/_____/_____
           r   cv   s

    b. surgical repair of the eyelid

    _____/_____/_____
           r   cv   s

    c. eyelid paralysis

    _____/_____/_____
           r   cv   s

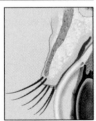

>16.3 **The eye lid**

3. **choroid/o**–combining form meaning **choroid layer**

The choroid layer is the middle layer of the wall of eyeball; contains many blood vessels

a. pertaining to choroid layer _____/_____
  <small>r</small>   <small>s</small>

b. choroid layer inflammation _____/_____
  <small>r</small>   <small>s</small>

4. **conjunctiv/o**–combining form meaning **conjunctiva**

The conjunctiva is a mucous membrane that protects anterior surface of eyeball and turns underneath to line eyelids

a. conjunctiva inflammation _____/_____
  <small>r</small>   <small>s</small>

b. pertaining to conjunctiva _____/_____
  <small>r</small>   <small>s</small>

5. **core/o**–combining form meaning **pupil**

The pupil is the opening in the center of the iris; becomes larger or smaller to control amount of light entering inside of eyeball

a. instrument to measure to pupil _____/____/_____
  <small>r</small>   <small>cv</small>   <small>s</small>

b. process of measuring pupil _____/____/_____
  <small>r</small>   <small>cv</small>   <small>s</small>

6. **corne/o**–combining form meaning **cornea**

The cornea is the anterior portion of the sclera; transparent to allow light through and curved to bend light rays so that they focus on retina

a. pertaining to cornea _____/_____
  <small>r</small>   <small>s</small>

>16.4 The cornea

7. **cycl/o**–combining form meaning **ciliary body**

The ciliary body is a ring of muscle around outer edge of lens; attached to lens by **suspensory ligaments;** pulls on edges of lens to change its shape to focus image onto retina

a. ciliary body paralysis _____/____/_____
  <small>r</small>   <small>cv</small>   <small>s</small>

b. cutting into ciliary body _____/_____
  <small>r</small>   <small>s</small>

8. **dacry/o**–combining form meaning **tear**

Tears are the watery fluid secreted by lacrimal glands that moisten and cleanse anterior surface of eyeball; **lacrimal glands** are located superior and lateral to eyeball and under orbital bone; tears collect in corner of eye and flow through **lacrimal canals** to **lacrimal sac**

a. tear stone _____/____/_____
  <small>r</small>   <small>cv</small>   <small>s</small>

b. tear flow _____/____/_____
  <small>r</small>   <small>cv</small>   <small>s</small>

c. tear gland inflammation

_____/_____/_____/_____
r   CV   r   s

d. tear sac inflammation

_____/_____/_____/_____
r   CV   r   s

---

9. **ir/o**–combining form meaning **iris**

    The iris is the colored portion of eye; made of muscle and contracts or relaxes to change size of pupil

    a. iris inflammation

_____/_____
r   s

---

10. **irid/o**–combining form meaning **iris**

    a. iris paralysis

_____/_____/_____
r   CV   s

    b. cutting into iris

_____/_____
r   s

---

11. **kerat/o**–combining form meaning **cornea**

    a. instrument to measure cornea

_____/_____/_____
r   CV   s

    b. process of measuring cornea

_____/_____/_____
r   CV   s

    c. surgical removal of cornea

_____/_____
r   s

    d. cornea inflammation

_____/_____
r   s

    e. cutting into cornea

_____/_____
r   s

    f. surgical repair of cornea

_____/_____/_____
r   CV   s

---

12. **lacrim/o**–combining form meaning **tears**

    a. pertaining to tears

_____/_____
r   s

    b. pertaining to nose and tears

_____/_____/_____/_____
r   CV   r   s

---

13. **ocul/o**–combining form meaning **eye**

    The eye is a complex sensory organ that allows us to see; hollow sphere; wall of eye composed of three layers: **sclera, choroid,** and **retina**

    a. pertaining to inside eye

_____/_____/_____
p   r   s

    b. abnormal condition of eye fungus

_____/_____/_____/_____
r   CV   r   s

    c. pertaining to eye

_____/_____
r   s

---

14. **ophthalm/o**–combining form meaning **eye**

    a. pertaining to eye

        _____/_____
                  r   s

    b. study of eye

        _____/_____/_____
                  r   cv   s

    c. one who studies eye

        _____/_____/_____
                  r   cv   s

    d. instrument for visually examining eye

        _____/_____/_____
                  r   cv   s

    e. process of visually examining eye

        _____/_____/_____
                  r   cv   s

    f. eye paralysis

        _____/_____/_____
                  r   cv   s

    g. dry eye state/condition

        _____/_____/_____
            r   r   s

---

15. **-opia**–suffix meaning **vision**

    a. without half of vision

        _____/_____/_____
                  p   p   s

    b. double vision

        _____/_____
                  r   s

---

16. **opt/o**–combining form meaning **vision**

    a. pertaining to vision

        _____/_____
                  r   s

    b. instrument to measure vision

        _____/_____/_____
                  r   cv   s

    c. process of measuring vision

        _____/_____/_____
                  r   cv   s

---

17. **phac/o**–combining form meaning **lens**

    The lens is a transparent structure lying behind iris and pupil; bends light rays passing through it so that they are focused on retina

    a. softening of lens

        _____/_____/_____
                  r   cv   s

    b. destruction of lens

        _____/_____/_____
                  r   cv   s

>**16.5 The lens**

    c. hardening of lens

        _____/_____/_____
                  r   cv   s

18. **pupill/o**–combining form meaning **pupil**

    a. pertaining to pupil

    _____/_____
                       _r_   _s_

    b. instrument to measure pupil

    _____/___/_____
               _r_   _cv_   _s_

19. **retin/o**–combining form meaning **retina**

The retina is the inner layer of eyeball; contains light receptors called **rods** and **cones;** rods function in dim light and see in gray tones, cones see color in bright light; area on posterior wall of eyeball, directly opposite lens, called **macula lutea;** small pit in center of macula called **fovea centralis** contains only cones and is point of clearest vision

    a. pertaining to retina

    _____/_____
             _r_   _s_

    b. retina disease

    _____/___/_____
          _r_   _cv_   _s_

    c. retina inflammation

    _____/_____
            _r_   _s_

    d. surgical fixation of retina using cold

    _____/___/_____/___/___
       _r_   _cv_   _r_   _cv_ _s_

20. **scler/o**–combining form meaning **sclera**

The sclera is the outermost layer of eye, commonly called *white of eye;* very fibrous and tough

    a. pertaining to sclera

    _____/_____
             _r_   _s_

    b. cutting into sclera

    _____/_____
             _r_   _s_

    c. softening of sclera

    _____/___/_____
          _r_   _cv_   _s_

    d. sclera inflammation

    _____/_____
             _r_   _s_

21. **ton/o**–combining form meaning **tension, pressure**

    a. instrument to measure pressure

    _____/___/_____
          _r_   _cv_   _s_

    b. process of measuring pressure

    _____/___/_____
          _r_   _cv_   _s_

22. **vitre/o**–combining form meaning **glassy**

This combining form refers to the gel-like shiny substance, **vitreous humor,** that fills large open cavity between lens and retina

    a. pertaining to glassy

    _____/_____
             _r_   _s_

Ophthalmology Vocabulary

The ophthalmology terms presented in this section include eponyms, modern English words, and those that contain Latin or Greek word parts but are not constructed solely from these word parts. When you recognize word parts within a term they will give you a hint about the word's meaning. In these instances, look for the word parts to follow the term.

Term	Explanation
accommodation (Acc)	Ability of eye to adjust to variations in distance
achromatopsia a– = without chrom/o = color	Profound inability to see in color from birth; also called *color blindness*

Term	Explanation	
amblyopia ambyl/o = dim **-opia** = vision	Loss of vision not due to any disease; not correctable with glasses; persons with amblyopia wear a patch over one eye to force affected eye to work; commonly called *lazy eye*	

>16.6 Young girls wearing eye patches under their glasses. The patch covers the strong eye to force the "lazy eye" to work
Source: Courtesy of the National Eye Institute, www.nei.nih.gov

astigmatism (Astigm)	Uneven bending of light rays caused by irregular curvature of cornea; image is fuzzy; corrected with cylindrical lenses

➕ TERMINOLOGY TIDBIT

The term *astigmatism* comes from the Greek word *stigma* meaning "point" combined with the prefix *a-* meaning "without." "Without a point" describes the fuzzy vision characteristic of astigmatism.

cataract	Lens becomes cloudy or opaque; results in whole vision field becoming blurry; treatment is usually surgical removal of cataract and replacement of lens with artificial lens

>16.7 Photograph of a woman with a cataract in her right eye

color vision tests	Use of multicolored charts to determine ability of patient to recognize color

>16.8 Color vision test. A person with red-green color blindness will not be able to see the green 27 embedded in the red colored circles

Term	Explanation
corneal abrasion **corne/o** = cornea **-al** = pertaining to	Scraping away of outer layer of cornea
cryoextraction **cry/o** = cold	Procedure to remove cataract from lens with extremely cold probe
diabetic retinopathy **retin/o** = retina **-pathy** = disease	Development of small hemorrhages and edema in retina as result of diabetes mellitus; dark spots appear in visual field; laser surgery can be necessary for treatment
fluorescein	Bright green fluorescent dye dropped onto surface of eyeball to highlight corneal abrasions
fluorescein angiography **angi/o** = vessel **-graphy** = process of recording	Procedure using intravenous bright green fluorescent dye, fluorescein, to examine movement of blood through blood vessels of eye
glaucoma	Condition resulting from increase in intraocular pressure, which, if untreated, can result in atrophy of optic nerve and blindness; patient notices that vision becomes blurry around edges; treated with medication and surgery

+ TERMINOLOGY TIDBIT

The term *glaucoma* comes from the Greek word *glaukos* meaning "grey-green." The inside of the eyeball appears grey-green when viewed through the pupil.

hyperopia **hyper–** = excessive **-opia** = vision	Visual condition in which person can see things in distance but has trouble reading material at close range; also known as *farsightedness;* corrected by convex lens

Hyperopia (farsightedness)

Corrected with biconvex lens

>**16.9** Hyperopia (farsightedness). In the uncorrected top figure, the image comes into focus behind the retina, making the image on the retina blurry. The bottom image shows how a biconvex lens corrects this condition

intraocular lens (IOL) implant
intra– = within
ocul/o = eye
-ar = pertaining to

Replacing defective natural lens with artificial lens following cataract extraction

Corneal incision
Lens and entire capsule removed
Pupil
Suspensory ligaments cut
Iris
Intraocular lens implanted in anterior chamber (in front of pupil and iris)

>16.10 (A) Damaged lens is removed and (B) prosthetic lens is implanted

A Cataract extraction **B Intraocular lens transplant**

---

laser-assisted in-situ keratomileusis (LASIK)
kerat/o = cornea

Correction of myopia using laser surgery to remove minute slices of corneal tissue

➕ TERMINOLOGY TIDBIT

The term *keratomileusis* comes from combining the Greek terms *kerato* meaning "cornea" and *smileusis* meaning "carving." This describes the procedure of using a laser to shave off minute pieces of the cornea.

---

laser retinal photocoagulation
retin/o = retina
-al = pertaining to
phot/o = light

Using laser to make pinpoint scars to stabilize detached or torn retina

---

macular degeneration

Deterioration of macula lutea of retina; patient notices loss of vision in center of visual field

---

myopia (MY)
-opia = vision

Visual condition in which person can see things close up but distance vision is blurred; also known as *nearsightedness;* corrected by concave lens

Myopia (nearsightedness)

Corrected with biconcave lens

>16.11 Myopia (nearsightedness). In the uncorrected top figure, the image comes into focus in front of the retina, making the image on the retina blurry. The bottom image shows how a biconcave lens corrects this condition

---

nyctalopia
-opia = vision

Poor vision at night or in dim light; commonly called *night blindness*

➕ TERMINOLOGY TIDBIT

The term *nyctalopia* comes from combining three Greek words: *nux* meaning "night," *alaos* meaning "blind," and *ops* meaning "eye."

---

nystagmus

Jerky-appearing involuntary eye movement

➕ TERMINOLOGY TIDBIT

The term *nystagmus* comes from the Greek word *nustagmos* meaning "nodding off." This compares the jerky back and forth eye movements to a nodding head.

Term	Explanation
optician opt/o = vision **-ician** = specialist	Health care professional trained to make corrective lenses and fit eyeglasses and contact lenses
phacoemulsification phac/o = lens	Use of high-frequency sound waves to break up cataract, which is then removed by suction with needle
photophobia phot/o = light **-phobia** = irrational fear	Excessive sensitivity to light leading to avoidance; not actual fear of light
photo-refractive keratectomy (PRK) phot/o = light kerat/o = cornea **-ectomy** = surgical removal	Use of laser to reshape cornea to improve visual acuity
radial keratotomy (RK) kerat/o = cornea **-otomy** = cutting into	Surgery with spokelike incisions in cornea to flatten it, done to correct nearsightedness
refractive error	Defect in ability of eye to bend light rays to focus image properly on fovea centralis (refraction); occurs in myopia and hyperopia
retinal detachment retin/o = retina **-al** = pertaining to	Occurs when retina becomes separated from choroid layer; this separation seriously damages blood vessels and nerves resulting in blindness

>16.12 Illustration of normal retina (A) and detached retina (B). Note "wavy" lines are caused by retina pulling away from the wall of the eyeball, losing its blood supply and dying

A Normal retina   **B** Detached retina

slit lamp microscope micro– = small **-scope** = instrument to view	Instrument used in ophthalmology for examining posterior surface of cornea

>16.13 Examination of the interior of the eye using a slit lamp microscope

Snellen chart	Chart used for testing visual acuity; contains letters of varying size and is given from distance of 20 feet; average person who can read at this distance is said to have 20/20 vision
strabismus	Weakness of external eye muscle; results in eyes looking in different directions at same time; can be corrected with glasses, eye exercises, and/or surgery; commonly called *cross eyed* if eye is turned toward the nose

>16.14 Illustration of child with strabismus in the right eye which turns in

TERMINOLOGY TIDBIT

The term *strabismus* comes from the Greek word *strabizein* meaning "to squint."

strabotomy **-otomy** = cutting into	Incision into eye muscles to correct strabismus
stye	Small purulent infection of sebaceous gland of eye treated with hot compresses and surgical incision; also called *hordeolum*
visual acuity test (VA)	Measurement of sharpness of patient's vision; usually, Snellen's chart is used for this test and patient identifies letters from distance of 20 feet; term, 20/20 vision, means person is able to see at 20 feet what normal person would expect to see at 20 feet; term such as 20/200 would indicate person's degree of myopia, that is, he or she must be 20 feet away from object to see it when "normal" person could see object from 200 feet away

USE ophthalmology abbreviations.

Ophthalmology Abbreviations

The list below presents common ophthalmology abbreviations.

Acc	accommodation	**Ophth.**	ophthalmology
Astigm	astigmatism	**OS**	left eye (oculus sinister)
c.gl.	correction with glasses	**OU**	both eyes (oculus uterque)
cyl	cylindrical lens	**PERRLA**	pupils equal, round, react to light and accommodation
D	diopter (lens strength)		
ECCE	extracapsular cataract extraction	**PRK**	photo-refractive keratectomy
ICCE	intracapsular cataract cryoextraction	**REM**	rapid eye movement
IOL	intraocular lens	**RK**	radial keratotomy
IOP	intraocular pressure	**s.gl.**	without correction or glasses
LASIK	laser-assisted in-situ keratomileusis	**VA**	visual acuity
MY	myopia	**VF**	visual field
OD	right eye (oculus dexter), doctor of optometry		

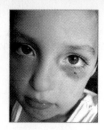

History of Present Illness

An 8-year-old boy was seen by an ophthalmologist in the ER following being struck in the right eye while playing basketball. Symptoms included pain, excessive tearing, decreased visual acuity, and photophobia.

Past Medical History

Fractured right femur in a bike accident at age 5. Hydrocele was surgically repaired shortly after birth with no further problems. Patient is taking no regular medications.

Family and Social History

Patient is a 3rd grade student. He is active in sports. Patient lives at home with his mother, father, and one older sister. All are healthy.

Physical Examination

Healthy-appearing 8-year-old male in obvious distress from inflamed right eye.

Diagnostic Tests

Snellen chart revealed visual acuity of 20/200 OD and 20/20 OS. A slit lamp microscope examination showed a conjunctival reddening in the right eye. Corneal examination after applying fluorescein dye revealed a 7-mm corneal abrasion. No ulcer was observed. Examination of the retina was unremarkable.

Diagnosis

Traumatic corneal abrasion in the right eye.

Plan of Treatment

1. Treat abrasion with antibiotic and pain with anesthetic eye drops
2. Use a lubricating ointment if his eye is too dry when he wakes up in the morning
3. Wear an eye patch if he is outside in the sun
4. See an ophthalmologist for a follow-up reexamination in 24 hrs

Critical Thinking Questions

Answer the following questions regarding this case study. Do not just copy words out of the case study, translate all medical terms. In order to answer some of these questions you may need to look up information from another chapter of this text, in a medical dictionary, or online. Answers are found at the back of the book.

1. List and describe the symptoms that brought this patient to the ER.

   _____

   _____

2. What is the common name for the bone this patient fractured at age 5?

   _____

   _____

3. Explain the results of the visual acuity examination.

   _____

   _____

4. Explain the purpose of using a fluorescein dye.

_____

_____

5. Fluorescein dye identified a corneal abrasion but no ulcer. Explain the difference between an abrasion and an ulcer.

_____

_____

6. Explain the purpose of each of the two medications used to treat the patient.

_____

_____

7. In addition to the medications, what additional recommendations were made?

_____

_____

Sound It Out

The following are some of the key terms from this chapter written as their phonetic spelling. Sound out each term and write it in the blank. Pronunciations for all terms are included in the audio glossary at www.mymedicalterminologylab.com <http://www.mymedicalterminologylab.com/>.

1. off-THAL-mik _____

2. KAIR-ah-toh-plass-tee _____

3. RET-in-al _____

4. koh-ROYD-al _____

5. ok-yoo-loh-my-KOH-sis _____

6. tone-OM-eh-ter _____

7. kon-junk-tih-VYE-tis _____

8. DAK-ree-oh-add-eh-NIGH-tis _____

9. op-TOM-eh-trist _____

10. ir-ih-DOT-oh-mee _____

11. dip-LOH-pee-ah _____

12. floo-oh-RESS-ee-in _____

13. ah-kroh-mah-TOP-see-ah _____

14. glau-KOH-mah _____

15. hem-ee-ah-NOP-ee-ah _____

16. ah-STIG-mah-tizm _____

17. blef-ah-rop-TOH-sis _____

18. high-per-OH-pee-ah _____

19. in-trah-OCK-yoo-lar _____

20. eye-RYE-tis _____

21. sklair-oh-mah-LAY-she-ah _____

22. off-thal-MOSS-koh-pee _____

23. kair-ah-TEK-toh-me _____

24. koh-ree-OM-eh-tree _____

25. cry-oh-RET-ih-noh-pek-see _____

26. off-THAL-mik _____

27. kair-ah-TYE-tis _____

28. am-blee-OH-pee-ah _____

29. kair-ah-TOT-oh-mee _____

30. LAK-rim-al _____

31. fak-oh-LYE-sis _____

32. my-OH-pee-ah _____

33. naz-oh-LAK-rim-al _____

34. KAT-ah-rakt _____

35. nik-tah-LOH-pee-ah _____

36. PYOO-pih-lair-ee _____

37. sigh-kloh-PLEE-jee-ah _____

38. KOR-nee-all _____

39. niss-TAG-mus _____

40. OCK-yoo-lar _____

41. op-TISH-an _____

42. fak-oh-skle-ROH-sis _____

43. AY-kwee-us _____

44. foh-toh-FOH-bee-ah _____

45. off-thal-moh-PLEE-jee-ah _____

46. SKLAIR-all _____

47. SIL-ee-ah _____

48. strah-BIZ-mus _____

49. hor-DEE-oh-lum _____

50. STIGH _____

Transcription Practice

Each sentence below is written in common English. Underline any words or phrases that can be replaced by a medical term. Then rewrite the entire sentence using medical terms. Answers can be found at the end of the text.

1. Dr. Cohen decided to use a procedure using an extremely cold probe to remove the patient's opaque lens rather than a procedure using high frequency sound waves.

   _____
   _____

2. Mr. Blair's nearsightedness was corrected by making spokelike incisions to flatten the cornea.

   _____
   _____

3. The head injury caused the inner layer of the eyeball to become separated from the choroids layer that required repair by using a device that emits an intense beam of light to make pinpoint scars.

_____

_____

4. Because the anterior portion of the sclera was abnormally curved, light rays were not evenly bent, resulting in a condition of distorted vision.

_____

_____

5. Examination of the eye with an instrument for viewing inside the eye did not reveal any reason for Mr. Mendez's fear of light.

_____

_____

6. Mrs. Capers made an appointment with the doctor of optometry because of an inflamed outer white layer of the eye and double vision.

_____

_____

7. The baby's mother was concerned about her infant when she noticed inflamed conjunctiva and excessive tear flow.

_____

_____

8. Mr. Carpenter decided that it was no longer safe for him to drive after he developed poor night vision and deterioration of the macula lutea.

_____

_____

9. A patient's sharpness of vision can be evaluated using a chart with letters of varying sizes.

_____

_____

10. A scrapping away of the outer layer of Karen's cornea occurred when sand became trapped under her contact lens that was identified by using bright green fluorescent dye.

_____

_____

Fill in the Blank

Fill in the blank to complete each of the following sentences.

1. _____ is the
   development of small hemorrhages and edema in the retina as a result of having diabetes mellitus.

2. _____ results from a chronic increase in intraocular pressure.

3. _____ was diagnosed using color vision tests.

4. Another word for stye _____.

5. Involuntary, jerky eye movements are called _____.

6. _____ is commonly referred to as *nearsightedness*.

7. A strabotomy is the surgical procedure that makes an incision in eye muscles to correct
   _____.

8. A _____ chart is used to test visual acuity.

9. _____ is commonly called *night blindness*.

10. In _____, light rays are bent unevenly due to an abnormally curved cornea.

Abbreviation Matching

Match each abbreviation with its definition.

_____ 1. OD   A. rapid eye movement

_____ 2. MY   B. intraocular lens

_____ 3. REM   C. diopter

_____ 4. s.gl.   D. cylindrical lens

_____ 5. D   E. right eye

_____ 6. ECCE   F. visual acuity

_____ 7. IOL   G. without correction or glasses

_____ 8. VA   H. age-related macular degeneration

_____ 9. ARMD   I. myopia

_____ 10. cyl   J. extracapsular cataract extraction

Labeling Exercise

Write the name of each structure on the numbered line. Also use this space to write the combining form where appropriate.

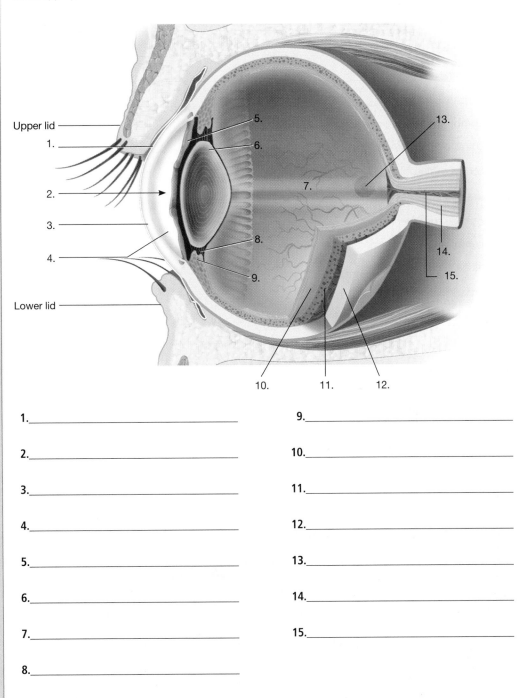

1. _____

2. _____

3. _____

4. _____

5. _____

6. _____

7. _____

8. _____

9. _____

10. _____

11. _____

12. _____

13. _____

14. _____

15. _____

Build Medical Terms

Use each of the following word parts to build the indicated medical terms.

The combining form ophthalm/o means eye.

1. study of eye _____

2. instrument to view inside eye _____

3. eye paralysis _____

4. pertaining to eye _____

The combining form kerat/o means cornea.

5. cornea surgical removal _____

6. cornea cutting into _____

7. instrument to measure cornea _____

8. cornea surgical repair _____

The combining form retin/o means retina.

9. retina disease _____

10. retina inflammation _____

The combining form blephar/o means eyelid.

11. eyelid surgical repair _____

12. eyelid paralysis _____

13. eyelid drooping _____

The suffix –opia means vision.

14. double vision _____

15. dim vision _____

mymedicalterminologylab

PEARSON

MyMedicalTerminologyLab is a premium online homework management system that includes a host of features to help you study. Registered users will find:

- Fun games and activities built within a virtual hospital
- Powerful tools that track and analyze your results—allowing you to create a personalized learning experience
- Videos, flashcards, and audio pronunciations to help enrich your progress
- Streaming lesson presentations and self-paced learning modules
- A space where you and your instructors can view and manage your assignments

Medical Term Analysis

*Examine each of the following terms. Begin by dividing it into its word parts and writing them in the indicated blanks (P = **prefix**, WR = **word root**; CF = **combining form**; S = **suffix**). Follow with the definition of each word part and then finally the meaning of the full term.*

1. **blepharoptosis**

   CF _____

   means _____

   S _____

   means _____

   Term Meaning: _____

   _____

2. **dacryoadenitis**

   CF _____

   means _____

   WR _____

   means _____

   S _____

   means _____

   Term Meaning: _____

   _____

3. **nasolacrimal**

   CF _____

   means _____

   WR _____

   means _____

   S _____

   means _____

   Term Meaning: _____

   _____

4. **intraocular**

   P _____

   means _____

   WR _____

   means _____

   S _____

   means _____

   Term Meaning: _____

   _____

5. **cryoretinopexy**

   CF _____

   means _____

   CF _____

   means _____

   S _____

   means _____

   Term Meaning: _____

   _____

6. **choroiditis**

   WR _____

   means _____

   S _____

   means _____

   Term Meaning: _____

   _____

7. keratoplasty

CF _____

means _____

S _____

means _____

Term Meaning: _____
_____

9. ophthalmoscope

CF _____

means _____

S _____

means _____

Term Meaning: _____
_____

8. optometry

CF _____

means _____

S _____

means _____

Term Meaning: _____
_____

10. phacosclerosis

CF _____

means _____

S _____

means _____

Term Meaning: _____
_____

Spelling

Some of the following terms are misspelled. Identify the incorrect terms and spell them correctly in the blank provided.

1. stie _____

2. nystagmus _____

3. hordoleum _____

4. miopia _____

5. nyctalopia _____

6. cryoextraction _____

7. dacrolith _____

8. oculomycosis _____

9. coreometer _____

10. strabismis _____

Photomatch Challenge

A person with no eye conditions would see the picture in the center. Examine each of the other photos and describe what the visual problem is. Then, referring to the Ophthalmology Vocabulary section for assistance, match each photo to its condition.

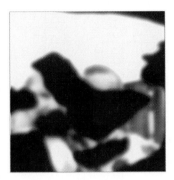

Source: National Eye Institute

1. Describe visual problem

_____

Pathology _____

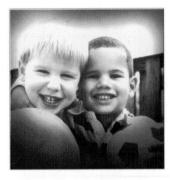

Source: National Eye Institute

2. Describe visual problem

_____

Pathology _____

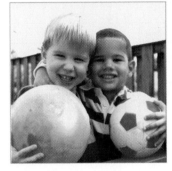

Source: National Eye Institute

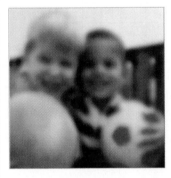

Source: National Eye Institute

3. Describe visual problem

_____

Pathology _____

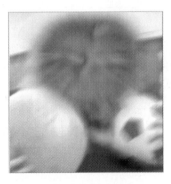

Source: National Eye Institute

4. Describe visual problem

_____

Pathology _____

Eye Conditions

- cataract
- diabetic retinopathy
- glaucoma
- macular degeneration

Crossword Puzzle

Use the definitions given to complete the crossword puzzle.

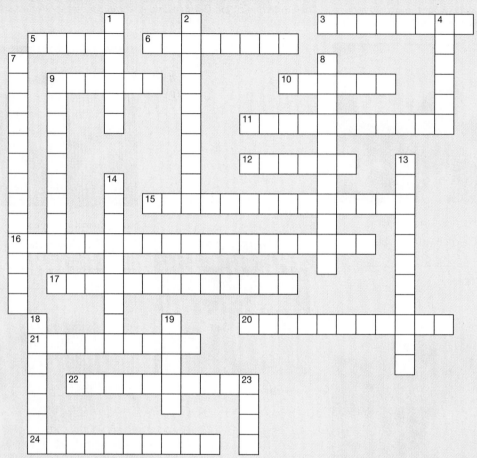

ACROSS

3 Condition caused by increased intraocular pressure
5 Eyelashes are also called _____
6 Specialist in making corrective lenses
9 Visual _____ measures sharpness of vision
10 Outer layer of eyeball
11 Fear of light
12 Slit lamp microscopy examines the _____
15 Procedure using cold to remove cataract
16 Use of sound waves to break up a cataract
17 Ability of eye to adjust to different distances
20 Condition caused by irregular curvature of cornea
21 Jerky involuntary eye movements
22 Condition caused by weakness of external eye muscle
24 Night blindness

DOWN

1 _____ keratotomy corrects myopia
2 Surgical procedure to correct strabismus
4 Nearsightedness
7 Color blindness
8 Bright green dye
9 Also called lazy eye
13 Mucous membrane protecting anterior eyeball
14 Farsightedness
18 A(n)_____ chart is used to test visual acuity
19 Opening in the iris
23 Also called hordeolum

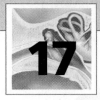

17

Otorhinolaryngology
The Ear, Nose, and Throat

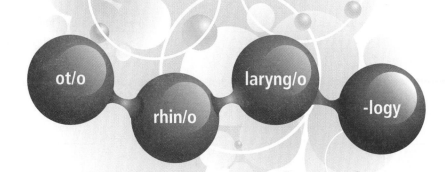

ot/o

rhin/o

laryng/o

-logy

A Brief Introduction to Otorhinolaryngology

 UNDERSTAND Understand the function of the ear, nose, and throat.

This medical specialty of **otorhinolaryngology (ENT)** focuses on a specific region of the body, the head, and the neck rather than on a whole body system, such as gastroenterology is to the gastrointestinal system or neurology is to the nervous system. As a group, the organs in the head and neck are responsible for two main functions: to house sensory receptors and to provide passageways for air, food, and drink.

These organs and their functions include the:

- **Ear**–hearing and equilibrium (balance)
- **Nose**–smell and entrance for air into the body
- **Pharynx**–carries air to the larynx and trachea, and food and drink to the esophagus
- **Larynx**–speech
- **Trachea**–brings air to the lungs

DESCRIBE the medical specialty of otorhinolaryngology.

Otorhinolaryngologists (ENTs, or ear, nose, and throat doctors) are physicians who specialize in diagnosing and treating conditions affecting these organs. A family physician or an internist can also treat these conditions, but the ENT physician is a specialist in treating problems with hearing, balance, swallowing, and voice as well as head and neck tumors and problems affecting the airways.

Otorhinolaryngology Combining Forms

The following list presents new combining forms important for building and defining otorhinolaryngology terms.

adenoid/o	adenoids	nas/o	nose
audi/o	hearing	ot/o	ear
audit/o	hearing	pharyng/o	pharynx (throat)
aur/o	ear	rhin/o	nose
cochle/o	cochlea	sinus/o	sinus
epiglott/o	epiglottis	tonsill/o	tonsils
laryng/o	larynx (voice box)	trache/o	trachea (windpipe)
myring/o	tympanic membrane (eardrum)	tympan/o	tympanic membrane (eardrum)

The following list presents combining forms that are not specific to the ear, nose, or throat but are also used for building and defining otorhinolaryngology terms.

gastr/o	stomach	neur/o	nerve
myc/o	fungus	py/o	pus

Suffix Review

These suffixes and prefixes were introduced in Chapters 2 and 3. They are being reviewed in this chapter because they are especially important suffixes in otorhinolaryngology terms.

-al	pertaining to	-ory	pertaining to
-algia	pain	-osis	abnormal condition
-ar	pertaining to	-osmia	smell
-eal	pertaining to	-otomy	cutting into
-ectomy	surgical removal	-phonia	voice
-gram	record	-plasty	surgical repair
-ic	pertaining to	-plegia	paralysis
-itis	inflammation	-rrhea	discharge, flow
-logist	one who studies	-rrhexis	rupture
-logy	study of	-sclerosis	hardening
-megaly	enlarged	-scope	instrument for viewing
-meter	instrument to measure	-scopy	process of viewing
-metry	process of measuring	-spasm	involuntary muscle contraction
-oma	tumor	-stenosis	narrowing

Prefix Review

a-	without	endo-	within
an-	without	pan-	all
de-	without	para-	alongside
dys-	difficult		

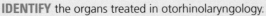
Organs Commonly Treated in Otorhinolaryngology

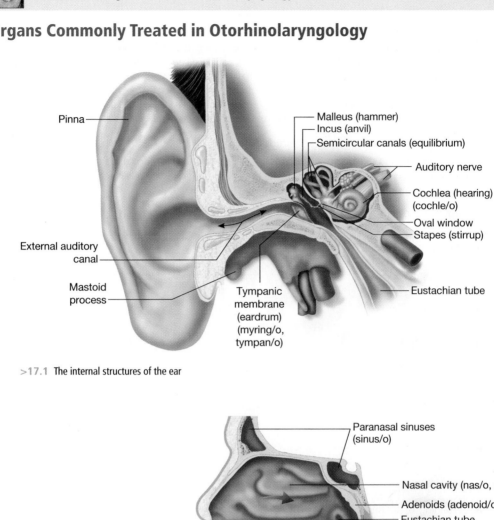

Pinna

Malleus (hammer)
Incus (anvil)
Semicircular canals (equilibrium)

Auditory nerve

Cochlea (hearing)
(cochle/o)

Oval window
Stapes (stirrup)

External auditory
canal

Mastoid
process

Tympanic
membrane
(eardrum)
(myring/o,
tympan/o)

Eustachian tube

>17.1 The internal structures of the ear

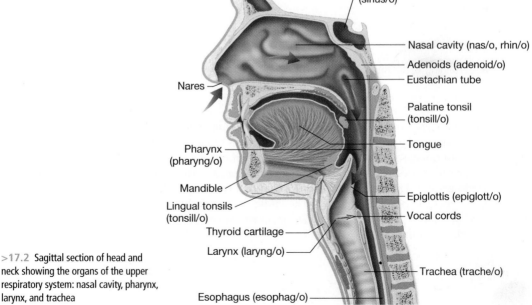

Paranasal sinuses
(sinus/o)

Nasal cavity (nas/o, rhin/o)
Adenoids (adenoid/o)
Eustachian tube

Nares

Palatine tonsil
(tonsill/o)

Tongue

Pharynx
(pharyng/o)

Mandible

Lingual tonsils
(tonsill/o)

Thyroid cartilage

Larynx (laryng/o)

Epiglottis (epiglott/o)
Vocal cords

Trachea (trache/o)

Esophagus (esophag/o)

>17.2 Sagittal section of head and
neck showing the organs of the upper
respiratory system: nasal cavity, pharynx,
larynx, and trachea

Building Otorhinolaryngology Terms

This section presents word parts most often used to build otorhinolaryngology terms. Following the explanation of the term, you have the opportunity to begin building your own vocabulary. Read the meaning for each term and then fill in the blanks to build a single medical term. Use the slashes to divide prefixes, word roots, combining vowels, and suffixes. To help you out you will find a key to the word parts underneath the blanks: r for word roots, p for prefix, cv for combining vowel, and s for suffix. Remember that not every term will contain all these word parts; it's up to you to decide which to use. As you gain experience, this process becomes easier. Answers can be found at the back of the book.

1. **adenoid/o**–combining form meaning **adenoids**

    The adenoids are one of three pairs of **tonsils** located in pharynx; also called **pharyngeal tonsils;** tonsils house large number of white blood cells that protect body by removing foreign invaders from air, food, and drink passing through pharynx

    a. surgical removal of adenoids   _____/_____
                                                   r   s

    b. adenoid inflammation   _____/_____
                                         r   s

2. **audi/o**–combining form meaning **hearing**

    a. study of hearing   _____/_____/_____
                                   r   cv   s

    b. one who studies hearing   _____/_____/_____
                                   r   cv   s

    c. process of measuring hearing   _____/_____/_____
                                   r   cv   s

    d. instrument to measure hearing   _____/_____/_____
                                   r   cv   s

    e. record of hearing   _____/_____/_____
                                   r   cv   s

3. **audit/o**–combining form meaning **hearing**

    a. pertaining to hearing   _____/_____
                                       r   s

4. **aur/o**–combining form meaning **ear**

    The ear is responsible for both **hearing** and **equilibrium** (balance); divided into **external ear, middle ear,** and **inner ear; pinna** (**auricle**) captures sound waves and funnels them into **external auditory canal;** sound waves strike **tympanic membrane** (eardrum) causing it to vibrate; three tiny bones (ossicles) in middle ear, the **malleus, incus,** and **stapes,** conduct this vibration across middle ear from tympanic membrane to **oval window;** oval window movement initiates vibrations in fluid inside inner ear; vibrating fluid bends hair cells in **cochlea,** which stimulates nerve endings; **auditory nerve** sends message to brain; inner ear also contains organs for equilibrium, **semicircular canals**

    a. pertaining to ear   _____/_____
                                     r   s

5. cochle/o–combining form meaning **cochlea**

The cochlea is part of the inner ear containing hair cells responsible for hearing; shaped like a coiled snail shell

>17.3 The cochlea

   a. pertaining to cochlea   _____/_____

                                                          r   s

---

6. epiglott/o–combining form meaning **epiglottis**

The epiglottis is a cartilage flap that sits above larynx; rotates to cover larynx with each swallow; prevents food or drink from entering larynx and trachea

>17.4 The epiglottis

   a. pertaining to epiglottis   _____/_____

                                                    r   s

   b. epiglottis inflammation   _____/_____

                                                  r   s

---

7. laryng/o–combining form meaning **larynx**

The larynx is commonly called the *voice box;* located between pharynx and trachea; contains **vocal cords** that vibrate as air passes through them to produce sound

   a. pertaining to larynx   _____/_____
                                               r   s

   b. larynx inflammation   _____/_____
                                             r   s

   c. process of visually examining larynx   _____/_____/_____
                                           r   CV   s

   d. instrument to visually examine larynx _____/_____/_____
                                           r   CV   s

   e. surgical removal of larynx   _____/_____
                                             r   s

   f. surgical repair of larynx   _____/_____/_____
                                           r   CV   s

   g. larynx paralysis   _____/_____/_____
                                           r   CV   s

   h. involuntary muscle contraction of larynx _____/_____/_____
                                           r   CV   s

---

8. myring/o–combining form meaning **tympanic membrane**

The tympanic membrane is commonly called the *eardrum*

   a. inflammation of eardrum   _____/_____
                                           r   s

   b. surgical removal of eardrum _____/_____
                                           r   s

   c. surgical repair of eardrum   _____/_____/_____
                                         r   CV   s

   d. hardening of eardrum   _____/_____/_____
                                         r   CV   s

   e. cutting into eardrum   _____/_____
                                         r   s

9. nas/o–combining form meaning **nose**

Air enters the nose through two openings called **nares,** passes through **nasal cavity,** and enters pharynx; divided down middle by cartilage plate called **nasal septum;** lined by **mucous membrane;** air is warmed, moisturized, and cleansed as it passes through; houses sensory receptors for sense of smell

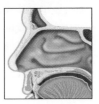

>17.5 The nose

a. pertaining to nose

_____/_____
r   s

b. pertaining to nose and stomach

_____/____/_____/_____
r   cv   r   s

c. pertaining to nose and throat

_____/____/_____/_____
r   cv   r   s

---

10. -osmia– suffix meaning **smell**

The sensory receptors for smell are located in roof of nasal cavity

a. without smell

_____/_____
p   s

---

11. ot/o–combining form meaning **ear**

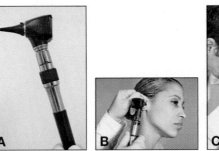
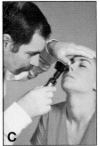
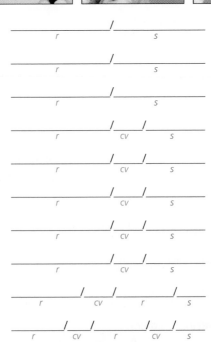

>17.6 An otoscope (A) can be used to examine both the ears (B) and nasal cavity (C)

a. pertaining to the ear

_____/_____
r   s

b. ear inflammation

_____/_____
r   s

c. ear pain

_____/_____
r   s

d. study of the ear

_____/____/_____
r   cv   s

e. one who studies the ear

_____/____/_____
r   cv   s

f. process of visually examining the ear

_____/____/_____
r   cv   s

g. instrument to visually examine the ear

_____/____/_____
r   cv   s

h. surgical repair of the ear

_____/____/_____
r   cv   s

i. abnormal condition or ear fungus

_____/____/_____/_____
r   cv   r   s

j. discharge of pus from the ear

_____/____/_____/____/_____
r   cv   r   cv   s

12. **pharyng/o**–combining form meaning **pharynx**

The pharynx is commonly called the *throat;* muscular tube receives air from nasal cavity and delivers it to larynx; also receives food from oral cavity and transports it to esophagus; location for three sets of tonsils (adenoids, **palatine tonsils,** and **lingual tonsils**); **Eustachian tube,** which opens with each swallow to equalize air pressure in middle ear, connects middle ear to pharynx

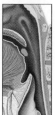

>17.7 The pharynx

   a. pertaining to the pharynx   _____/_____
                                                               r   *s*

   b. pharynx inflammation   _____/_____
                                                             r   *s*

   c. surgical repair of pharynx   _____/____/_____
                                                              r   *cv*   *s*

   d. involuntary muscle contraction of pharynx   _____/____/_____
                                                              r   *cv*   *s*

   e. cutting into pharynx   _____/_____
                                                              r   *s*

13. **-phonia**–suffix meaning **voice**

   a. without voice   _____/_____
                                              p   *s*

   b. difficult voice   _____/_____
                                            p   *s*

14. **rhin/o**–combining form meaning **nose**

   a. nose inflammation   _____/_____
                                          r   *s*

   b. surgical repair of nose   _____/____/_____
                                          r   *cv*   *s*

   c. discharge from nose   _____/____/_____
                                         r   *cv*   *s*

   d. abnormal condition of having nose fungus   _____/____/_____/____
                                            r   *cv*   *r*   *s*

15. **sinus/o**–combining form meaning **sinuses**

The **paranasal sinuses** (para- = alongside) are air-filled cavities located within facial bones and connected to nasal cavity; lined with mucous membrane; act as echo chamber for sound production

   a. sinus inflammation   _____/_____
                                         r   *s*

   b. inflammation of all sinuses   ____/_____/_____
                                     p   *r*   *s*

   c. nose and sinus inflammation   _____/____/_____/____
                                        r   *cv*   *r*   *s*

16. tonsill/o–combining form meaning **tonsils**

    a. pertaining to tonsils

                                _____ / _____
                                               r   *s*

    b. tonsil inflammation

                                  _____ / _____
                                             r   *s*

    c. surgical removal of tonsils

                                  _____ / _____
                                             r   *s*

---

17. trache/o–combining form meaning **trachea**

The trachea is commonly called the *windpipe;* tube that carries air from larynx to lungs; lined with mucous membrane that warms, moisturizes, and cleanses air

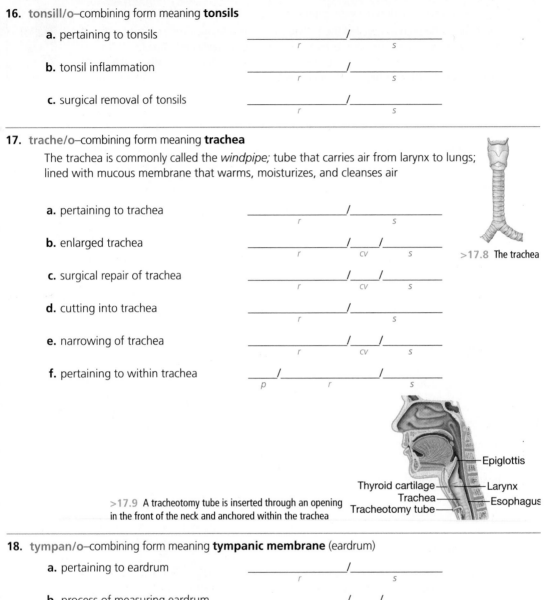

    a. pertaining to trachea

        _____ / _____
                r   *s*

    b. enlarged trachea

        _____ / ____ / _____
                r   *cv*   *s*

    >17.8 The trachea

    c. surgical repair of trachea

        _____ / ____ / _____
                r   *cv*   *s*

    d. cutting into trachea

        _____ / _____
                r   *s*

    e. narrowing of trachea

        _____ / ____ / _____
                r   *cv*   *s*

    f. pertaining to within trachea

        ____ / _____ / _____
          p   *r*   *s*

—Epiglottis

Thyroid cartilage—   —Larynx
Trachea—
Tracheotomy tube—   —Esophagus

>17.9 A tracheotomy tube is inserted through an opening in the front of the neck and anchored within the trachea

---

18. tympan/o–combining form meaning **tympanic membrane** (eardrum)

    a. pertaining to eardrum

        _____ / _____
                r   *s*

    b. process of measuring eardrum

        _____ / ____ / _____
                r   *cv*   *s*

    c. instrument to measure eardrum

        _____ / ____ / _____
                r   *cv*   *s*

    d. eardrum record

        _____ / ____ / _____
                r   *cv*   *s*

    e. eardrum surgical repair

        _____ / ____ / _____
                r   *cv*   *s*

    f. eardrum rupture

        _____ / ____ / _____
                r   *cv*   *s*

    g. cutting into eardrum

        _____ / _____
                r   *s*

Otorhinolaryngology Vocabulary

The otorhinolaryngology terms presented in this section include eponyms, modern English words, and those that contain Latin or Greek word parts but are not constructed solely from these word parts. When you recognize word parts within a term they will give you a hint about the word's meaning. In these instances, look for the word parts to follow the term.

Term	Explanation
acoustic neuroma **neur/o** = nerve **-oma** = tumor	Benign tumor of auditory nerve sheath; symptoms include tinnitus, headache, vertigo, and progressive hearing loss
cochlear implant **cochle/o** = cochlea **-ar** = pertaining to	Hearing device surgically placed under skin behind ear; converts sound signals into magnetic impulses to stimulate auditory nerve

+ TERMINOLOGY TIDBIT

The term *cochlea* comes from the Latin word *cochlea* meaning "snail shell." This describes coiled shape of the cochlea.

>17.10 Photograph of a child with a cochlear implant. This device sends electrical impulses directly to the brain

Term	Explanation
croup	Acute respiratory condition common in infants and children; symptoms include barking cough
deafness	Inability to hear or having some degree of hearing impairment
decongestant **de-** = without	Medication to reduce nasal and sinus stuffiness and congestion
diphtheria	Bacterial upper respiratory infection; characterized by formation of thick membranous film across throat and high mortality rate; rare now due to diphtheria, pertussis, tetanus (DPT) vaccine

+ TERMINOLOGY TIDBIT

The term *diphtheria* comes from the Greek word *diphthera* meaning "leather hide." This describes the thick membranous film that forms across the throat.

Term	Explanation
endotracheal (ET) intubation **endo-** = within **trache/o** = trachea **-al** = pertaining to	Inserting tube through mouth and into trachea; creates open upper respiratory airway

>17.11 Endotracheal intubation. (A) A lighted scope is used to identify the trachea from the esophagus. (B) The tube is placed through the pharynx and into the trachea. (C) The scope is removed, leaving the tube in place

A   Epiglottis   B   C

Trachea

Esophagus

Term	Explanation
epistaxis	Nosebleed
falling test	Group of tests to evaluate balance and equilibrium; for example, balancing on one foot, heel to toe walking, and walking forward with eyes open; test is repeated with patient's eyes closed; swaying and falling with eyes closed can indicate an equilibrium malfunction
hearing aid	Device used by persons with impaired hearing to amplify sound; also called an *amplification device*
Ménière disease	Acute or chronic inner ear condition; can lead to a progressive hearing loss; symptoms include vertigo, hearing loss, and tinnitus
nasal cannula nas/o = nose -al = pertaining to	Two-pronged plastic device for delivering oxygen directly into nose; one prong is inserted into each naris

+ TERMINOLOGY TIDBIT

The term *cannula* comes from the Latin word *canna* meaning "reed." Reeds are hollow and can be used to like a snorkel to breathe while underwater. This describes the hollow tube shape of a cannula.

>17.12 (A) Two–pronged nasal cannula and (B) patient using a nasal cannula

Term	Explanation
otitis externa (OE) ot/o = ear -itis = inflammation	External ear infection; commonly caused by fungus; also called *otomycosis;* common name is *swimmer's ear*
otitis interna ot/o = ear -itis = inflammation	Inflammation of inner ear; can affect both hearing and equilibrium; also called *inner ear infection*
otitis media (OM) ot/o = ear -itis = inflammation	Bacterial or viral infection of middle ear; common in children; often preceded by upper respiratory infection during which pathogens move from pharynx to middle ear through eustachian tube; commonly referred to as a *middle ear infection*

Fluid collecting in middle ear cavity

Inflamed eardrum

Eustachian tube swollen shut

>17.13 Otitis media. Note inflamed eardrum, swollen Eustachian tube, and fluid accumulating in middle ear cavity

pertussis

Bacterial infection of upper respiratory system; rare now due to diphtheria, pertussis, tetanus (DPT) vaccine; commonly called *whooping cough* due to "whoop" sound made when coughing

+ TERMINOLOGY TIDBIT

The term *pertussis* comes from the Latin word *tussis* meaning "cough." Pertussis, or whooping cough, is recognized by its characteristic cough.

---

pressure-equalizing tube (PE tube)

Small tube surgically placed in eardrum; assists in draining trapped fluid and equalizing pressure between middle ear cavity and atmosphere

Eardrum

>17.14 Illustration of a PE tube in place through the eardrum

Pressure-equalizing tube through eardrum

Trapped fluid in middle ear cavity

Rinne and Weber tuning fork tests

Tests to assess both function of auditory nerve and ability of ear structures to conduct sound waves to inner ear; physician holds tuning fork against or near bones on side of patient's head

>17.15 Physician placing a tuning fork behind a patient's ear as part of the Rinne and Weber tuning fork tests

---

tinnitus

Ringing in the ears

+ TERMINOLOGY TIDBIT

The term *tinnitus* comes from the Latin word *tinnire* meaning "to ring, tinkle." It is used to describe a ringing sensation in the ear.

---

vertigo

Dizziness

+ TERMINOLOGY TIDBIT

The term *vertigo* comes from the Latin word *verto* meaning "whirling." Typically a person with vertigo perceives the world as spinning around in a circle.

 USE otorhinolaryngology abbreviations.

Otorhinolaryngology Abbreviations

The following list presents common otorhinolaryngology abbreviations.

AD	right ear	**HEENT**	head, eyes, ears, nose, throat
AS	left ear	**OE**	otitis externa
AU	both ears	**OM**	otitis media
DPT	diphtheria, pertussis, tetanus	**Oto**	otology
EENT	eyes, ears, nose, throat	**PE tube**	pressure-equalizing tube
ENT	ear, nose, and throat	**T&A**	tonsillectomy and adenoidectomy
ET	endotracheal	**URI**	upper respiratory infection

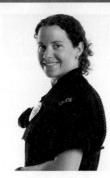

History of Present Illness

A 30-year-old female reports a history of chronic fatigue and headaches for at least 10 years. Headaches are centered above her eyes and occasionally radiate into the teeth of her upper jaw. Recently she became concerned when she noted that she was unable to smell fish she was cooking. She denies fever or cough.

Past Medical History

Patient has no history of hypertension, dental problems, or neurological problems. No known allergies. No prior hospitalizations except for birth of child.

Family and Social History

Patient is a police officer. She is married with one healthy child. She does not drink alcohol but does smoke one to one and half packs of cigarettes per day. Family history is noncontributory.

Physical Examination

Well-developed and well-nourished female who appears her stated age and is in no obvious distress. Temperature is 99°F, blood pressure is 115/65, pulse is 93 bpm, and breathing rate is 14 breaths per minute. There is tenderness over her brow ridge bilaterally. Examination with otoscope revealed normal-appearing tympanic membranes and no evidence of otitis externa or otitis media. There was no cervical lymphadenopathy.

Diagnostic Tests

Sinus cultures were positive for bacteria and negative for fungus.

Diagnosis

Pansinusitis, potentially chronic based on patient's chronic symptoms

Plan of Treatment

1. Long-term course of oral antibiotic
2. Corticosteroid nose spray
3. Repeat culture in 3 months
4. Strongly recommend patient seek medical assistance to stop smoking
5. Refer to allergist to investigate whether she has allergies, which can have contributed to development of chronic infections

Critical Thinking Questions

Answer the following questions regarding this case study. Do not just copy words out of the case study; translate all medical terms. To answer some of these questions, you may need to look up information from another chapter of this text, in a medical dictionary, or online. Answers are found at the back of the book.

1. Explain the history of this patient's present illness in your own words.

    _____

    _____

2. What is the medical term for the inability to smell?

    _____

    _____

3. Which of the following conditions was NOT mentioned in her past medical history?
   a. Problems with brain, spinal cord, or nerves
   b. Problems with the thyroid gland
   c. High blood pressure
   d. Problems with the teeth

4. Refer to the immunology chapter and explain what cervical lymphadenopathy means.
   _____
   _____

5. What does "pan-" mean in pansinusitis?
   _____
   _____

6. Go to National Institutes of Health Medline Plus Medical Encyclopedia at http://www.nlm.nih.gov/medlineplus/encyclopedia.html. Click on the "V," scroll down the list, and click on "Vital Signs." Compare this patient's vital signs to the normal ranges for the average healthy adult and note whether any of her vital signs are outside the normal ranges.
   _____
   _____

7. What is a culture? Explain the results of the sinus culture.
   _____
   _____

8. Describe what you think the purpose of each treatment is.
   _____
   _____

Sound It Out

The following are some of the key terms from this chapter written as their phonetic spelling. Sound out each term and write it in the blank. Pronunciations for all terms are included in the audio glossary at www.mymedicalterminologylab.com <http://www.mymedicalterminologylab.com/>.

1. oh-TAL-jee-ah _____
2. ah-NOZ-mee-ah _____
3. MAL-ee-us _____
4. aw-dee-OM-eh-ter _____
5. KOK-lee-ar _____
6. dif-THEAR-ee-ah _____
7. fair-IN-goh-spazm _____
8. my-RIN-goh-skle-ROH-sis _____
9. dis-FOH-nee-ah _____
10. ADD-eh-noy-DEK-toh-mee _____

11. en-doh-TRAY-kee-al _____

12. OH-toh-plas-tee _____

13. ep-ih-GLOT-iss _____

14. AW-dih-tor-ee _____

15. ING-kus _____

16. lair-in-GEE-all _____

17. lair-in-JYE-tis _____

18. ee-kwih-LIB-ree-um _____

19. lair-RING-goh-plee-gee-ah _____

20. lair-RING-go-scope _____

21. mir-IN-goh-plass-tee _____

22. fair-IN-GOT-oh-me _____

23. NAIR-eez _____

24. VER-tih-goh _____

25. TIM-pan-oh-gram _____

26. NAY-zoh-GAS-trik _____

27. tim-pah-NOM-eh-tree _____

28. OSS-ih-kls _____

29. KROOP _____

30. oh-TYE-tis _____

31. oh-toh-pye-oh-REE-ah _____

32. oh-TOSS-koh-pee _____

33. pan-sigh-nus-EYE-tis _____

34. ep-ih-STAKS-is _____

35. per-TUH-is _____

36. AW-ral _____

37. FAIR-inks _____

38. oh-TOL-oh-jist _____

39. PIN-ah _____

40. rye-NYE-tis _____

41. rye-noh-REE-ah _____

42. STAY-peez _____

43. tin-EYE-tus _____

44. ton-sih-LEK-toh-mee _____

45. ton-sil-EYE-tis _____

46. TRAY-kee-oh-MEG-ah-lee _____

47. AW-dee-oh-gram _____

48. tray-kee-oh-steh-NOH-sis _____

49. rye-noh-my-KOH-sis _____

50. tim-pan-oh-REK-sis _____

Transcription Practice

Each of the following sentences is written in common English. Underline any words or phrases that can be replaced by a medical term. Then rewrite the entire sentence using medical terms. Answers are found at the end of the text.

1. The new parents were quite concerned when their baby developed an acute respiratory condition with a barking cough.

   _____

   _____

2. Meilin's inability to hear was caused by a benign tumor of the auditory nerve sheat

3. The DPT vaccination protects children against a bacterial upper respiratory infection characterized by formation of thick membranous film across the throat and whooping cough.

4. The physician ordered supplemental oxygen to be delivered by a two-pronged plastic device directly in the nose.

5. His physician became concerned when Mr. Janssen developed dizziness and ringing in the ears.

6. Carmen's physician recommended to her parents that she have tubes surgically placed in the eardrums because of her repeated bacterial infections of the middle ear.

7. The paramedics had to quickly determine whether the patient's condition required a cutting into the trachea or a tube placed through the mouth and into the trachea.

8. Ursula went to see a specialist in the study of the ear, nose, and throat because of her repeated nosebleeds.

9. For his inability to hear, Tariq needed a hearing device surgically placed under the skin behind the ear rather than a device that amplifies sound.

10. After examining the external auditory canal with an instrument for examining the ear, it was obvious Jackson had swimmer's ear caused by a fungal infection.

Fill in the Blank

Fill in the blank to complete each of the following sentences.

1. The ear is responsible for the sense of _____ and _____.

2. The _____ prevents food and drink from entering the larynx.

3. The _____ is commonly called the *voice box*.

4. The pharyngeal tonsils are also called the _____.

5. Sound waves traveling down the external auditory canal strike the _____.

6. The _____ nerve sends hearing messages to the brain.

7. Air enters the nasal cavity through two holes called the _____.

8. The common name for epistaxis is _____.

9. A hearing aid is also referred to as a(n) _____.

10. The three small ossicles in the middle ear are the _____, _____, and _____.

Abbreviation Matching

Match each abbreviation with its definition.

_____ **1.** URI	**A.**	left ear
_____ **2.** OM	**B.**	otology
_____ **3.** AS	**C.**	tonsillectomy and adenoidectomy
_____ **4.** HEENT	**D.**	diphtheria, pertussis, tetanus
_____ **5.** Oto	**E.**	upper respiratory infection
_____ **6.** PE tube	**F.**	right ear
_____ **7.** AD	**G.**	head, eyes, ears, nose, throat
_____ **8.** T&A	**H.**	endotracheal
_____ **9.** ET	**I.**	otitis media
_____ **10.** DPT	**J.**	pressure-equalizing tube

Labeling Exercise

Write the name of each structure on the numbered line. Also use this space to write the combining form where appropriate.

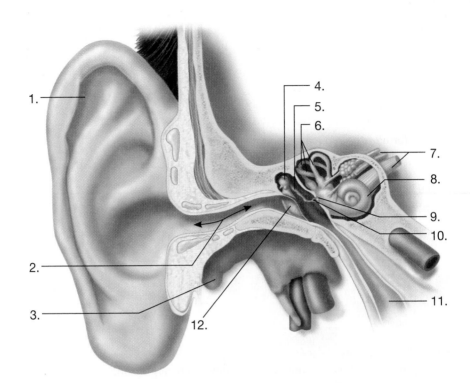

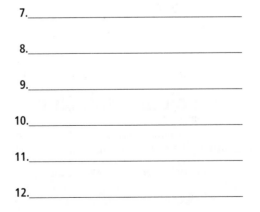

1._____

2._____

3._____

4._____

5._____

6._____

7._____

8._____

9._____

10._____

11._____

12._____

Build Medical Terms

Use each of the following word parts to build the indicated medical terms.

The combining form *ot/o* means ear.

1. study of ear _____

2. ear fungus abnormal condition _____

3. surgical repair of ear _____

4. ear inflammation _____

5. process of viewing ear _____

The combining form *pharyng/o* means pharynx.

6. involuntary muscle contraction of pharynx _____

7. pertaining to the pharynx _____

The suffix *-phonia* means voice.

8. without voice _____

9. difficult voice _____

The combining form *trache/o* means trachea.

10. trachea narrowing _____

11. trachea cutting into _____

12. enlarged trachea _____

The combining form *tympan/o* means tympanic membrane (eardrum).

13. eardrum surgical repair _____

14. instrument to measure the eardrum _____

15. eardrum rupture _____

PEARSON
mymedicalterminologylab

MyMedicalTerminologyLab is a premium online homework management system that includes a host of features to help you study. Registered users will find:

- Fun games and activities built within a virtual hospital
- Powerful tools that track and analyze your results—allowing you to create a personalized learning experience
- Videos, flashcards, and audio pronunciations to help enrich your progress
- Streaming lesson presentations and self-paced learning modules
- A space where you and your instructors can view and manage your assignments

Medical Term Analysis

Examine each of the following terms. Begin by dividing it into its word parts and writing them in the indicated blanks (P = prefix, WR = word root; CF = combining form; S = suffix). Follow with the definition of each word part and then finally the meaning of the full term.

1. **tympanotomy**

   WR _____

   means _____

   S _____

   means _____

   Term Meaning: _____

   _____

2. **cochlear**

   WR _____

   means _____

   S _____

   means _____

   Term Meaning: _____

   _____

3. **nasogastric**

   CF _____

   means _____

   WR _____

   means _____

   S _____

   means _____

   Term Meaning: _____

   _____

4. **endotracheal**

   P _____

   means _____

   WR _____

   means _____

   S _____

   means _____

   Term Meaning: _____

   _____

5. **rhinomycosis**

   CF _____

   means _____

   WR _____

   means _____

   S _____

   means _____

   Term Meaning: _____

   _____

6. **tonsillectomy**

   WR _____

   means _____

   S _____

   means _____

   Term Meaning: _____

   _____

7. anosmia

P _____

means _____

S _____

means _____

Term Meaning: _____

_____

8. laryngoplegia

CF _____

means _____

S _____

means _____

Term Meaning: _____

_____

9. pansinusitis

P _____

means _____

WR _____

means _____

S _____

means _____

Term Meaning: _____

_____

10. myringosclerosis

CF _____

means _____

S _____

means _____

Term Meaning: _____

_____

Spelling

Some of the following terms are misspelled. Identify the incorrect terms and spell them correctly in the blank provided.

1. audiology _____

2. epitaxis _____

3. diptheria _____

4. otopyorhea _____

5. tracheostenosis _____

6. tympanotomy _____

7. vertigo _____

8. canula _____

9. tinnitus _____

10. pertusiss _____

Photomatch Challenge

Match each upper respiratory condition with its name Word Bank.

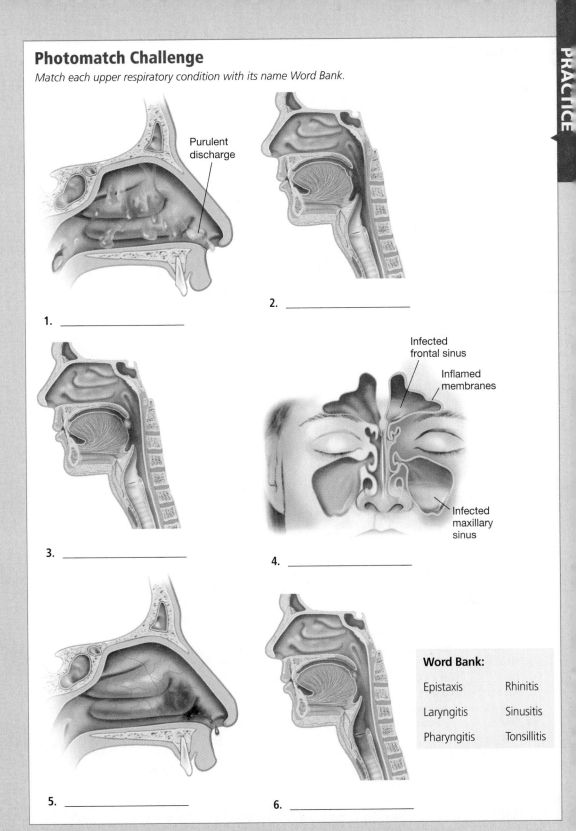

Purulent
discharge

1. _____

2. _____

3. _____

Infected
frontal sinus

Inflamed
membranes

Infected
maxillary
sinus

4. _____

5. _____

6. _____

Word Bank:

Epistaxis	Rhinitis
Laryngitis	Sinusitis
Pharyngitis	Tonsillitis

Crossword Puzzle

Use the definitions given to complete the crossword puzzle.

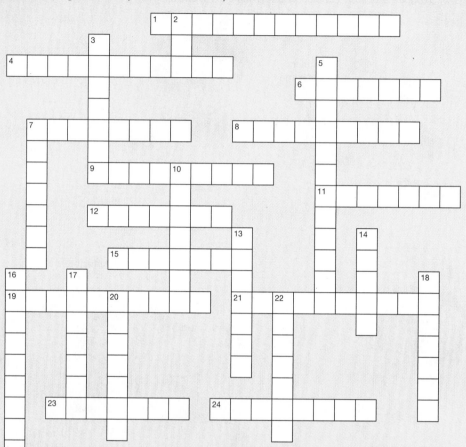

ACROSS

1. Term meaning process of viewing voice box
4. Term meaning eardrum record
6. Dizziness
7. Another name for pharyngeal tonsils
8. Term meaning study of hearing
9. Nosebleed
11. Otitis _____ is also called swimmer's ear
12. Nasogastric refers to the nose and _____
15. Inner ear structure shaped like snail shell
19. The _____ tube connects middle ear to pharynx
21. Condition forms thick membranous film
23. _____ test evaluates balance and equilibrium
24. Ringing in the ears

DOWN

2. Paranasal sinuses are filled with _____
3. Another term for equilibrium
5. Medication to reduce nasal stuffiness
7. Term meaning without voice
10. Anatomical name for windpipe
13. Common name for tympanic membrane
14. Rinne and _____ tuning fork test
16. Whooping cough
17. Term meaning ear pain
18. PE tubes are placed in the _____
20. A nasal _____ delivers oxygen directly into nose
22. Anatomical name for throat

Word Parts

Combining Forms

Form	Meaning	Form	Meaning
abdomin/o	abdomen	choledoch/o	common bile duct
acr/o	extremities	chondr/o	cartilage
aden/o	gland	chori/o	chorion
adenoid/o	adenoids	choroid/o	choroid layer
adip/o	fat	clavicul/o	clavicle (collar bone)
adren/o	adrenal glands	coagul/o	clotting
adrenal/o	adrenal glands	coccyg/o	coccyx (tailbone)
albumin/o	albumin	cochle/o	cochlea
alveol/o	alveolus; air sac	col/o	colon
ambly/o	dull or dim	colon/o	colon
amni/o	amnion	colp/o	vagina
an/o	anus	coni/o	dust
angi/o	vessel	conjunctiv/o	conjunctiva
anter/o	front (side of body)	core/o	pupil
aort/o	aorta	corne/o	cornea
append/o	appendix	coron/o	heart
appendic/o	appendix	corpor/o	body
arteri/o	artery	cortic/o	cortex
arteriol/o	arteriole	cost/o	rib
arthr/o	joint	crani/o	skull
atel/o	incomplete	crin/o	secrete
ather/o	fatty substance, plaque	cry/o	cold
atri/o	atrium	crypt/o	hidden
audi/o	hearing	cubit/o	elbow
audit/o	hearing	cutane/o	skin
aur/o	ear	cyan/o	blue
azot/o	nitrogen waste	cycl/o	ciliary body
bacteri/o	bacteria	cyst/o	bladder
balan/o	glans penis	cyst/o	sac
bas/o	base	cyt/o	cell
bi/o	life	dacry/o	tears
blephar/o	eyelid	derm/o	skin
brachi/o	arm	dermat/o	skin
bronch/o	bronchus	dipl/o	double
bronchi/o	bronchus	dist/o	farthest (away from beginning of structure)
bronchiol/o	bronchiole	diverticul/o	diverticulum
burs/o	bursa	dors/o	back (side of body)
carcin/o	cancer	duoden/o	duodenum
cardi/o	heart	electr/o	electricity
carp/o	carpals (wrist)	embol/o	plug
caud/o	tail	embry/o	embryo
cephal/o	head	encephal/o	brain
cerebell/o	cerebellum	enter/o	intestine
cerebr/o	cerebrum	eosin/o	rosy red
cervic/o	neck, cervix	epididym/o	epididymis
chol/eo	bile	epiglott/o	epiglottis
cholangi/o	bile duct		
cholecyst/o	gallbladder		

Form	Meaning	Form	Meaning
episi/o	vulva	hydr/o	water
erythr/o	red	hyster/o	uterus
esophag/o	esophagus	ile/o	ileum
femor/o	femur (thigh bone)	ili/o	ilium (part of pelvis)
femor/o	femur, thigh bone	immun/o	protection
fet/o	fetus	infer/o	below, lower
fibr/o	fibrous	inguin/o	groin
fibul/o	fibula (thinner lower leg bone)	ir/o	iris
gastr/o	stomach	irid/o	iris
genit/o	genitals	isch/o	to keep back
glomerul/o	glomerulus	ischi/o	ischium (part of pelvis)
glute/o	buttocks	jejun/o	jejunum
glycos/o	sugar, glucose	kerat/o	keratin, hard, hornlike, cornea
glycos/o	sugar	kyph/o	hump
gynec/o	woman, female	lacrim/o	tears
hem/o	blood	lapar/o	abdomen
hemat/o	blood	laryng/o	larynx (voice box)
hepat/o	liver	later/o	side
hidr/o	sweat	leuk/o	white
humer/o	humerus (upper arm bone)	lip/o	fat
		lith/o	stone
		lob/o	lobe
		lord/o	bent backward
		lumb/o	low back
		lymph/o	lymph

lymphaden/o	lymph node	path/o	disease	splen/o	spleen
lymphangi/o	lymph vessel	pelv/o	pelvis	spondyl/o	vertebra
mamm/o	breast	phac/o	lens	stern/o	sternum (breast bone)
mandibul/o	mandible (lower jaw)	phag/o	eating	steth/o	chest
mast/o	breast	phalang/o	phalanges (fingers and toes)	super/o	above, upper
maxill/o	maxilla (upper jaw)			system/o	system
medi/o	middle	pharyng/o	pharynx (throat)	tars/o	tarsals (ankle)
mediastin/o	mediastinum	phleb/o	vein	ten/o	tendon
medull/o	medulla oblongata	phot/o	light	tendin/o	tendon
melan/o	melanin, black	pineal/o	pineal gland	testicul/o	testes
men/o	menses, menstruation	pituitar/o	pituitary gland	testicul/o	testicle
mening/o	meninges	pleur/o	pleura	thalam/o	thalamus
metacarp/o	metacarpus (hand bones)	pneum/o	lung, air	thorac/o	chest
		pneumon/o	lung	thromb/o	clot
metatars/o	metatarsus (foot bones)	polyp/o	polyps	thym/o	thymus
		pont/o	pons	thym/o	thymus gland
metr/o	uterus	poster/o	back (side of body)	thyr/o	thyroid gland
muscul/o	muscle	proct/o	rectum and anus	thyroid/o	thyroid gland
my/o	muscle	prostat/o	prostate gland	tibi/o	tibia (shin, larger lower leg bone)
myc/o	fungus	proxim/o	nearest (to beginning of structure)		
myel/o	bone marrow			ton/o	tension, pressure
myel/o	spinal cord	pub/o	pubis (part of pelvis)	tonsill/o	tonsils
myring/o	tympanic membrane (eardrum)	pulmon/o	lung	toxic/o	poison
		pupill/o	pupil	trache/o	trachea (windpipe)
nas/o	nose	py/o	pus	trache/o	trachea, windpipe
nat/o	birth	pyel/o	renal pelvis	trich/o	hair
nephr/o	kidney	radi/o	radius (part of forearm)	tympan/o	tympanic membrane (eardrum)
neur/o	nerve				
neutr/o	neutral	rect/o	rectum	uln/o	ulna (part of forearm)
noct/i	night	ren/o	kidney	ungu/o	nail
o/o	egg	retin/o	retina	ur/o	urine
ocul/o	eye	rhin/o	nose	ureter/o	ureter
olig/o	scanty	sacr/o	sacrum	urethr/o	urethra
onych/o	nail	salping/o	fallopian tubes, uterine tubes	urin/o	urine
oophor/o	ovary			uter/o	uterus
ophthalm/o	eye	scapul/o	scapula (shoulder blade)	vagin/o	vagina
opt/o	eye, vision			valv/o	valve
or/o	mouth	scler/o	hardening	valvul/o	valve
orbit/o	eye socket	scler/o	sclera	varic/o	dilated vein
orch/o	testes	scoli/o	crooked, bent	vas/o	blood vessel
orchi/o	testes	seb/o	sebum, oil	vas/o	vas deferens
orchid/o	testes	semin/i	semen	vascul/o	blood vessels
orth/o	straight	septic/o	infection	ven/o	vein
oste/o	bone	sigmoid/o	sigmoid colon	ventr/o	belly (side of body)
ot/o	ear	sinus/o	sinus	ventricul/o	ventricle
ovari/o	ovary	son/o	sound	venul/o	venule
ox/i	oxygen	sperm/o	sperm	vertebr/o	vertebra, back bone
pancreat/o	pancreas	spermat/o	sperm	vesicul/o	seminal vesicle
parathyroid/o	parathyroid gland	sphygm/o	pulse	vitre/o	glassy
patell/o	patella (knee cap)	spin/o	spine	xanth/o	yellow
patell/o	patella, kneecap	spir/o	breathing	xer/o	dry

Prefixes

a-	without	hetero-	different	para-	alongside
an-	without	homo-	same	per-	through
ante-	before, in front of	hyper-	excessive, more than normal	peri-	around
anti-	against	hypo-	below, insufficient, less than normal	poly-	many, much
auto-	self			post-	after
brady-	slow	infra-	below, under	pre-	before
de-	without	inter-	between	primi-	first
di-	two	intra-	inside, within	quadri-	four
dys-	painful, difficult	micro-	small	retro-	behind
endo-	within, inner	mono-	one	sub-	beneath, under
epi-	above, upon	multi-	many	supra-	above
eu-	normal	neo-	new	tachy-	fast
ex-	outward	nulli-	none	trans-	across
extra-	outside of	pachy-	thick	ultra-	excess
hemi-	half	pan-	all		

Suffixes

-ac	pertaining to	-gram	record, picture	-oma	tumor, mass
-al	pertaining to	-graphy	process of recording	-opia	vision
-algia	pain	-graph	instrument for recording	-opsy	view of
-an	pertaining to	-gravida	pregnancy	-ory	pertaining to
-ar	pertaining to	-iac	pertaining to	-ose	pertaining to
-ary	pertaining to	-iasis	abnormal condition	-osis	abnormal condition
-asthenia	weakness	-iatric	medical specialty	-osmia	smell
-atic	pertaining to	-iatrist	physician	-ostomy	surgically create an opening
-cele	hernia, protrusion	-iatry	treatment, medicine		
-centesis	puncture to withdraw fluid	-ia	state, condition	-otomy	cutting into
		-ician	specialist	-ous	pertaining to
-clasia	surgical breaking	-ic	pertaining to	-oxia	oxygen
-cle	small	-ine	pertaining to	-para	to bear (offspring)
-cyesis	pregnancy	-ior	pertaining to	-partum	childbirth
-cyte	cell	-ism	state of, condition	-pathy	disease
-cytosis	abnormal cell condition (too many)	-ist	specialist	-penia	too few
		-itis	inflammation	-pepsia	digestion
-derma	skin condition	-kinesia	movement	-pexy	surgical fixation
-desis	surgical fixation	-lith	stone	-phagia	eat, swallow
-dipsia	thirst	-logist	one who studies	-phasia	speech
-dynia	pain	-logy	study of	-phil	attracted to
-eal	pertaining to	-lysis	destruction	-phobia	fear
-ectasis	dilated, expansion	-malacia	abnormal softening	-phonia	voice
-ectomy	surgical removal	-manometer	instrument for measuring pressure	-plasm	formation
-edema	swelling			-plasty	surgical repair
-emesis	vomit	-megaly	enlargement, large	-plegia	paralysis
-emia	blood condition	-meter	instrument for measuring	-pnea	breathing
-esthesia	feeling, sensation			-poiesis	formation
-genesis	produces, generates	-metry	process of measuring	-porosis	porous
-genic	producing			-ptosis	drooping
-gen	that which produces	-nic	pertaining to	-ptysis	spitting
-globin	protein	-oid	resembling	-rrhage	bursting forth
-globulin	protein	-ole	small		

-rrhagia	bursting forth	-spasm	involuntary muscle contraction	-toxic	poison
-rrhaphy	suture	-stasis	stopping	-tripsy	crushing
-rrhea	discharge, flow	-stenosis	narrowing	-trophic	development
-rrhexis	rupture	-therapy	treatment	-trophy	nourishment, development
-sclerosis	hardened condition	-thorax	chest	-ule	small
-scope	instrument to view	-tic	pertaining to	-uria	urine condition
-scopy	process of visually examining	-tome	instrument to cut		

Abbreviations and Symbols

Introduction

Abbreviations and symbols are commonly used when writing medical documents because they are convenient and save time. However, they can certainly be confusing. For example, DC may mean discontinue or discharge. Use of the incorrect abbreviation can result in problems for a patient as well as insurance records and processing. If you ever think that an abbreviation may be misinterpreted, spell out the word instead.

It is never acceptable to use one's own abbreviations or symbols. All health care facilities have a list of approved abbreviations and symbols, and it is extremely important to become familiar with and follow this list closely. Just as importantly, there is also a list that should never be used. Abbreviations and symbols that have been shown to be misleading are placed on this list.

This appendix presents basic abbreviations and symbols used in medical documents. They have been grouped together into categories for ease of learning. However, abbreviations are so essential to learning medical terminology that throughout this book, they are included immediately following terms. In addition, a list of common abbreviations for each medical specialty is given in each chapter.

Abbreviations for Health Care Providers, Services, or Units

AuD	Doctor of Audiology
BSN	Bachelor of Science in Nursing
CCS	Certified Coding Specialist
CCU	Coronary Care Unit
CLS	Clinical Laboratory Scientist
CLT	Clinical Laboratory Technician
CMA	Certified Medical Assistant
CNA	Certified Nurse Aide
COTA	Certified Occupational Therapy Assistant
CRT	Certified Respiratory Therapist
CV	Cardiovascular
DC	Doctor of Chiropractic
DDM	Doctor of Dental Medicine
DDS	Doctor of Dental Surgery
Derm	Dermatology
DI	Diagnostic imaging
DO	Doctor of Osteopathy
DPT	Doctor of Physical Therapy
DTR	Dietetic Technician, Registered
ED	Emergency Department
EMT-B	Emergency Medical Technician–Basic
EMT-I	Emergency Medical Technician–Intermediate
EMT-P	Emergency Medical Technician–Paramedic
ENT	Ear, Nose, and Throat
ER	Emergency Room
GI	Gastrointestinal
GU	Genitourinary
GYN	Gynecology
ICU	Intensive Care Unit
LPN	Licensed Practical Nurse
LVN	Licensed Vocational Nurse

MD	Medical Doctor
MLT	Medical Laboratory Technician
MSN	Master of Science in Nursing
MSW	Medical Social Worker
MT	Medical Technologist
NICU	Neonatal Intensive Care Unit
NP	Nurse Practitioner
OB	Obstetrics
OD	Doctor of Optometry
OPD	Outpatient Department
Ophth	Ophthalmology
OR	Operating room
Orth, Ortho	Orthopedics
OT	Occupational Therapy; Occupational Therapist
OTA	Occupational Therapy Assistant
Path	Pathology
Peds	Pediatrics
PharD	Doctor of Pharmacy
PT	Physical Therapy; Physical Therapist
PTA	Physical Therapy Assistant
RD	Registered Dietitian
RDH	Registered Dental Hygienist
Rehab	Rehabilitation Unit
RHIA	Registered Health Information Administrator
RN	Registered Nurse
RPh	Registered Pharmacist
RRT	Registered Respiratory Therapist, Registered Radiologic Technologist

RR	Recovery Room
X-ray	Radiology

Abbreviations Indicating Time or Frequency

ā	before
ac	before meals
ad lib	as desired
am, AM	morning
ante	before
bid	twice a day
d	day
noc, noct	night
p̄	after
pc	after meals
pm, PM	evening
prn	as needed
q	every
qh	every hour
qid	four times a day
STAT, stat	at once/immediately
tid	three times a day
yr	year

Abbreviations for Units of Measurement

cg	centigram
cm	centimeter
dr	dram
ft	foot, feet
g	gram
gm	gram
gr	grain
gt	drop
gtt	drops
h	hour
hr	hour

in	inch
kg	kilogram
L	liter
lb	pound
m	meter
mcg	microgram
mEq	milliequivalent
mg	milligram
min	minutes
mL	milliliter
mm	millimeter
oz	ounce
pt	pint
qt	quart
sec	seconds
T, tbsp	tablespoon
t, tsp	teaspoon
yd	yard

Patient Chart Abbreviations

ADLs	activities of daily living
AK	above knee
AMA	against medical advice
amb	ambulate, walk
BK	below knee
BR	bathroom; bed rest
BRP	bathroom privileges
CA	cancer; chronological age
CBR	complete bed rest
CC	chief complaint
c/o	complains of
DOA	dead on arrival
DOB	date of birth
DNR	do not resuscitate
Dx	diagnosis
Ex	examination
FH	family history
f/u	follow up
h/o	history of
H&P	history and physical
HEENT	head, eye, ear, nose, throat
Hx	history
I&O	intake and output
LA	left arm
LE	lower extremity
LL	left leg
MH	marital history; mental health
MS	mental status
NKA	no known allergies
PE	physical exam
PERRLA	pupils equal, round, reactive to light and accommodation
PI	present illness

PMH	past medical history
pt	patient
RA	right arm
RL	right leg
r/o, R/O	rule out
ROM	range of motion
SH	social history
s/p	status post (previous disease condition)
Sx	symptoms, signs
Tx	treatment
UE	upper extremity
WDWN	well developed, well nourished

Vital Signs Abbreviations

BP	blood pressure
BPM, bpm	beats per minute
ht	height
NTP	normal temperature and pressure
P	pulse
R	respirations
RR	respiratory rate
T	temperature
TPR	temperature, pulse, and respirations
VS, V/S	vital signs
wt	weight

Pharmacy Abbreviations

APAP	acetaminophen (Tylenol™)
ASA	aspirin
cap(s)	capsule(s)
Chemo	chemotherapy
disp	dispense
dtd	give of such a dose
ī	one
ID	intradermal
īī	two
īīī	three
IM	intramuscular
inj	injection
IV	intravenous
no sub	no substitute
non rep	do not repeat
npo, NPO	nothing by mouth
NS	normal saline
OD, od	overdose
oint	ointment
OTC	over the counter
PCA	patient-controlled administration

PDR	Physician's Desk Reference
po, PO	by mouth
Rx	prescription, treatment
Sig	label as follows/directions
sl	under the tongue
sol	solution
s̄s̄	one-half
subcut	subcutaneous
SuQ	subcutaneous
suppos, supp.	suppository
tab(s)	tablet
top	apply topically

Miscellaneous Abbreviations

aq	aqueous (water)
ant	anterior
AP	anteroposterior
cont	continue
DC, dc, d/c	discontinue
DISC, disc	discontinue
et	and
ETOH	ethanol
HIPPA	Health Insurance Portability and Accountability Act
L, Ⓛ	left
lat	lateral
mets	metastases
neg	negative
PA	posteroanterior
per	by
p/o	postoperative
pos	positive
post	posterior
post-op	after operation
prep	prepare for
PTA	prior to admission
R, Ⓡ	right
ROS	review of systems
TO	telephone order
VO	verbal order
w/c	wheelchair
WNL	within normal limits
w/u	work up
y/o	years old

Chemical Abbreviations

Ba	barium
C	carbon
$C_6H_{12}O_6$	glucose
Ca	calcium
CO_2	carbon dioxide
Cl	chlorine

Fe	iron			1°	primary
H	hydrogen			2°	secondary
HCl	hydrochloric acid			3°	tertiary
HCO_3^-	bicarbonate			%	percent
Hg	mercury			°C	degrees Celcius
H_2O	water			°F	degrees Fahrenheit
I	iodine			≈	approximately
K	potassium			Δ	change
Mg	magnesium			α	alpha
N	nitrogen			β	beta
Na	sodium			×	times
NaCl	sodium chloride (salt)			'	inch
O_2	oxygen			"	feet
Pb	lead				

Symbols

c̄	with
s̄	without
=	equal
≠	not equal
+	positive
−	negative
±	plus or minus
↑	increase
↓	decrease
#	pounds, number
♀	female
♂	male
→	from–to (in the direction of)

Abbreviations to Be Avoided

Abbreviations make writing notes faster but they also create the possibility of being misunderstood. For this reason, the Joint Commission on Accreditation of Healthcare Organizations (JCAHO) and the Institute for Safe Medication Practices (ISMP) publishes lists of error-prone abbreviations that are not to be used. The following table presents these abbreviations and what should be used instead. The Joint Commission (TJC) has determined that the first six abbreviations (marked with an*) must appear on an accredited institution's "Do Not Use" list of abbreviations.

Abbreviation	Intended Meaning	Potential Problem	Recommendation
U*	Unit	Mistaken for "0," "4," or "cc"	Write "unit"
IU*	International unit	Mistaken for "IV" or "10"	Write "international unit"
qd and qod*	Daily and every other day	Mistaken for each other or for "qid"	Write "daily" and "every other day"
Using a zero after a decimal point*	X.0 mg	Decimal point is missed	Never write a zero by itself after a decimal point (X mg is correct)
Not using a zero before a decimal point (0.X)*	.X mg	Decimal point is missed	Always write a zero before a decimal point (0.X mg)
MS, MSO_4, and $MgSO_4$*	Morphine sulfate, magnesium sulfate	Mistaken for each other	Write "morphine sulfate" or "magnesium sulfate"
µg	microgram	Mistaken for "mg"	Write "mcg"
hs	Half-strength or at bedtime	Meanings can be mistaken for each other	Write "half-strength" or "at bedtime"
tiw	Three times a week	Mistaken for "three times a day" or "twice weekly"	Write "3 times weekly"
SC or SQ	Subcutaneous	Mistaken for "SL" or "5 every"	Write "SubQ," "subcut," or "subcutaneous"
D/C	discharge	Mistaken to mean "discontinue"	Write "discharge"

Abbreviation	Intended Meaning	Potential Problem	Recommendation
cc	Cubic centimeter	Mistaken for "U" (units)	Since a cubic centimeter is equal to a milliliter, write "mL"
AS, AD, AU and OS, OD, OU	Left ear, right ear, both ears and left eye, right eye, both eyes	Mistaken for each other (for example "AS" and "OS")	Write "left ear," "right ear," "both ears," "left eye," "right eye," and "both eyes"
bt	bedtime	Mistaken for "bid"	Write "bedtime"
IJ	injection	Mistaken for "IV"	Write "injection"
IN	Intranasal	Mistaken for "IM" or "IV"	Write "intranasal" or "NAS"
od or OD	once daily	Mistaken for "right eye (OD)" or "overdose"	write "daily"
OJ	orange juice	Mistaken for "right eye (OD)"	write "orange juice"
per os	by mouth	"os" can be mistaken to mean "left eye"	write "PO," "orally," or "by mouth"
qhs	every bedtime	Mistaken for "qhr"	Write "bedtime"
qn	every night	Mistaken for "qh"	Write "nightly"
q1d	every day	Mistaken for "qid"	Write "daily"
q6PM	every day at 6PM	Mistaken to mean "every 6 hours"	Write "daily at 6 PM"
ss	sliding scale or one-half	Mistaken for each other and for "55"	Write "sliding scale," "one-half," or "1/2"
SSRI and SSI	sliding scale regular insulin and sliding scale insulin	Mistaken for "selective-serotonin reuptake inhibitor" and "strong solution of iodine"	Write "sliding scale (insulin)"
īd	one daily	Mistaken for "tid"	Write "one daily"
ʒ	dram	Mistaken for "3"	Write "dram"
@	at	Mistaken for "2"	Write "at"
< and >	lesser than and greater than	Mistakenly read as the opposite symbol	Write "lesser than" and "greater than"
x3d	for three days	Mistaken to mean "for 3 doses"	Write "for three days"
&	and	Mistaken for "2"	Write "and"
°	hour	Mistaken for "0"	Write "hr," "h," or "hour"
+	and	Mistaken for "4"	Write "and"

Selected English/Spanish Glossary*

English	Spanish	English	Spanish
abdomen (belly)	vientre	concussion	concusión; conmoción
acute	agudo	convulsion	convulsión; ataque
AIDS (Acquired Immune Deficiency Syndrome)	SIDA (Sindrome de Immune Deficiencia Adquirida)	cough	tos
		croup	crup
allergy	alergia	CT scan	tomografía axial computarizada
anemia	anemia; sangre delgada		
angina	angina	dark	oscuro
ankle	tobillo	dead	muerto
anxiety	ansiedad	deaf	sordo(a)
appendix	apéndice	deep breath	rispirar profundo
arm	brazo	deficient	deficiente
artery	arteria	dermatology	dermatología
arthritis	artritis	diabetes	diabetes
asphyxia	asfixia; sofocación	diagnosis	diagnóstico
asthma	asma; ansia	dialysis	diálisis
back	espalda; lomo	diarrhea	diarrea; estómago suelto
bad	malo	difficulty in breathing	dificultad de la respiración
benign	benigno; de poca gravedad	diphtheria	difteria
better	major	dizziness	mareo; vértigo
black	negro	double vision	visión doble; ver doble
bladder	vejiga	dry	seco
blood	sangre	dysuria	disuria; emisión de la orina
blood pressure	presión sanguínea; presión arterial	ear	oreja; oído
blood test	prueba de sangre	earache	dolor de oído
blue	azul	edema	edema
body	cuerpo	elbow	codo
bone	hueso	endocrinology	endocrinología
brain	cerebro	epilepsy	epilepsia
breast	pecho; seno	equilibrium	equilibrio
breathe	respirar; inhalar	esophagus	esófago
bronchitis	bronquitis; catarro de pecho	excessive	excesivo; desmesurado
bruise	contusión; morado	exhale	exhalar
burning	ardiente	external	externo
cancer	cáncer	eye	ojo
capillary	capilar	fainting	desmayo
cardiology	cardiología	fast	rápido(a)
cartilage	cartílago	fatigue	fatiga; cansancio
cataract	catarata	fever	fiebre; calentura
cheek	mejilla; cachete	finger	dedo de la mano
chest	pecho; tórax	foot	pie
chickenpox	varicela; viruela loca	forearm	antebrazo
cholesterol	colesterol	fracture	fractura
chronic	crónico	gallbladder	vesócula biliar
clavicle	clavícula	gallstones	cálculos biliar
closed	cerrado	gastroenterology	gastroenterología
clot	coágulo; trombo	genital	genital
cold	frío; catarro	gland	glándula
common cold	resfriado común	glaucoma	glaucoma

*Note that a full English/Spanish translator is included on MyMedicalTerminologyLab.

English	Spanish	English	Spanish
good	bueno	malignant	maligno; pernicioso
gray	gris	mandible	mandíbula
green	verde	maxilla	maxilar
gums	encías	measles	sarampión
gynecology	ginecología	middle	medio
hand	mano	mouth	boca
hard	duro	mumps	paperas; parotiditis
head	cabeza	murmur	soplo; murmullo del corazón
headache	dolor de cabeza	muscle	músculo
healthy	sana	muscle spasm	espasmo muscular
hearing	audición; oído	narrow	estrecho
heart	corazón	nausea	náusea; mareo
hematology	hematología	navel	ombligo
hemorrhage	hemorragia; desangramiento	neck	cuello; pescuezo
hepatitis	hepatitis	nephrology	nefrología
hip	cadera	nerve	nervio
hormone	hormona	neurology	neurologia
hot	caliente; calor	nose	nariz
hypertension	hipertensión; presión arterial alta	nosebleed	hemorragia nasal
immunology	immunología	obstetrics	obstericia
incision	corte; incisión	oncology	oncología
infection	infección	open	abierto
inflammation	inflamación	ophthalmology	oftalmología
influenza	gripe; influenza	orange-yellow	cirrho
inhale	inhalar	orthopedics	ortopedia
injection	inyección; piquete	otorhinolaryngology	otorrinolaringología
inner	interior	ovary	ovario
insulin	insulina	oxygen	oxígeno
internal	interno	pain	dolor
intestine	intestino; tripa	palpitation	palpitación
intravenous	intravenoso	pancreas	páncreas
itching	comezón; picazón	paralysis	parálisis
jaundice	ictericia	parathyroid	paratiroideo
joint	articulación; coyuntura	pathology	patología
kidney	riñón	pelvis	pelvis
kidney stone	cálculo renales	penis	pene
knee	rodilla; gozne	phlegm	flemón; inflamación difusa
large	grande	pituitary	pituitaria
larynx	laringe	pneumonia	neumonía; inflamación de los pulmones
left	izquierdo(a)	pregnancy	embarazo
leg	pierna	prostate gland	próstata
ligament	ligarnento	pulmonology	neumólogía
lips	labios	pulse	pulso
liver	hígado	purple	morado
lump	bolita; abultamiento; nudo; protuberancia	rash	salpullido; sarpullido; erupción cutánea
lung	pulmón; bofe	rectum	recto; guía de atrás
lymph node	nódulo; ganglio linfático	red	rojo
lymphatic	linfático	redness	enrojecimiento; piel colorada
		respiration	respiración

English	Spanish	English	Spanish
rib	costilla	thorax	tórax
right	derecha	throat	garganta
sacrum	sacro; rabadilla	thyroid	tiroides
scapula	escápula; hueso de la espaldilla	toe	dedo del pié
shoulder	hombro	tongue	lengua
sick	enfermo(a); mal(a)	tonsil	tonsila; amigdala
side	costado	tonsillitis	tonsilitis; amigdalitis
skeleton	esqueleto	trachea	tráquea
skin	piel; cuero; pellejo; cutis	treatment	tratamiento
skull	cráneo; calavera	tremor	temblor
slow	lento(a); pausado(a)	tuberculosis	tuberculosis
small	pequeño(a)	ulcer	úlcera
soft	blando(a)	ultrasound	ecografía; ultrasonido
sore throat	dolor de garganta	unconscious	inconsciente
spasm	espasmo	urethra	uretra; canal
spine	espinazo	urinalysis	análisis de orina
spleen	bazo	urination	urinacion
sprain	torcedura; falseamiento; falseado	urine	orina; pipí
sternum	esternón	urology	urología
stiff	tieso(a); rígido(a)	uterus	útero
stomach	estómago	vaccination	vacunación
stroke	apoplejía; embolia; derrame cerebral	vagina	vagina
strong	fuerte	vein	vena
surgery	cirugía	vertebral column	columna vertebral
swallow	ingerir; pasar; tragar	vision	visión
sweating	sudar	vomit	vómito
swelling	hinchar	weakness	debilidad
symptom	síntoma	white	blanco
teeth	dientes	whooping cough	tos ferina
temperature	temperatura	worse	peor
tendon	cuello	wound	herida
test	puerba	wrist	muñeca
testes	testículos; huevos; bolas	x-ray	radiografia; rayos equis
tetanus	tétano	yellow	amarillo
thigh	muslo		

Answer Keys

Chapter 1

Practice Exercises

A. Recognizing Types of Medical Terms

1. Latin/Greek;   2. modern English;   3. eponym;   4. Latin/Greek;   5. Latin/Greek;
6. eponym;   7. modern English;   8. eponym;   9. modern English;   10. Latin/Greek

B. Forming Plurals

1. bursae;   2. diverticula;   3. adenoma;   4. ganglia;   5. indices;   6. diagnosis;
7. alveolus

C. Practice Defining Medical Terms

1. word root, combining vowel, suffix, softening of the brain;   2. prefix, word root, suffix, pertaining to underneath the skin;   3. word root, combining vowel, suffix, surgical fixation of the uterus;   4. prefix, word root, suffix, inflammation of all the sinuses;   5. word root, combining vowel, suffix, to suture a vessel;   6. prefix, word root, suffix, pertaining to between the ventricles

D. Practice Building Medical Terms

1. laryngoplasty;   2. arthroscope;   3. subscapular;   4. ophthalmology;   5. neuroma;
6. intramuscular

Chapter 2

Practice Exercises

A. Recognizing Categories of Suffixes

1. paralysis, disease/abnormal condition;   2. process of measuring, diagnostic;   3. cell, general;
4. cutting into, surgical;   5. stone, disease/abnormal condition;   6. instrument for viewing, diagnostic;   7. chest, general;   8. process of recording, diagnostic;   9. vomiting, disease/abnormal condition;   10. surgical breaking, surgical;   11. destruction, disease/abnormal condition;   12. surgical removal, surgical

B. Matching

1. E;   2. L;   3. F;   4. H;   5. C;   6. D;   7. I;   8. A;   9. K;   10. G;   11. B;   12. J

C. Choosing the Correct Adjective Forms

1. cardiac;   2. ovarian;   3. duodenal;   4. ventricular;   5. pulmonary;   6. esophageal;
7. gastric;   8. uterine;   9. venous;   10. hepatic

D. Build Medical Terms

1. gastrectomy;   2. gastroscope;   3. gastroscopy;   4. gastralgia or gastrodynia;   5. cystolith;
6. cystoscope;   7. cystoscopy;   8. cystostomy;   9. cystic;   10. angioplasty;   11. angioma;
12. angiography;   13. angiogram;   14. angiostenosis;   15. arteriosclerosis;   16. arteriospasm;
17. arteriorrhexis;   18. arteriole;   19. arthritis;   20. arthroscope;   21. arthroscopy;
22. arthroplasty;   23. arthrocentesis;   24. dermatology;   25. dermatologist;   26. dermatitis;
27. dermatorrhaphy;   28. dermatosis;   29. hepatitis;   30. hepatoma;   31. hepatomegaly;
32. hepatocyte;   33. hepatic;   34. rhinorrhea;   35. rhinoplasty;   36. rhinorrhagia;

37. bronchitis;   38. bronchoscope;   39. bronchoscopy;   40. tracheostomy;   41. tracheotomy;   42. tracheocele;   43. tracheomalacia;   44. tracheal;   45. colostomy;   46. colectomy;   47. colopexy;   48. nephrology;   49. nephrologist;   50. nephromalacia;   51. nephrosis;   52. nephropathy;   53. nephropexy;   54. thoracotomy;   55. thoracocentesis;   56. thoracodynia or thoracalgia;   57. neurology;   58. neurologist;   59. neuroplasty;   60. neurotripsy;   61. neuralgia or neurodynia;   62. myorrhaphy;   63. myopathy;   64. myalgia or myodynia;   65. myotome;   66. myograph;   67. myogram;   68. myography

E. Crossword Puzzle

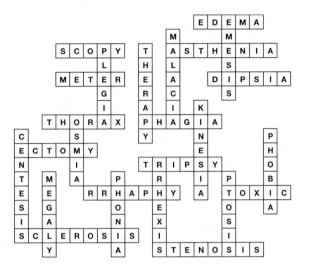

Chapter 3

Practice Exercises

A. Recognizing Categories of Prefixes

1. painful/difficult, disease/abnormality;   2. below, direction/body position;   3. none, number;   4. slow, disease/abnormality;   5. without, disease/abnormality;   6. new, time;   7. between, direction/body position;   8. after, time;   9. large, number;   10. around/near, direction/body position;   11. above/upon, direction/body position;   12. against, disease/abnormality

B. Matching

1. G;   2. D;   3. L;   4. A;   5. J;   6. K;   7. E;   8. B;   9. F;   10. H;   11. I;   12. C

C. Build Medical Terms

1. tachycardia;   2. bradycardia;   3. endocarditis;   4. pericarditis;   5. pancarditis;   6. intracellular;   7. extracellular;   8. multicellular;   9. unicellular;   10. intradermal;   11. subdermal;   12. epidermal;   13. homograft;   14. heterograft;   15. autograft;   16. bilateral;   17. unilateral;   18. preoperative;   19. postoperative;   20. intraoperative;   21. primipara;   22. nullipara;   23. multipara;   24. aphagia;   25. dysphagia;   26. polyphagia;   27. apepsia;   28. dyspepsia;   29. bradypepsia;   30. atrophy;   31. dystrophy;   32. hemiplegia;   33. quadriplegia;   34. monoplegia;   35. apnea;   36. eupnea;   37. tachypnea;   38. bradypnea;   39. hyperpnea;   40. hypopnea;   41. infrascapular;   42. suprascapular;   43. subscapular;   44. anuria;   45. polyuria;   46. dysuria

D. Crossword Puzzle

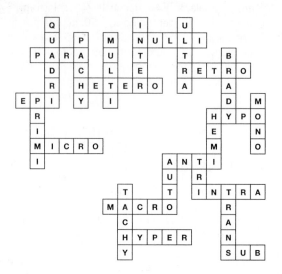

Chapter 4

Building Direction Terms

1. anterior;   2. caudal;   3. cephalic;   5. distal;   6. dorsal;   7. inferior;   8. lateral;   9. medial;
10. posterior;   12. proximal;   14. superior;   16. ventral

Building Body Surface Terms

1. abdominal;   2. antecubital;   4. brachial;   5. cervical;   6. cranial;   7. femoral;   8. genital;
9. gluteal;   10. inguinal;   12. nasal;   13. orbital;   14. oral;   15. otic;   17. patellar;
18. pelvic;   21. thoracic;   22. scapular;   23. sternal;   27 vertebral

Practice Exercises

A. Directional Terms

1. posterior or dorsal;   2. cephalic or superior;   3. caudal or inferior;   4. superficial;   5. proximal;
6. ventral or anterior;   7. superior or cephalic;   8. medial;   9. lateral;   10. anterior or ventral;
11. distal;   12. deep;   13. inferior or caudal;   14. dorsal or posterior;   14. prone

B. Fill in the Blank

1. spinal;   2. pleura;   3. dorsal;   4. kidney;   5. thoracic;   6. peritoneum;   7. brain;
8. heart;   9. pelvic;   10. meninges;   11. abdominal;   12. mediastinum

C. Labeling Exercise—External Surface Anatomy

1. Cranial;   2. Cervical;   3.Thoracic;   4. Brachial;   5. Abdominal;   6. Pelvic;   7. Genital;
8. Femoral;   9. Trunk;   10. Scapular;   11. Vertebral;   12. Gluteal

D. Matching - Planes and Sections

1. A;   2. F;   3. B;   4. A, B;   5. A;   6. E;   7. C;   8. C;   9. D

E. Matching–Organs and Clinical Divisions of the Abdominopelvic Cavity

1. A;   2. D;   3. C;   4. C;   5. E;   6. A;   7. B;   8. D;   9. C;   10. F;   11. C;   12. E;   13. B

F. Labeling Exercise—Anatomical Divisions of the Abdominopelvic Cavity

1. Right hypochondriac region;   2. Right lumbar region;   3. Right iliac region;   4. Epigastric region;   5. Umbilical region;   6. Hypogastric region;   7. Left hypochondriac region;
8. Left lumbar region;   9. Left iliac region

G. Crossword Puzzle

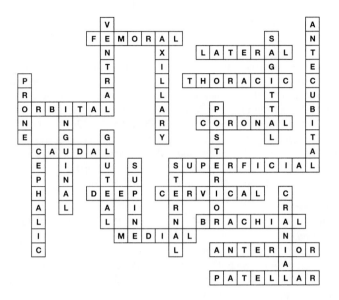

Chapter 5

Word Building

1. a. adenectomy; b. adenitis; c. adenoma; d. adenopathy; e. adenomegaly;   2. a. adipose;
b. adipocyte; c. adipoma;   3. a. cutaneous; b. subcutaneous; c. percutaneous;   4. a. cyanosis;
b. cyanotic;   5. a. ichthyoderma; b. scleroderma; c. xanthoderma; d. xeroderma; e. pachyderma;
f. erythroderma; g. pyoderma; h. leukoderma;   6. a. dermatitis; b. dermatology; c. dermatologist; d. dermatosis; e. dermatoplasty; f. dermatomycosis; g. dermatopathy; h. dermatosclerosis;
7. a. dermal; b. epidermal; c. intradermal; d. hypodermic; e. transdermal;   8. a. hidrosis;
b. anhidrosis; c. hidradenitis; d. hyperhidrosis;   9. a. keratoderma; b. keratosis; c. keratogenic;
10. a. lipectomy; b. lipoid; c. lipoma; d. lipocyte;   11. a. melanoma; b. melanocyte; c. melanotic;
12. a. onychectomy; b. onychitis; c. onychomalacia; d. onychomycosis; e. onychophagia;
f. hyperonychia;   13. a. pyogenic; b. pyorrhea;   14. a. seborrhea;   15. a. trichomycosis;
b. trichophagia;   16. a. ungual; b. subungual

Case Study

1. First appeared as painful, reddened, raised spots with pus in them
2. Antibiotic pills taken by mouth, ointments to reduce inflammation rubbed into the skin, swirling water baths to clean the ulcers
3. diabetes mellitus
4. a
5. C&S–C means culture, growing the bacteria in a petri dish to identify what kind of bacteria it is. S means sensitivity, determining which antibiotic will best kill the bacteria. In this case, penicillin will not kill it, so vancomycin is recommended

6. *Staph* is common bacteria found on the skin and in nose and throat. Can become a serious infection if it gets down into the layers of the skin or invades the bloodstream, urinary tract, lungs, and heart. Some strains of staph have become resistant to many common antibiotics.
7. Gangrene occurs when tissue does not have sufficient circulation to keep the tissue healthy. As a result, the tissue dies
8. Antibiotics to fight the infection given into a vein, treatments in a whirlpool bath to clean up the ulcers, go to surgery to remove the dead and infected tissue

Practice Exercises

A. Sound It Out

1. onychomycosis; 2. cryosurgery; 3. abrasion; 4. adipoma; 5. contusion; 6. cyst; 7. alopecia; 8. anhidrosis; 9. biopsy; 10. cauterization; 11. cellulitis; 12. chemabrasion; 13. varicella; 14. ulcer; 15. ecchymosis; 16. debridement; 17. abscess; 18. dermatome; 19. epidermal; 20. erythema; 21. fissure; 22. cyanosis; 23. gangrene; 24. hypodermic; 25. impetigo; 26. pustule; 27. vesicle; 28. adenopathy; 29. keratin; 30. lipoma; 31. nodule; 32. macule; 33. lesion; 34. urticaria; 35. melanocyte; 36. scleroderma; 37. necrosis; 38. papule; 39. xeroderma; 40. psoriasis; 41. hidradenitis; 42. percutaneous; 43. dermatology; 44. pyogenic; 45. onychophagia; 46. seborrhea; 47. subcutaneous; 48. tinea; 49. ungual; 50. leukoderma

B. Transcription Practice

1. The dermatologist took a biopsy to determine that the patient has a nevus rather than malignant melanoma.
2. A culture and sensitivity was performed to determine how best to treat the infected ulcer.
3. The patient had a very large boil (or furuncle) surrounded by a large area of cellulitis.
4. Ms. Marks was lucky, when she tripped off the curb she received only abrasions and contusions.
5. Mr. Brown's chronic exposure to toxins at work had left him with xeroderma, ichthyoderma, and pachyderma.
6. After years of onychophagia, the patient developed onychomalacia and onychomycosis that required onychectomy.
7. To repair the areas of 3rd degree burns a skin graft was necessary.
8. Mr. Strong was concerned that the lump he could feel under his skin was an adenoma, but it turned out to only be a lipoma/adipoma, and it was removed with a lipectomy/adipectomy.
9. The plastic surgeon helped Mr. Marsh decide whether to use chemabrasion or dermabrasion for his face lift.
10. New medical students often have difficulty telling the difference between a macule, a papule, and a cyst.

C. Labeling Exercises

1. Epidermis; 2. Dermis; 3. Subcutaneous layer; 4. Sweat gland (hidr/o); 5. Sensory receptors; 6. Sebaceous gland (seb/o); 7. Arrector pili muscle; 8. Hair (trich/o); 9. Nerve; 10. Vein; 11. Artery

D. Build Medical Terms

1. a. xeroderma; b. erythroderma; c. pyoderma; d. scleroderma; e. pachyderma; 2. a. hidradenitis; b. anhidrosis; 3. a. melanocyte; b. melanoma; 4. a. dermatopathy; b. dermatoplasty; c. dermatology; 5. a. onychomalacia; onychomycosis; c. onychectomy

E. Spelling

1. impetigo, 2. correctly spelled; 3. wheal; 4. correctly spelled; 5. correctly spelled; 6. tinea; 7. petechiae; 8. gangrene; 9. correctly spelled; 10. necrosis

F. Fill in the Blank

1. fissure, laceration;   2. herpes simplex;   3. dermabrasion.   4.   3rd degree;   5. macule;
6. debridement;   7. ecchymosis;   8. biopsy;   9. papule or nodule, pustule;   10. decubitus ulcer

G. Abbreviation Matching

1. E;   2. I;   3. H;   4. G;   5. J;   6. B;   7. A;   8. D;   9. F;   10. C

H. Med Term Analysis

1. aden/o, gland, -megaly, enlarged, enlarged gland;   2. adip, fat, -cyte, cell, fat cell;
3. cyan/o, blue, -osis, abnormal condition, abnormal condition of blue;   4. hypo-, under, derm, skin, -ic, pertaining to, pertaining to under skin;   5. kerat/o, hard or horn-like, -genic, producing, producing hard, horn-like;   6. lip, fat, -ectomy, surgical removal, surgical removal of fat;
7. py/o, pus, -rrhea, discharge or flow, pus discharge;   8. erythr/o, red, -derma, skin condition, red skin condition;   9. trich/o, hair, myc, fungus, -osis, abnormal condition, abnormal condition of hair fungus;   10. sub-, under, cutane, skin, -ous, pertaining to, pertaining to under the skin

I. Photomatch Challenge

1. cyst;   2. fissure;   3. macule;   4. pustule;   5. ulcer;   6. vesicle

J. Crossword Puzzle

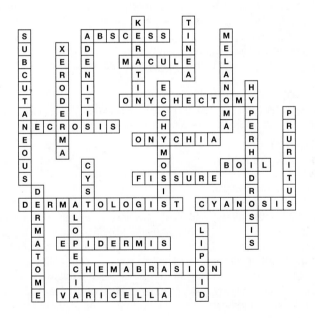

Chapter 6

Word Building

1. a. iliac; b. subiliac;   2. a. carpal; b. costal; c. intercostal; d.; femoral; e. humeral; f. ischial; g. metacarpal; h. metatarsal; i. radial; j. sacral; k. sternal; l. substernal; m. tarsal; n. tibial; o. vertebral; p. intervertebral;   3. a. clavicular; b. fibular; c. mandibular; d. submandibular; e. patellar; f. scapular; g. subscapular; h. ulnar;   4. a. arthrocentesis; b. arthroclasia; c. arthrodesis; d. arthrography; e. arthrogram; f. arthritis; g. arthroscopy; h. arthroscope; i. arthroplasty; j. arthralgia;   5. a. maxillary; b. supramaxillary;   6. a. bursal; b. bursitis; c. bursectomy;   7. a. chondral; b. chondritis; c. chondrectomy; d. chondromalacia;

e. chondroma; f. chondroplasty;   8. a. cranial; b. intracranial; c. craniotomy; d. cranioplasty;
9. a. coccygeal; b. phalangeal;   10. a. pubic; b. suprapubic;   11. a. bradykinesia;
b. dyskinesia; c. hyperkinesia;   12. a. muscular; b. intramuscular;   13. a. myeloma;
b. myelogenic; c. myelopathy;   14. a. myalgia; b. myasthenia; c. electromyogram;
d. electromyography; e. myopathy; f. myorrhaphy; g. myorrhexis;   15. a. ostealgia;
b. osteocyte; c. osteogenic; d. osteoarthritis; e. osteochondritis; f. osteochondroma;
g. osteoclasia; h. osteomyelitis; i. osteopathy; j. osteotome; k. osteomalacia; l. osteoporosis;
16. a. spondylosis; b. spondylitis;   17. a. tenalgia; b. tenodynia; c. tenodesis;
d. tenorrhaphy;   18. a. tendinous; b. tendinitis; c. tendinoplasty; d. tendinosis

Case Study

1. *Osteoporosis*–means "porous bones"; the thinning and loss of bone density that occurs
   slowly over time as more minerals such as calcium are removed from the bone than are
   deposited; very common in postmenopausal women
   Compression fracture–loss of height of a vertebral body; osteoporosis makes bones less
   strong , and they collapse easily
2. Answers will vary. Example of a correct answer is Actonel–slows bone loss and increases bone mass
3. RL–right leg; fx–fracture; T10–10th thoracic vertebra; NSAIDs–non-steroidal anti-inflammatory
   drug; # - pound; hr–hour; LE–lower extremity; DTRs–deep tendon reflexes; MRI–magnetic resonance imaging; L4-5–between 4th and 5th lumbar vertebrae; HNP–herniated nucleus pulposus
4. b
5. myocardial infarction–heart attack; renal failure–kidney's stop filtering waste from blood; Alzheimer
   disease–progressive dementia; spina bifida–vertebrae do not fully form around spinal cord
6. X-ray–radiation is passed through the body to produce an image by exposing a photographic
   plate–it showed spondylosis but no arthritis
   MIR–image created by strong magnetic field and radiowaves–showed herniated nucleus
   pulposus at L4-5
7. pain relief, traction, back strengthening exercises
8. Use of thin catheter tube inserted into intervertebral disk through skin to suck out pieces of
   herniated or ruptured disk; or laser is used to vaporize disk

Practice Exercises

A. Sound It Out

1. osteocyte;   2. fibromyalgia;   3. bradykinesia;   4. chondroplasty;.   5. maxillary;
6. coccygeal;   7. electromyogram;   8. orthosis;   9. synovial;   10. femoral;   11. humerus;
12. sacrum;   13. arthroplasty;   14. iliac;   15. intervertebral;   16. intramuscular;
17. kyphosis;   18. lordosis;   19. mandibular;   20. phalangeal;   21. bursitis;
22. metacarpal;   23. ulnar;   24. fibular;   25. myeloma;   26. arthrocentesis;
27. craniotomy;   28. myorrhexis;   29. osteomyelitis;   30. scoliosis;   31. patellar;
32. tenorrhaphy;   33. prosthesis;   34. tenodesis;   35. pubic;   36. radial;   37. metatarsal;
38. ischium;   39. radiography;   40. scapula;   41. spondylosis;   42. sternum;
43. cartilage;   44. chondroma;   45. tendinoplasty;   46. osteoporosis;   47. tenodynia;
48. contracture;   49. pubis;   50. tibial

B. Transcription Practice

1. The comminuted fracture required open reduction and internal fixation.
2. Radiography revealed a femoral osteochondroma.
3. The patient's chronic bursitis eventually required a bursectomy.
4. Mary's hand deformities from rheumatoid arthritis were improved by wearing an orthosis.
5. When Otto's osteoarthritis in his knee prevented him from walking he had a total knee
   arthroplasty.

6. What first appeared to be an oblique fracture turned out to be a spiral fracture.
7. A bone scan was necessary to identify the stress fracture.
8. Jean's vertebral osteoporosis was diagnosed by dual energy absorptiometry.
9. The child's dyskinesia caused the physician to suspect muscular dystrophy.
10. The ankle strain was severe enough to require a tenodesis.

C. Labeling Exercises

1. Maxilla–upper jaw (maxill/o);   2. Mandible–lower jaw (mandibul/o);   3. Sternum–breast bone (stern/o);   4. Rib (cost/o);   5. Vertebrae (spondyl/o, vertebr/o);   6. Sacrum (sacr/o); 7. Coccyx–tailbone (coccyg/o);   8. Cranium–skull (crani/o);   9. Clavicle–collar bone (clavicul/o); 10. Scapula–shoulder blade (scapul/o);   11. Humerus (humer/o);   12. Radius–forearm (radi/o); 13. Ulna–forearm (uln/o);   14. Carpals–wrist bones (carp/o);   15. Metacarpus–hand bones (metacarp/o);   16. Phalanges–finger bones (phalang/o);   17. Ilium (ili/o);   18. Pubis (pub/o); 19. Ischium (ischi/o);   20. Femur–thigh bone (femor/o);   21. Patella–knee cap (patell/o); 22. Tibia–shin bone (tibi/o);   23. Fibula (fibul/o);   24. Tarsals–ankle bones (tars/o); 25. Metatarsus–foot bones (metatars/o);   26. Phalanges–toe bones (phalang/o)

D. Build Medical Terms

1. arthrocentesis;   2. arthritis;   3. arthroscope;   4. arthroplasty;   5. arthrography; 6. myasthenia;   7. myorrhaphy;   8. hyperkinesia;   9. bradykinesia;   10. osteotome; 11. osteoporosis;   12. osteogenic;   13. chondromalacia;   14. chondroma;   15. chondroplasty

E. Fill in the Blank

1. closed;   2. osteoporosis;   3. kyphosis;   4. orthosis;   5. Carpal tunnel syndrome; 6. prosthesis;   7. Greenstick;   8. ligaments, tendons;   9. internal fixation;   10. spasm

F. Abbreviation Matching

1. D;   2. G;   3. F;   4. J;   5. A;   6. C;   7. I;   8. B;   9. H;   10. E

G. Med Term Analysis

1. arthr/o, joint, -desis, surgical fixation, surgical fixation of joint;   2. burs, bursa, -ectomy, surgical removal, surgical remove bursa;   3. electr/o, electricity, my/o, muscle, -gram, record, record of muscle electricity;   4. intra-, within, crani, skull, -al, pertaining to, pertaining to within the skull; 5. oste/o, bone, myel, red bone marrow, -itis, inflammation, inflammation of bone and red bone marrow;   6. ten, tendon, -algia, pain, tendon pain;   7. spondyl, vertebra, -osis, abnormal condition, vertebra abnormal condition;   8. sub-, below, stern, sternum, -al, pertaining to, pertaining to below the sternum;   9. inter-, between, vertebr, vertebrae, -al, pertaining to, pertaining to between vertebrae;   10. supra-, above, maxill, maxilla, -ary, pertaining to, pertaining to above the maxilla

H. Spelling

1. correctly spelled;   2. bursectomy;   3. correctly spelled;   4. correctly spelled;   5. correctly spelled;   6. correctly spelled;   7. chondrectomy;   8. coccygeal;   9. dyskinesia;   10. spondylosis

I. Photomatch Challenge

1. transverse fracture;   2. oblique fracture;   3. spiral fracture;   4. comminuted fracture; 5. greenstick fracture;   6. compression fracture

J. Crossword Puzzle

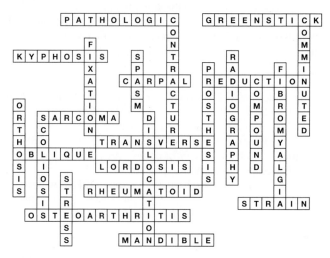

Chapter 7

Word Building

1. a. angiogram; b. angiography; c. angioma; d. angioplasty; e. angiospasm f. polyangiitis
2. a. aortic; b. aortoplasty   3. a. arterial; b. arteriogram; c. arteriography; d. arteriorrhaphy; e. arteriorrhexis; f. arteriostenosis; g. arteriole   4. a. arteriolar   5. a. atherosclerosis; b. atherectomy   6. a. atrial; b. interatrial; c. atrioventricular   7. a. cardiac; b. cardiodynia; c. electrocardiogram; d. electrocardiography; e. cardiologist; f. cardiology; g. cardiomegaly; h. cardiomyopathy; i. cardiorrhexis; j. cardiospasm; k. pericardial; l. endocardial; m. myocardial
8. a. coronary   9. a. embolectomy; b. embolism   10. a. ischemia   11. a. phlebitis; b. phlebotomy; c. phlebogram; d. phlebography   12. a. arteriosclerosis   13. a. stethoscope
14. a. thrombotic; b. thrombosis; c. thromboangiitis; d. thrombophlebitis; e. thrombogenic; f. thrombolysis   15. a. valvoplasty; b. valvotomy; c. valvule   16. a. valvular; b. valvulitis
17. a. varicosis; b. varicose   18. a. vascular; b. cardiovascular   19. a. vasospasm
20. a. venous; b. venogram; c. venography; d. intravenous; e. venule   21. a. ventricular; b. interventricular   22. a. venular

Case Study

1. SOB—shortness of breath, having difficulty breathing, especially with activity; angina pectoris—chest pain associated with cardiac ischemia
2. CHF—congestive heart failure, the inability of the heart to pump blood forcefully enough through the body; swelling in the feet.
3. *Digoxin*, or digitalis, is a drug given to people with congestive heart failure to make their hearts beat stronger.
4. The heart is beating too fast (153 beats per minute), but there is no abnormality in the heart beat and no evidence of a heart attack.
5. *Edema* is tissue swelling. She has edema in both feet and her abdomen. She does not have edema in her hands or face.
6. b
7. Final diagnosis is mitral valve prolapse. This means the valve between the left atrium and left ventricle is too loose to close tightly, allowing blood to flow backward into the atrium. This diagnosis is best supported by the echocardiogram, which showed the regurgitation (backflow) of blood into the atrium.
8. The patient is scheduled to undergo valvoplasty, or the surgical repair of the mitral valve with an artificial valve.

Practice Exercises

A. Sound It Out

1. vasospasm;   2. angioplasty;   3. intravenous;   4. cardiomyopathy;   5. arrhythmia;
6. arteriography;   7. atherosclerosis;   8. atrioventricular;   9. atrium;   10. bradycardia;
11. venular;   12. cardiac;   13. mitral;   14. cardiovascular;   15. aortic;   16. coronary;
17. defibrillation;   18. electrocardiography;   19. ultrasonography;   20. ischemia;
21. embolism;   22. angioma;   23. endarterectomy;   24. fibrillation;   25. pericardial;
26. auscultation;   27. hypertension;   28. cardiorrhexis;   29. hypotension;   30. infarct;
31. venous;   32. myocardial;   33. phlebitis;   34. endocarditis;   35. phlebogram;   36. septum;
37. venipuncture;   38. sphygmomanometer;   39. tachycardia;   40. interventricular;
41. thrombolysis;   42. valvular;   43. varicose;   44. aneurysm;   45. plaque;   46. cardiomegaly;
47. polyangiitis;   48. ventricular;   49. thrombosis;   50. stethoscope

B. Transcription Practice

1. Dr. Jones suspected his patient had had a myocardial infarction, so he ordered an electrocardiogram and cardiac enzymes.
2. The paramedics applied defibrillation because fibrillation was detected.
3. The patient developed bradycardia and required surgery to implant a pacemaker.
4. Susan wore a Holter monitor for 24 hours to further evaluate her angina pectoris.
5. The patient had a Doppler ultrasonography to assess whether she had heart valve prolapse or heart valve stenosis.
6. During auscultation, the nurse detected a heart murmur caused by mitral valve prolapse.
7. The patient suffered an infarct when an embolus broke off a plaque.
8. A cardiac catheterization was ordered in order to determine whether the patient requires a percutaneous transluminal coronary angioplasty.
9. The patient experiences angina pectoris because of severe coronary artery disease.
10. This patient's hypertension eventually caused him to develop congestive heart failure.

C. Spelling

1. tachycardia;   2. correctly spelled;   3. correctly spelled;   4. auscultation;   5. atherosclerosis;
6. correctly spelled;   7. correctly spelled;   8. aneurysm;   9. angioma;   10. correctly spelled

D. Labeling Exercis

1. Left atrium (atri/o);   2. Aortic valve (valvul/o, valv/o);   3. Mitral valve (valvul/o, valv/o);
4. Left ventricle (ventricul/o);   5. Endocardium;   6. Myocardium;   7. Aorta (aort/o);   8. Right atrium (atri/o);   9. Pulmonary valve (valvul/o, valv/o);   10. Bicuspid valve (valvul/o, valv/o);
11. Right ventricle (ventricul/o)

E. Build Medical Terms

1. cardiology;   2. cardiomegaly;   3. cardiorrhexis;   4. cardiogram;   5. valvoplasty;
6. valvotomy;   7. arteriosclerosis;   8. atherosclerosis;   9. angioma;   10. angiospasm;
11. arteriorrhaphy;   12. arterial;   13. arteriography;   14. thrombophlebitis;   15. thrombolysis

F. Fill in the Blank

1. aneurysm;   2. cardiac arrest;   3. stethoscope;   4. Holter monitor;   5. congenital septal defect;   6. venipuncture;   7. vegetation;   8. clot-busters;   9. heart murmur;
10. cardiopulmonary resuscitation

G. Abbreviation Matching

1. D;   2. H;   3. F;   4. B;   5. G.   6. I;   7. A;   8. J;   9. E;   10. C

H. Medical Term Analysis

1. aort/o, aorta, –plasty, surgical repair, surgical repair of the aorta;   2. embol, plug, –ectomy, surgical removal, surgical removal of a plug;   3. cardi/o, heart, my/o, muscle, –pathy, disease, disease of heart muscle;   4. endo–, within, cardi, heart, –al, pertaining to, pertaining to within the heart;   5. thromb/o, clot, angi, vessel, –itis, inflammation, inflammation of vessel with clots; 6. ather/o, fatty substance, –sclerosis, hardening, hardening with fatty substance;   7. valvul, valve, –otomy, cutting into, cutting into of valve;   8. inter–, between, ventricul, ventricle, –ar, pertaining to, pertaining to between ventricles;   9. cardi/o, heart, vascul, blood vessel, –ar, pertaining to blood vessels of the heart;   10. steth/o, chest, –scope, instrument to view, instrument to view chest

I. Photomatch Challenge

1. C;   2. B;   3. D;   4. A;   5. slow, E;   6. fast, F

J. Crossword Puzzle

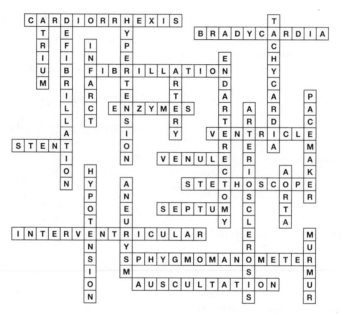

Chapter 8

Word Building

1. a. erythrocyte; b. leukocyte; c. thrombocyte; d. monocyte;   3. lymphocyte   2. a. erythrocytosis; b. leukocytosis; c. thrombocytosis   3. a. anemia; b. hyperglycemia; c. hypoglycemia; d. hyperlipemia   4. a. hematology; b. hematologist; c. hematic; d. hematoma; e. hematopathology; f. hematocytopenia; hematopoiesis   5. a. hemocyte; b. hemoglobin; c. hemostasis; d. hemorrhage; e. hemolysis; f. hemocytolysis; g. hemocytoma; h. hemocytometer; i. hemocytometry   6. a. erythropenia; b. leukopenia; c. thrombocytopenia; d. pancytopenia; e. eosinopenia; neutropenia   7. a. eosinophil; b. basophil; c. neutrophil   8. a. erythropoiesis; b. leukopoiesis; thrombopoiesis   9. a. thrombolysis; b. thrombectomy; c. thrombosis

Case Study

1. fatigue and dyspnea (shortness of breath) with even light activity; 3 episodes of sinusitis (sinus inflammation) and pharyngitis (throat inflammation) in past 6 months; easy bruising; 2 episodes of epistaxis (nose bleed) in last week
2. a complete blood count (CBC); consists of red blood cell count (RBC), white blood cell count (WBC), hemoglobin (Hgb), hematocrit (Hct), white blood cell differential, and platelet count
3. pancytopenia; fatigue and dyspnea because of low red cell count; recurring infections because of low white cell count; bruising and epistaxis because of low platelet count
4. appendix removed at age 12; gallbladder removed at age 35; has been pregnant 3 times with 2 children born and 1 child died before it was a viable age
5. she could be exposed to toxic chemicals in her job working with pesticides
6. the patient's results are probably much higher than yours
7. A *biopsy* removes a small sample of tissue for examination under a microscope for the purpose of making a diagnosis. This patient had her bone marrow biopsied; the biopsy revealed a low number of blood cells in the marrow and that are normal in appearance
8. Blood transfusion–treats symptoms; long-term antibiotics treats symptoms; medication to stimulate the bone marrow treats underlying cause; bone marrow transplant treats underlying cause; washing hands and avoiding sick people treats symptoms

Practice Exercise

A. Sound It Out

1. hematocrit;   2. anticoagulant;   3. leukopoiesis;   4. coagulate;   5. embolus;
6. hemocytometer;   7. eosinopenia;   8. hematic;   9. anemia;   10. hematopathology;
11. basophil;   12. hematopoiesis;   13. erythrocyte;   14. hemocytolysis;   15. thrombolysis;
16. hemoglobin;   17. autotransfusion;   18. hemolysis;   19. erythropenia;   20. hyperlipemia;
21. leukemia;   22. erythrocytosis;   23. leukocyte;   24. hematologist;   25. leukocytosis;
26. hemocytoma;   27. thrombosis;   28. hemostasis;   29. lymphocyte;   30. monocyte;
31. hemocytometry;   32. eosinophil;   33. neutrophil;   34. pancytopenia;   35. hematoma;
36. phlebotomy;   37. erythropoiesis;   38. plasma;   39. hemorrhage;   40. platelets;
41. septicemia;   42. thalassemia;   43. hypoglycemia;   44. thrombectomy;
45. neutropenia;   46. thrombocyte;   47. thrombocytosis;   48. hemophilia;
49. leukopenia;   50. thrombopoiesis

B. Transcription Practice

1. The formed elements of blood are erythrocytes, leukocytes, and platelets (thrombocytes).
2. The patient had a bone marrow aspiration to determine whether she had leukemia.
3. The blood vessel was blocked by an embolus.
4. Elena received thrombolytic therapy during her heart attack.
5. Because he had diabetes, Ted monitored his blood for hyperglycemia.
6. The patient suffered hemorrhage and hematoma as a result of the auto accident.
7. The hematologist determined that Genevieve had developed pernicious anemia.
8. Following heart surgery, Tran received an autotransfusion.
9. A complete blood count revealed that Marco had pancytopenia.
10. Because septicemia was suspected, a blood culture and sensitivity was ordered.

C. Abbreviation Matching

1. G; 2. J;   3. E;   4. A;   5. I;   6. H;   7. D;   8. B;   9. F;   10. C

D. Fill in the Blanks

1. aplastic;   2. embolus;   3. thrombolytic;   4. too many;   5. venipuncture;   6. culture and sensitivity;   7. hematocrit;   8. leukemia;   9. vitamin B12;   10. blood poisoning

E. Labeling Exercise

1. Plasma;   2. Erythrocytes (erythr/o);   3. Platelets;   4. Neutrophil (neutr/o);   5. Lymphocyte (lymph/o);   6. Monocyte;   7. Basophil (bas/o);   8. Eosinophil (eosin/o)

F. Build Medical Terms

1. erythrocyte;   2. leukocyte;   3. thrombocyte;   4. hematology;   5. hematopoiesis;
6. hematic;   7. hematoma;   8. hyperglycemia;   9. anemia;   10. hemostasis;
11. hemorrhage;   12. hemolysis;   13. eosinophil;   14. basophil;   15. neutrophil

G. Medical Term Analysis

1. erythr/o, red, -cytosis, abnormal cell condition, abnormal red cell condition;   2. hemat/o, blood, -logist, one who studies, one who studies blood;   3. hemat/o, blood, path/o, disease, -logy, study of, study of blood diseases;   4. hyper-, excessive, lip, fat, -emia, blood condition, blood condition of excessive sugar;   5. hem/o, blood, cyt/o, cell, -meter, instrument to measure, instrument to measure blood cells;   6. leuk/o, white, -poiesis, formation, white formation;
7. lymph/o, lymph, -cyte, cell, lymph cell;   8. hem/o, blood, -globin, protein, blood protein;
9. pan-, all, cyt/o, cells, -penia, too few, too few of all cells;   10. thromb, clot, -ectomy, surgical removal, surgical removal of clot

H. Spelling

1. hypoglycemia;   2. correctly spelled;   3. correctly spelled;   4. septicemia;   5. correctly spelled;   6. platelet;   7. polycythemia vera;   8. correctly spelled;   9. correctly spelled;
10. erythropoiesis

I. Photomatch Challenge

1. C;   2. D;   3. E;   4. F;   5. B;   6. A

J. Crossword Puzzle

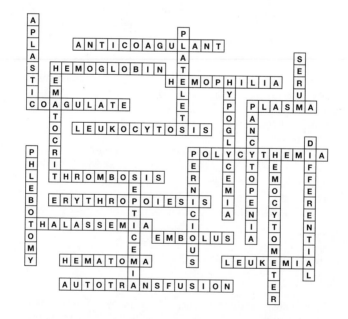

Chapter 9

Word Building

1. a. adenoidectomy; b. adenoiditis   2. a. immunologist; b. immunology; c. immunoglobulin;
   d. immunogenic; e. immunotherapy   3. a. lymphatic; b. lymphoma; c. lymphedema;
   d. lymphocyte; e. lymphocytic; f. lymphocytoma; g. lymphogenic; h. lymphoid; i. lymphostasis
4. a. lymphadenectomy; b. lymphadenopathy; c. lymphadenography; d. lymphadenogram;
   e. lymphadenitis; f. lymphadenosis   5. a. lymphangiitis; b. lymphangiopathy; c. lymphangioma;
   d. lymphangiography; e. lymphangiogram; f. lymphangiectomy; g. lymphangiectasis;
   h. lymphangioplasty   6. a. pathogenic; b. pathogen; c. pathology; d. pathologist
7. a. phagocyte; b. phagocytic   8. a. splenic; b. splenitis; c. splenoid; d. splenoma;
   e. splenectomy; f. splenomegaly; g. splenomalacia; h. splenopexy; i. splenorrhaphy
9. a. thymic; b. thymectomy; c. thymoma   10. a. tonsillar; b. tonsillectomy; c. tonsillitis

Case Study

1. As a heroin addict, he probably shared needles; unsafe sex practices and blood transfusion
2. yeast
3. thrush, weight loss, recurring infections (sinusitis and bronchitis), diarrhea, night sweats,
   extreme fatigue, unexplained fevers, muscular wasting, fever, enlarged cervical and inguinal
   lymph nodes
4. ELISA; Western blot is considered more precise than ELISA
5. ARC is early in the infection and the symptoms are milder; AIDS is the later stages of infection
   in which the immune system is no longer able to resist infections and the person is prone to
   opportunistic infections
6. Infections that occur when the immune system is compromised; PCP and Kaposi sarcoma
7. Zidovudine keeps virus from reproducing; Epivir prevents virus from multiplying; Viracept
   slows growth of virus
8. If the CD4 count is low, the immune system is not able to work very well and patient is
   at higher risk of opportunistic infection; if it remains OK, then the HIV medications are
   working

Practice Exercises

A. Sound It Out

1. lymphoma;   2. allergy;   3. immunogenic;   4. lymphadenopathy;   5. immunoglobulin;
6. pathology;   7. lymphatic;   8. immunotherapy;   9. inflammation;   10. lymph;
11. splenomegaly;   12. lymphadenectomy;   13. antihistamine;   14. lymphadenitis;
15. corticosteroids;   16. lymphadenography;   17. adenoidectomy;   18. lymphangiectomy;
19. lymphangiitis;   20. lymphangiogram;   21. splenoma;   22. lymphangioma;
23. sarcoidosis;   24. lymphocytic;   25. thymic;   26. lymphoid;   27. lymphostasis;
28. mononucleosis;   29. pathogen;   30. splenoid;   31. pathogenic;   32. phagocyte;
33. lymphocytoma;   34. urticaria;   35. phagocytic;   36. splenectomy;   37. tonsillectomy;
38. splenitis;   39. immunologist;   40. splenomalacia;   41. elephantiasis;   42. lymphedema;
43. splenopexy;   44. thymectomy;   45. tonsillar;   46. vaccination;   47. thymoma;
48. adenoiditis;   49. lymphogenic;   50. tonsils

B. Transcription Practice

1. Marcie's repeated bouts of tonsillitis required her to have a tonsillectomy and
   adenoidectomy.
2. The lymphangiogram revealed a lymphangioma.

3. The immunologist is a physician who treats autoimmune diseases.
4. Jamar had a history of anaphylactic shock in response to bee stings.
5. Mykos had to take immunosuppressants after his kidney transplant.
6. Joyce's allergy to pollen was treated with antihistamines.
7. The AIDS patient developed *Pneumocystis carinii* pneumonia.
8. Jennifer's allergic reactions consisted of hives and urticaria.
9. Shona's hand pain turned out to be caused by systemic lupus erythematosus.
10. Carlos' lymphadenopathy turned out to be Hodgkin disease.

C. Build Medical Terms

1. lymphadenectomy;   2. lymphadenogram;   3. lymphadenopathy;   4. immunoglobulin;
5. immunologist;   6. splenomegaly;   7. splenoid;   8. splenic;   9. tonsillitis;   10. tonsillectomy;
11. tonsillar;   12. lymphangiitis;   13. lymphangioplasty;   14. lymphangiography;
15. lymphangioma

D. Labeling Exercises

1. Lymphatic vessel (lymphangi/o);   2. Lymph nodes (lymphaden/o);   3. Tonsils (tonsill/o,
adenoid/o);   4. Thymus gland (thym/o);   5. Spleen (splen/o)

E. Spelling

1. urticaria;   2. spelled correctly;   3. spelled correctly;   4. spelled correctly;   5. lymphadenosis;
6. immunosuppressants;   7. splenomalacia;   8. tonsillitis;   9. spelled correctly;   10. spelled
correctly

F. Fill in the Blank

1. allergist;   2. autoimmune;   3. lymph vessels, edema;   4. wheals;   5. Corticosteroids;
6. AIDS-related complex;   7. immunizations;   8. skin;   9. Anaphylactic shock;   10. Western
blot test

G. Abbreviation Matching

1. G;   2. C;   3. J;   4. H;   5. D;   6. A;   7. E;   8. I;   9. B;   10. F

H. Med Term Analysis

1. adenoid, adenoids, -itis, inflammation, adenoid inflammation;   2. lymph/o, lymph, -genic,
producing, lymph producing;   3. immun/o, immunity or protection, -therapy, treatment, immunity treatment;   4. lymph/o, lymph, cyt, cell, -oma, tumor, lymph cell tumor;   5. phag/o, eating,
cyt, cell, -ic, pertaining to, pertaining to eating cell;   6. lymphaden/o, lymph node, -pathy, disease, lymph node disease;   7. path/o, disease, -logy, study of, study of disease;   8. lymphangi,
lymph vessel, -ectasis, dilated, dilated lymph vessel;   9. thym, thymus gland, -ectomy, surgical
removal, surgical removal of thymus gland;   10. lymph, lymph, -edema, swelling, lymph
swelling

I. Photomatch Challenge

1. B;   2. E;   3. A;   4. F;   5. D;   6. C

J. Crossword Puzzle

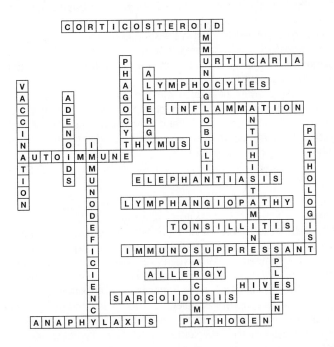

Chapter 10

Word Building

1. a. alveolar   2. a. bronchial; b. bronchiole; c. bronchiectasis   3. a. bronchiolar
4. a. bronchogram; b. bronchography; c. bronchitis; d. bronchoscope; e. bronchoscopy;
f. bronchospasm; g. bronchogenic   5. a. pneumoconiosis   6. a. cyanosis   7. a. lobar;
b. lobectomy   8. a. mediastinal; b. mediastinotomy   9. a. orthopnea   10. a. anoxia
11. a. oximeter; b. oximetry   12. a. pleural; b. pleurocentesis; c. pleurodynia; d. pleuralgia;
e. pleuritis   13. a. apnea; b. dyspnea; c. eupnea; d. hyperpnea; e. hypopnea; f. bradypnea;
g. tachypnea   14. a. pneumogram; b. pneumograph; c. pneumography; d. pneumothorax
15. a. pneumonic; b. pneumonocentesis; c. pneumonectomy; d. pneumonotomy
16. a. pulmonary; b. pulmonology; c. pulmonologist   17. a. hemoptysis   18. a. spirogram;
b. spirometer; c. spirometry   19. a. thoracalgia; b. thoracodynia; c. thoracic; d. thoracotomy;
e. thoracocentesis; f. thoracostomy   20. a. hemothorax; b. pyothorax; c. pneumothorax
21. a. tracheal; b. tracheoplasty; c. tracheostomy; d. tracheotomy; e. tracheitis; f. endotracheal

Case Study

1. d. pain in the chest region
2. *endometriosis*–presence of endometrial tissue outside the uterus; she had the uterus removed
   cholelithiasis–gallbladder stones; she had her gallbladder removed
   lumbar compression fracture due osteoporosis–collapse of vertebra because her bones were brittle
3. No, it is not important; it does not include lung problems. Her brother has high blood pressure, her mother had a stroke (blood vessel disease), and her father had diabetes mellitus (problem with blood sugar levels because the pancreas fails to produce enough insulin).
4. rales (crackling sound during inhalation), but no rhonchi (whistling sound during inhalation or exhalation)

5. In a sputum culture and sensitivity, a sputum specimen is placed in a culture medium in an attempt to grow and then identify the type of bacteria present and what antibiotic is effective in killing it. This test did not reveal any bacteria in her sputum.
Sputum cytology examines the cells in the sputum for the presence of cancer. This test did identify cancerous cells in this patient's sputum.
6. Chest radiograph, AP view, is a plain chest x-ray taken from the front to the back. It showed a suspicious looking cloudy area in her lung.
Chest CT scan is an x-ray image formed with the assistance of a computer to have a cross-sectional view of the chest. It shows more detail and revealed that the cloudy area was a tumor.
7. thoracic surgeon to open up her chest and remove one lobe of her lung;
oncologist (cancer specialist) to determine whether the cancer has spread and whether she needs to have chemotherapy treatments

Practice Exercise

A. Sound It Out

1. tracheotomy; 2. apnea; 3. ventilator; 4. asthma; 5. bradypnea; 6. bronchiolar; 7. bronchitis; 8. bronchodilator; 9. hemothorax; 10. alveolar 11. bronchogenic; 12.pneumonectomy; 13. bronchoscope; 14. asphyxia; 15. bronchospasm; 16. cyanosis; 17. dyspnea; 18. emphysema; 19. oxygen; 20. atelectasis; 21. eupnea; 22. hemoptysis; 23. hyperventilation; 24. phlegm; 25. pulmonary; 26. pneumograph; 27. influenza; 28. lobectomy; 29. mediastinal; 30. endotracheal; 31. oximeter; 32. croup; 33. aspirate; 34. pleural; 35. bronchography; 36. pleurisy; 37. pulmonology; 38. pneumocentesis; 39. pneumoconiosis; 40. pneumothorax; 41. tuberculosis; 42. purulent; 43. thoracic; 44. pyothorax; 45. spirometry; 46. sputum; 47. pleurocentesis; 48. anoxia; 49. thoracotomy; 50. tracheoplasty

B. Transcription Practice

1. During auscultation, the physician heard rales when the patient inhaled.
2. It was unclear from the chest x-ray whether the patient had hemothorax or pyothorax.
3. The results of the arterial blood gases revealed hypoxia.
4. The patient underwent a lobectomy after the discovery of bronchogenic carcinoma.
5. Mr. Scott's hypopnea was so severe because he had cyanosis.
6. Carlyn went to the pulmonologist when she noticed hemoptysis several mornings in a row.
7. The physician ordered a sputum culture and sensitivity because Lars was coughing up purulent sputum.
8. The patient underwent pulmonary function tests using a spirometer and an oximeter.
9. The patient had chronic obstructive pulmonary disease causing him to have dyspnea and a chronic cough.
10. Pulmonary angiography was ordered to determine whether there was a pulmonary embolism.

C. Spelling

1. pneumoconiosis; 2. correctly spelled; 3. correctly spelled; 4. ventilator; 5. purulent; 6. correctly spelled; 7. correctly spelled; 8. hyperpnea; 9. correctly spelled; 10. alveolar

D. Labeling Exercise

1. Trachea (trache/o); 2. Apex; 3. Lobe (lob/o); 4. Hilum; 5. Right lung (pneum/o, pneumon/o, pulmon/o) 6. Base; 7. Mediastinum (mediastin/o); 8. Bronchus (bronch/o, bronchi/o); 9. Left lung (pneum/o, pneumon/o, pulmon/o) 10. Chest (thorac/o, steth/o); 11. Diaphragm

E. Build Medical Terms

1. bronchogram; 2. bronchoscopy; 3. bronchospasm; 4. pneumonocentesis; 5. pneumonectomy; 6. pneumonic; 7. pneumonotomy; 8. atelectasis; 9. bronchiectasis; 10 tracheostomy; 11. tracheoplasty; 12. tracheitis; 13. apnea; 14. tachypnea; 15. dyspnea

F. Fill in the Blanks

1. asthma;   2. bronchoscopy;   3. emphysema;   4. cystic fibrosis;   5. trachea;   6. spirometer;   7. hyperventilation;   8. infant respiratory distress syndrome;   9. pneumothorax;   10. pulmonary embolism

G. Abbreviation Matching

1. D;   2. H;   3. F;   4. A;   5. J;   6. B;   7. I;   8. E;   9. G;   10. C

H. Medical Term Analysis

1. thorac/o, chest, -centesis, puncture to withdraw fluid, puncture chest to withdraw fluid;   2.cyan, blue, -osis, abnormal condition, abnormal condition of being blue;   3. pneum/o, air, -thorax, chest, air in the chest;   4. endo-, within, trache, trachea, -al, pertaining to, pertaining to within the trachea;   5. pneum/o, lung, coni, dust, -osis, abnormal condition, abnormal condition of lung dust;   6.ox/i, oxygen, -meter, instrument to measure, instrument to measure oxygen;   7. orth/o, straight, -pnea, breathing, straight breathing;   8. pleur/o, pleura, -dynia, pain, pleura pain;   9. bronchi, bronchus, -ectasis, expansion, bronchus expansion;   10. lob, lobe, -ectomy, surgical removal, surgical removal of lobe

I. Photomatch Challenge

1. pleural effusion;   2. pneumothorax;   3. asthma;   4. atelectasis;   5. pneumonia;   6. emphysema

J. Crossword Puzzle

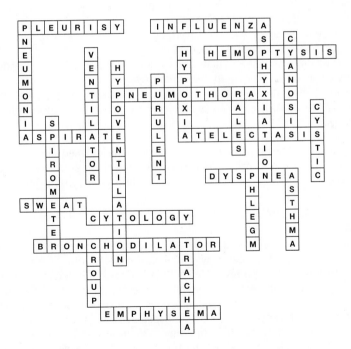

Chapter 11

Word Building

1. a. anal   2. a. appendicitis   3. a. appendectomy   4. a. cholelithiasis; b. cholelithotripsy   5. a. cholangiogram; b. cholangiography   6. a. cholecystitis; b. cholecystectomy; c. cholecystogram; d. cholecystography   7. a. choledocholithiasis; b. choledocholithotripsy   8. a. colostomy; b. colitis; c. colorectal   9. a. colonoscope; b. colonoscopy; c. colonic   10. a. diverticulitis; b. diverticulosis; c. diverticulectomy   11. a. duodenal; b. duodenostomy   12. a. hematemesis; b. hyperemesis   13. a. enteritis; b. enteric   14. a. esophageal; b. esophagoplasty; c. esophagitis; d. esophagoscope; e. esophagoscopy   15. a. gastric; b. gastritis; c. gastroenteritis; d. gastrectomy; e. gastrostomy; f. gastroscope; g. gastroscopy; h. gastrodynia; i. gastralgia; j. gastroenterologist; k. gastroenterology   16. a. hepatitis; b. hepatic; c. hepatoma   17. a. ileal; b. ileostomy   18. a. jejunal; b. jejunostomy   19. a. laparotomy; b. laparoscope; c. laparoscopy   20. a. pancreatic; b. pancreatitis   21. a. apepsia; b. dyspepsia; c. bradypepsia   22. a. aphagia; b. dysphagia; c. polyphagia   23. a. polyposis; b. polypectomy   24. a. proctoptosis; proctoscope; c. proctoscopy; d. proctologist; e. proctology   25. a. rectocele; b. rectal   26. a. sigmoidoscope; b. sigmoidoscopy

Case Study

1. increasing upper abdominal pain for past 8 months, sharp upper abdominal pain about 30 minutes after eating
2. milk and ice cream; spicy foods; over-the-counter antacids (Tums, Rolaids, Zantac)
3. blood test for *Helicobacter pylori*, a bacteria that can cause stomach ulcers; this test was positive, meaning the bacteria are present; *esophagogastroduodenoscopy,* a visual examination of the esophagus, stomach, and first section of intestine showed the stomach was inflamed, but there was no evidence of bleeding or an ulcer
4. in the middle of the upper abdomen overlying much of the stomach; *radiate* means the pain travels from one area of the body to another
5. difficulty swallowing/eating, burning sensation under the breast bone, feeling like he is going to throw up, actually throwing up, pain in the lower abdomen, vomiting blood, dark tarry stools, loose watery stools
6. because his family has had serious GI problems, his mother had cancer of the colon, and his brother had liver disease
7. c
8. Patient was put on two medications, one to reduce the inflamed stomach and one to kill the bacterial infection. If he is not better in 3 months, the physician will repeat the visual exam of the esophagus, stomach, and first section of intestine to see what is happening.

Practice Exercises

A. Sound It Out

1. sigmoidoscope;   2. apepsia;   3. rectocele;   4. gastritis;   5. ascites;   6. cholangiogram;   7. cirrhosis;   8. colitis;   9. colonoscopy;   10. colorectal;   11. diverticulum;   12. anal;   13. duodenostomy;   14. polyposis;   15. cholecystectomy;   16. dyspepsia;   17. aphagia;   18. enteric;   19. esophagoplasty;   20. vomit;   21. esophagoscopy;   22. gastroenteritis;   23. jaundice;   24. gastroscope;   25. hematemesis;   26. appendicitis;   27. hemorrhoids;   28. dysentery;   29. choledocholithiasis;   30. hyperemesis;   31. bradypepsia;   32. ileostomy;   33. jejunal;   34. laparoscopy;   35. laparotomy;   36. melena;   37. nausea;   38. pancreatic;   39. dysphagia;   40. polypectomy;   41. gastrectomy;   42. polyphagia;   43. hepatic;   44. volvulus;   45. proctoptosis;   46. rectal;   47. rectum;   48. sigmoidoscopy;   49. appendix;   50. proctologist

B. Transcription Practice

1. Mr. Mercado was noted to have jaundice, leading to a diagnosis of hepatitis.
2. Mrs. Mendez underwent an esophagogastroduodenoscopy (EGD) that revealed peptic ulcer disease.
3. Mr. Brown's severe diverticulitis resulted in his having a diverticulectomy.
4. The patient presented in the ER with severe nausea and hematemesis.
5. The physician ordered a barium enema (BE, or lower GI series) because of concern that the patient could have polyposis.
6. Because of her cholelithiasis, Ms. Katopolis had a laparotomy and cholecystectomy.
7. Common symptoms of gastroesophageal reflux disease (GERD) include dysphagia and gastrodynia/gastralgia.
8. The patient was found to have an ileus and required a jejunostomy.
9. The BM (or feces) was tested for occult blood and ova and parasites (O&P).
10. To evaluate Mr. Habib's melena, his gastroenterologist performed a proctoscopy, a sigmoidoscopy, and a colonoscopy.

C. Labeling Exercise

1. Liver (hepat/o); 2. Gallbladder (cholecyst/o); 3. Colon (col/o, colon/o); 4. Appendix (appendic/o, append/o); 5. Esophagus (esophag/o); 6. Stomach (gastr/o); 7. Pancreas (pancreat/o); 8. Duodenum (duoden/o); 9. Ileum (ile/o); 10. Jejunum (jejun/o); 11. Sigmoid colon (sigmoid/o); 12. Rectum (rect/o, proct/o); 13. Anus (an/o); 14. Intestine (enter/o)

D. Build Medical Terms

1. gastritis; 2. gastrectomy; 3. gastroscope; 4. gastralgia or gastrodynia; 5. gastrodynia or gastralgia; 6. proctoptosis; 7. rectocele; 8. cholecystitis; 9. cholecystectomy; 10. duodenostomy; 11. colostomy; 12. gastrostomy; 13. apepsia; 14. dyspepsia; 15. bradypepsia

E. Abbreviation Matching

1. H; 2. D; 3. G; 4. I; 5. C; 6. A; 7. B; 8. F; 9. J; 10. E

F. Fill in the Blank

1. total parenteral nutrition; 2. stomach, lower esophagus, duodenum; 3. vomit; 4. barium swallow; 5. liver, gallbladder; 6. ascites; 7. ileus; 8. ulcerative colitis; 9. spastic colon; 10. gastric bypass

G. Spelling

1. correctly spelled; 2. esophageal; 3. pancreatitis; 4. correctly spelled; 5. gastritis; 6. correctly spelled; 7. correctly spelled; 8. cirrhosis; 9. volvulus; 10. correctly spelled

H. Medical Term Analysis

1. esophag/o, esophagus, -plasty, surgical repair, surgical repair of esophagus; 2. append, appendix, -ectomy, surgical removal, surgical removal of appendix; 3. choledoch/o, common bile duct, lith/o, stone, -tripsy, surgical crushing, surgical crushing of stone in common bile duct; 4. hyper-, excessive, -emesis, vomiting, excessive vomiting; 5. gastr/o, stomach, enter, intestine, -itis, inflammation, inflammation of stomach and intestine; 6. hepat, liver, -oma, tumor, liver tumor; 7. diverticul, blind pouch, -osis, abnormal condition, abnormal condition of blind pouches; 8. ile, ileum, -ostomy, create artificial opening, create artificial opening in ileum; 9. lapar/o, abdomen, -scope, instrument to view, instrument to view inside abdomen; 10. poly-, many or excessive, -phagia, eating, excessive eating

I. Photomatch Challenge

1. diverticulosis or diverticulitis; 2. colostomy; 3. laparoscopy; 4. polyposis; 5. cholelithiasis; 6. appendicitis

J. Crossword Puzzle

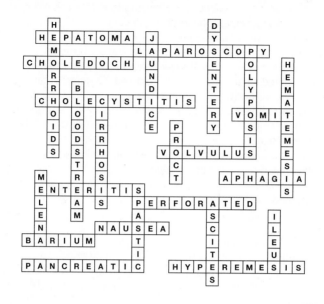

Chapter 12

Word Building

1. a. balanitis; b. balanorrhea 2. a. cystalgia; b. cystocele; c. cystectomy; d. cystitis; e. cystoscopy; f. cystogram; g. cystography; h. cystoscope; i. cystic; j. cystolith 3. a. epididymitis; b. epididymal 4. a. lithotripsy; b. ureterolithiasis; c. nephrolithiasis; d. cystolithiasis 5. a. nephrectomy; b. nephritis; c. nephromegaly; d. nephroma; e. nephroptosis; f. nephrotomy; g. nephropathy; h. nephropexy; i. nephrosclerosis; j. glomerulonephritis; k. nephrolith; l. nephrosis 6. a. orchidectomy 7. a. orchiopexy; b. orchialgia 8. a. anorchism; b. orchitis; c. cryptorchism 9. a. cystostomy; b. nephrostomy; c. ureterostomy; d. pyelostomy; e. urethrostomy; f. vasovasostomy 10. a. prostatectomy; b. prostatitis; c. prostatic 11. a. pyelonephritis; b. pyelogram; c. pyelography 12. a. renal; b. renogram; c. renography 13. a. seminal; b. seminuria 14. a. spermatogenesis; b. spermatolysis; c. spermatic; d. spermatocyte 15. a. aspermia; b. oligospermia 16. a. testicular 17. a. ureteritis; b. ureterostenosis; c. ureteral 18. a. urethroplasty; b. urethralgia; c. urethritis; d. urethroscope; e. urethroscopy; f. urethrostenosis; g. urethrotomy; h. urethral 19. a. glycosuria; b. nocturia; c. oliguria; d. pyuria; e. anuria; f. dysuria; g. hematuria; h. polyuria; i. albuminuria; j. azoturia; k. bacteriuria 20. a. urinary; b. urinometer 21. a. urology; b. urologist; c. uremia 22. a. vasectomy; b. vasorrhaphy 23. a. vesiculitis; b. vesiculectomy; c. vesicular

Case Study

1. He has nocturnal hesitancy (difficulty initiation urination during the night) and frequency (urinating more often but without any increase in the overall volume of urine). He does not have urinary incontinence (inability to hold back urination) or erectile dysfunction (inability to achieve an erection).
2. d. prostatic cancer
3. Vital signs are routine measures of general health. They include temperature, pulse, respiration rate, and blood pressure.
4. urinalysis (UA), digital rectal exam (DRE), prostate-specific antigen (PSA), computed tomography scan (CT scan), culture and sensitivity (C&S), erectile dysfunction (ED), myocardial infarction (MI), percutaneous transluminal coronary angioplasty (PTCA), hypertension (HTN), biopsy (Bx), red blood cells (RBC)

5. A urinalysis is a physical and chemical examination of the urine. It is checked for pH, specific gravity, and the presence of substances such as blood and sugar. This patient did have blood present in his urine, but no bacteria were found.

6. An *oncologist* is a physician specializing in diagnosing and treating cancer. The oncologist did not recommend that this patient have any radiation or chemotherapy treatments because the cancer showed no signs of having left the prostate gland. However, the patient is to continue having a PSA done every 3 months.

7. The two tests were diagnostic images: a bone scan and a CT scan. A *metastasis* is the spread of the initial cancerous tumor to another site in the body.

8. A *myocardial infarction* is a heart attack; part of the heart muscle dies because of lack of blood supply. A *percutaneous transluminal coronary angioplasty* is a treatment procedure that uses a balloon to expand a blocked coronary artery and improve blood flow to the heart muscle.

Practice Exercises

A. Sound It Out

1. ureterostenosis; 2. balanorrhea; 3. urology; 4. cryptorchism; 5. urinometer; 6. aspermia; 7. cystocele; 8. testosterone; 9. nephroma; 10. dysuria; 11. enuresis; 12. epididymitis; 13. glomerulus; 14. vesiculitis; 15. hematuria; 16. chlamydia; 17. hemodialysis; 18. gonorrhea; 19. pyelonephritis; 20. cystolith; 21. nephrosis; 22. lithotripsy; 23. meatus; 24. phimosis; 25. nephrosclerosis; 26. glycosuria; 27. nocturia; 28. oligospermia; 29. orchidectomy; 30. orchiopexy; 31. polyuria; 32. spermatolysis; 33. prostatitis; 34. ureter; 35. pyuria; 36. renography; 37. seminal; 38. spermatogenesis; 39. testicular; 40. urethral; 41. calculus; 42. trichomoniasis; 43. uremia; 44. cystectomy; 45. urethroscope; 46. vasectomy; 47. urinalysis; 48. varicocele; 49. nephromegaly; 50. nephropexy

B. Transcription Practice

1. A cystoscopy revealed the presence of cystolith and the patient underwent a lithotripsy.
2. When noting the balanorrhea and balanitis, the physician knew she needed to determine if the patient had acquired an sexually transmitted disease.
3. A retrograde pyelogram confirmed the diagnosis of pyelonephritis.
4. A semen analysis performed 6 weeks after the vasectomy confirmed aspermia.
5. The patient's polycystic kidney disease had resulted in renal failure, necessitating the use of hemodialysis.
6. The results of the urinalysis showed that there was pyuria, bacteriuria, and glycosuria.
7. After the patient developed anuria a renogram revealed that the patient had developed nephrosclerosis.
8. The elderly gentleman required a circumcision for phimosis.
9. The patient required a ureterostomy following a cystectomy for bladder cancer.
10. Bob developed nephrolithiasis and underwent extracorporeal shockwave lithotripsy.

C. Abbreviation Matching

1. J; 2. G; 3. F; 4. B; 5. A; 6. E; 7. I; 8. H; 9. D; 10. C

D. Labeling Exercise

1. Kidney (ren/o, nephr/o); 2. Ureter (ureter/o); 3. Renal artery; 4. Renal vein 5. Urinary bladder (cyst/o); 6. Urethra (urethr/o)

E. Build Medical Terms

1. nephrology; 2. nephromegaly; 3. nephropathy; 4. nephroptosis; 5. nephropexy; 6. spermatolysis; 7. spermatic; 8. cystogram; 9. cystoscopy; 10. prostatitis; 11. prostatectomy; 12. hematuria; 13. nocturia; 14. dysuria; 15. glycosuria

F. Fill in the Blank

1. varicocele;   2. benign prostatic hypertrophy;   3. testosterone;   4. number, swimming strength, shape;   5. voiding cystourethrography;   6. circumcision;   7. Hesitancy;   8. Prostate specific antigen;   9. blood urea nitrogen;   10. calculus

G. Spelling

1. epididymitis;   2. nephrolithiasis;   3. correctly spelled;   4. pyelography;   5. correctly spelled;   6. correctly spelled;   7. hydrocele;   8. trichomoniasis;   9. correctly spelled;   10. correctly spelled

H. Medical Term Analysis

1. balan, glans penis, -itis, inflammation, inflammation of glans penis;   2. vas, vas deferens, -ectomy, surgical removal, surgical removal of vas deferens;   3. py, pus, -uria, urine condition, urine condition of pus;   4. ureter, ureter, -ostomy, create a surgical opening, create a surgical opening in ureter;   5. nephr/o, kidney, lith, stone, -iasis, abnormal condition, abnormal condition of kidney stones;   6. ur/o, urine, -logy, study of, study of urine;   7. testicul, testes, -ar, pertaining to, pertaining to the testes;   8. crypt, hidden, orch, testes, -ism, condition, condition of hidden testes;   9. prostat, prostate gland, -ectomy, surgical removal, surgical removal of prostate gland;   10. cyst/o, bladder, -scope, instrument to view, instrument to view bladder

I. Photomatch Challenge

1. epididymitis;   2. varicocele;   3. undescended testicle;   4. orchitis;   5. testicular cancer;   6. hydrocele

J. Crossword

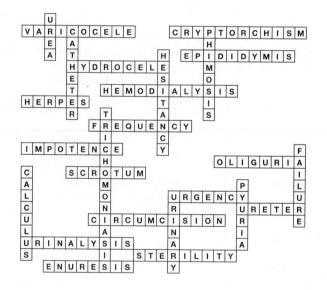

Chapter 13

Word Building

1. a. amniotic; b. amniotomy; c. amniorrhea; d. amniocentesis; e. amniorrhexis   2. a. cervical; b. cervicectomy; c. cervicitis; d. endocervicitis; e. cervicoplasty   3. a. chorionic; b. choriocarcinoma   4. a. colposcope; b. colposcopy; c. colpectomy; d. colporrhaphy   5. a. embryonic; b. embryogenic; c. embryology   6. a. episiorrhaphy; b. episioplasty; c. episiotomy   7. a. fetal; b. fetometry; c. fetoscope; d. fetoscopy   8. a. nulligravida; b. primigravida; c. multigravida   9. a. gynecology; b. gynecologist   10. a. hysteropexy; b. hysterorrhexis; c. hysterectomy; d. hysterography; e. hysterogram   11. a. laparotomy; b. laparoscope; c. laparoscopy   12. a. mammary; b. mammogram; c. mammography; d. mammoplasty   13. a. mastalgia; b. mastitis; c. mastectomy   14. a. amenorrhea; b. dysmenorrhea; c. oligomenorrhea; d. menorrhagia   15. a. endometritis; b. metrorrhea; c. metrorrhagia   16. a. natal; b. neonatal; c. neonatology; d. neonatologist   17. a. oocyte; b. oogenesis   18. a. oophoritis; b. oophorectomy; c. oophoropexy   19. a. ovarian; b. ovariosalpingitis   20. a. nullipara; b. primipara; c. multipara   21. a. antepartum; b. postpartum   22. a. salpingectomy; b. salpingitis; c. salpingography; d. salpingogram; e. salpingocyesis   23. a. uterine; b. uteroplasty; c. uteroscope; d. uteroscopy; e. intrauterine   24. a. vaginal; b. vaginitis; c. transvaginal

Case Study

1. patient is postmenopausal; she had not had any menstrual periods for three years; mild to moderate uterine cramps, lower abdominal pain, and painful intercourse
2. prn = as needed; grav2 = two pregnancies; para2 = two live births; D&C = dilation of cervix and curettage of endometrial lining; EMB = endometrial biopsy, removing a piece of tissue to examine under a microscope
3. migraine–takes pain medicine as needed; asthma–takes a bronchodilator; hyperlipemia–using no treatment
4. cervical cancer; she has endometrial cancer, not cervical cancer
5. Blood tests, Hgb = hemoglobin, measures amount of hemoglobin present in blood; HCT = hematocrit, measures volume of red blood cells in blood; anemic because of loss of blood from the continuous vaginal bleeding
6. Stage I: tumor confined to body of uterus; Stage II: tumor extends to the cervix; Stage III: tumor has spread to the pelvic region; Stage IV: extensive pelvic tumors or tumors have spread to distant organs
7. *hysteroscopy* is a visual examination of the inside of the uterus with a fiberoptic camera; tumor area was very small, so the D&C missed it
8. *lymphadenectomy* means surgical removal of lymph nodes; they will be examined for cancer cells to see whether the cancer has spread

Practice Exercises

A. Sound It Out

1. amenorrhea;   2. amniocentesis;   3. amnion;   4. atresia;   5. cervicoplasty;   6. cervix;   7. choriocarcinoma;   8. chorion;   9. colporrhaphy;   10. colposcopy;   11. conization;   12. cystocele;   13. dysmenorrhea;   14. embryo;   15. endocervicitis;   16. endometriosis;   17. episiotomy;   18. fetometry;   19. fetus;   20. fistula;   21. gynecology;   22. hysterectomy;   23. hysterography;   24. intrauterine;   25. laparoscopy;   26. laparotomy;   27. mammogram;   28. mastectomy;   29. mastitis;   30. menorrhagia;   31. multipara;   32. neonatal;   33. nulligravida;   34. obstetrics;   35. oligomenorrhea;   36. oophorectomy;   37. ovaries;   38. ovariosalpingitis;   39. ovum;   40. placenta;   41. postpartum;   42. primigravida;   43. rectocele;   44. salpingocyesis;   45. transvaginal;   46. uteroplasty;   47. uterus;   48. vagina;   49. vaginitis;   50. vulva

B. Transcription Practice

1. Mrs. Scott's dysmenorrhea was treated with a dilation and curettage.
2. Over time Mrs. Martinez had developed a vesicovaginal fistula.
3. The neonatologist assisted with the cesarean section.
4. Jean's infertility was the result of scarring caused by pelvic inflammatory disease.
5. A hysterectomy became necessary because of extensive endometriosis.
6. The new patient at the one who studies women's office was primigravida and nullipara.
7. Maria was happy to find out she had fibrocystic breast disease and not breast cancer.
8. Ectopic pregnancy (or salpingocyesis).
9. Following an abnormal Pap smear, Tawanda's cervical cancer was diagnosed by conization.
10. A laparoscopy was conducted to examine the patient for ovarian cancer.

C. Build Medical Terms

1. hysteropexy;   2. hysterectomy;   3. hysterorrhexis;   4. hysterogram;   5. fetal;
6. fetometry;   7. antepartum;   8. postpartum;   9. amenorrhea;   10. dysmenorrhea;
11. oligomenorrhea;   12. menorrhagia;   13. mastalgia;   14. mastitis;   15. mastectomy

D. Spelling

1. hysterectomy;   2. spelled correctly;   3. spelled correctly;   4. spelled correctly;
5. premenstrual;   6. antepartum;   7. menorrhagia;   8. spelled correctly;   9. amniotomy;
10. spelled correctly

E. Fill in the Blank

1. fallopian, uterine;   2. gynecology, obstetrics;   3. endometrium, myometrium;   4. chorionic villus sampling;   5. fetal heart rate, fetal heart tone;   6. hemolytic disease of the newborn;
7. fistula;   8. tubal ligation;   9. cervix;   10. stillbirth

F. Labeling Exercises

1. Milk gland;   2. Nipple;   3. Areola;   4. Milk duct;   5. Fat;   6. Uterus (metr/o, hyster/o, uter/o);   7. Vagina (colp/o, vagin/o);   8. Fallopian (uterine) tube (salping/o);   9. Ovum (o/o);
10. Ovary (oophor/o, ovari/o);   11. Myometrium;   12. Endometrium;   13. Cervix (cervic/o)

G. Med Term Analysis

1. oophor/o, ovary, -pexy, surgical fixation, surgical fixation of the ovary;   2. colp/o, vagina, -scope, instrument for viewing, instrument for viewing the vagina;   3. chori/o, chorion, carcin, cancer, oma, tumor, chorion cancerous tumor;   4. intra-, inside, uter, uterus, -ine, pertaining to, pertaining to inside the uterus;   5. trans-, across, vagin, vagina, -al, pertaining to, pertaining to across the vagina;   6. embry/o, embryo, -nic, pertaining to, pertaining to the embryo;   7. o/o, egg, -cyte, cell, egg cell;   8. cervic/o, cervix, -plasty, surgical repair, surgical repair of cervix;
9. ovari/o, ovary, salping, fallopian tube, -itis, inflammation, inflammation of ovary and fallopian tube;   10. episi, vulva, -otomy, cutting into, cutting into the vulva

H. Abbreviation Matching

1. F;   2. C;   3. I;   4. A;   5. H;   6. B;   7. J;   8. D;   9. G;   10. E

I. Photomatch Challenge

1. hysterectomy;   2. amniocentesis;   3. right salpingo-oophorectomy;
4. bilateral hysterosalpingo-oophorectomy;   5. laparoscopy;   6. bilateral salpingo-oophorectomy

J. Crossword Puzzle

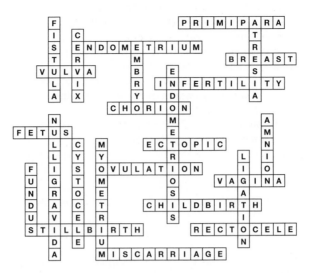

Chapter 14

Word Building

1. a. cerebellar; b. cerebellitis   2. a. meningocele; b. meningomyelocele   3. a. cerebral;
b. cerebrospinal; c. cerebritis; d. cerebromalacia; e. cerebrosclerosis; f. cerebrovascular;
g. cerebrotomy   4. a. encephalic; b. electroencephalogram; c. electroencephalography;
d. encephalalgia; e. encephalitis; f. encephalopathy; g. encephaloma; h. encephalomalacia;
i. encephalosclerosis   5. a. anesthesia; b. hyperesthesia   6. a. medullary   7. a. meningeal;
b. meningitis; c. meningomyelitis   8. a. myelogram; b. myelography; c. myelitis; d. myelomalacia;
e. myeloneuritis; f. myelopathy; g. myelosclerosis; h. myelotomy   9. a. neural; b. neuralgia;
c. neurectomy; d. neurology; e. neurologist; f. neuroma; g. neuropathy; h. neuroplasty;
i. polyneuritis; j. neurorrhaphy   10. a. aphasia; b. dysphasia   11. a. monoplegia; b. diplegia;
c. quadriplegia; d. hemiplegia; e. neuroplegia   12. a. pontine; b. pontocerebellar;
c. pontomedullary   13. a. thalamic; b. thalamotomy

Case Study

1. aphasia, hemiplegia;   2. transient ischemic attack;   3. c;   4. nonsteroidal anti-inflammatory
drugs taken for her arthritis;   5. emergency room, magnetic resonance imaging, intensive care
unit, physical therapy, occupational therapy;   6. because she was found on the floor and had
probably fallen;   7. each side of the brain controls the opposite side of the body

Practice Exercises

A. Sound It Out

1. meningitis;   2. anticonvulsant ;   3. neuroma;   4. aphasia ;   5. cerebromalacia;   6. cerebellar;
7. encephalosclerosis;   8. cerebellum;   9. cerebral;   10. concussion;   11. encephalitis;
12. dementia;   13. anesthesia;   14. cerebrospinal;   15. dysphasia;   16. electroencephalogram;
17. myelopathy;   18. encephalic;   19. neurectomy;   20. epilepsy;   21. hemiplegia;
22. thalamus;   23. hydrocephalus;   24. medullary;   25. meningeal;   26. quadriplegia;
27. thalamic;   28. meningocele;   29. neurorrhaphy;   30. migraine;   31. cerebrum ;
32. myelin;   33. neurology;   34. myelography;   35. cerebrotomy;   36. myelotomy;
37. neural;   38. neuralgia;   39. neuron;   40. meninges;   41. pontine;   42. neuroplasty;
43. paralysis;   44. encephaloma;   45. polyneuritis;   46. myelitis;   47. pons;   48. seizure;
49. cerebrovascular;   50. syncope

B. Transcription Practice

1. Jon took anticonvulsants to control his epileptic seizures.
2. As a result of the cerebrovascular accident, Mr.van Pelt was in a coma.
3. The auto accident victim developed quadriplegia following a spinal cord injury.
4. During the transient ischemic attack, Mr. Edelstein had aphasia.
5. Ilina's monoplegia was caused by multiple sclerosis.
6. Antonio went to the neurologist because he was having migraines.
7. A positron emission tomography was completed to see whether the tumor was in the cerebrum or the cerebellum.
8. A lumbar puncture was performed to analyze cerebrospinal fluid for signs of encephalitis.
9. Mr. Larsen's severe leg pain was caused by polyneuritis.
10. The elderly gentle man with Alzheimer disease eventually developed dementia.

C. Labeling Exercises

1. Brain (encephal/o);   2. Cranial nerve (neur/o);   3. Spinal cord (myel/o);   4. Spinal nerve (neur/o)

D. Build Medical Terms

1. neuralgia;   2. neuroma;   3. neurology;   4. neuroplasty;   5. neuropathy;   6. thalamic;
7. thalamotomy;   8. diplegia;   9. hemiplegia;   10. meningeal;   11. meningitis;
12. myelogram;   13. myelomalacia;   14. myelosclerosis;   15. myelitis

E. Fill in the Blank

1. motor neurons;   2. concussion, contusion;   3. syncope;   4. cerebrum, cerebellum, thalamus, brain stem;   5. meninges;   6. cerebral palsy;   7. grand mal;   8. Myasthenia gravis;
9. Parkinson;   10. shingles

F. Abbreviation Matching

1. H;   2. C;   3. J;   4. A;   5. F;   6. B;   7. I;   8. D;   9. G;   10. E

G. Med Term Analysis

1. cerebell, cerebellum, -ar, pertaining to, pertaining to the cerebellum;   2. mening/o, meninges, -cele, protrusion, protrusion of the meninges;   3. cerebr/o, cerebrum, spin, spine, -al, pertaining to, pertaining to the cerebrum and spine;   4. an-, without, -esthesia, sensation, without sensation;   5. mening/o, meninges, myel, spinal cord, -itis, inflammation, inflammation of meninges and spinal cord;   6. encephal, brain, -oma, tumor, brain tumor;   7. dys-, difficult, -phasia, speech, difficult speech;   8. neur/o, nerve, -logy, study of, study of nerves,   9. pont/o, pons, medull, medulla oblongata, -ary, pertaining to, pertaining to the pons and medulla oblongata;   10. cerebr, cerebrum, -otomy, cutting into, cutting into the cerebrum

H. Spelling

1. neurorrhaphy;   2. correctly spelled;   3. correctly spelled;   4. meningitis;   5. quadriplegia;
6. correctly spelled;   7. electroencephalography;   8. correctly spelled;   9. myasthenia gravis;
10. correctly spelled

I. Photomatch Challenge

1. cerebrum, cerebrum softening;   2. thalamus, cutting into thalamus;   3. cerebellum, cerebellum inflammation;   4. spinal cord, record of spinal cord;   5. pons, pertaining to the pons;
6. medulla oblongata, pertaining to medulla oblongata

J. Crossword Puzzle

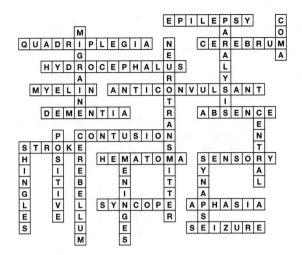

Chapter 15

Word Building

1. a. adenocarcinoma; b. adenocyte; c. adenoid; d. adenomalacia   2. a. adrenal; b. adrenomegaly
3. a. adrenalectomy; b. adrenalitis; c. adrenalopathy   4. a. endocrinology; b. endocrinologist;
c. endocrinoma; d. endocrinopathy   5. a. hyperglycemia; b. hypoglycemia   6. a. glycosuria
7. a. oophoritis; b. oophoroplasty; c. oophorotomy; d. oophorectomy   8. a. orchiectomy;
b. orchiopexy; c. orchiotomy   9. a. ovarian; b. ovariocentesis; c. ovariorrhexis   10. a. pancreatic;
b. pancreatectomy; c. pancreatitis; d. pancreatotomy   11. a. parathyroidal; b. parathyroidectomy;
c. hyperparathyroidism; d. hypoparathyroidism   12. a. pinealectomy   13. a. hypopituitarism;
b. hyperpituitarism   14. a. polydipsia; b. polyuria   15. a. testicular   16. a. thymic; b. thymectomy;
c. thymitis; d. thymoma   17. a. thyromegaly; b. thyrotomy   18. a. thyroidal; b. thyroiditis;
c. thyroidectomy; d. hyperthyroidism; e. hypothyroidism

Case Study

1. hypertension, high blood pressure; elevated heart rate, heart beating too fast; heart palpitations, pounding heart beat; diaphoresis, profuse sweating; hand tremors, uncontrollable
shaking of the hands; extreme anxiety, feeling of dread
2. a
3. less than 120/80, 12–18 breaths per minute, 60–80 beats per minute
4. emergency room, electrocardiogram, chest X-ray, beats per minute, blood pressure
5. difficulty breathing
6. *malignant* is cancerous, life-threatening tumor that tends to spread throughout the body;
benign is not cancerous
7. to verify that the tumor is a pheochromocytoma and to determine whether the tumor is
cancerous
8. adrenalectomy

Practice Exercises

A. Sound It Out

1. thyromegaly; 2. adenomalacia; 3. adrenomegaly; 4. antidiuretic; 5. aldosterone;
6. corticosteroids; 7. pancreatitis; 8. cretinism; 9. parathyroidectomy; 10. dwarfism;
11. acromegaly; 12. endocrinology; 13. epinephrine; 14. exophthalmos; 15. glucagon;
16. adrenalectomy; 17. glycosuria; 18. goiter; 19. orchiectomy; 20. hyperpituitarism;
21. insulin; 22. melatonin; 23. myxedema; 24. hypoparathyroidism; 25. gigantism;
26. oophoroplasty; 27. hypothyroidism; 28. polyuria; 29. orchiopexy; 30. ovarian;
31. oxytocin; 32. pancreas; 33. pancreatectomy; 34. hyperglycemia; 35. pancreatic;
36. endocrinopathy; 37. pheochromocytoma; 38. pinealectomy; 39. triiodothyronine;
40. polydipsia; 41. prolactin; 42. testicular; 43. tetany; 44. thymitis; 45. thymosin;
46. adrenal; 47. thyroidectomy; 48. thyrotoxicosis; 49. oophorectomy; 50. thyroxine

B. Transcription Practice

1. Gladys' glucose tolerance test confirmed the diagnosis of diabetes mellitus.
2. When Dr. Nguyen noted exophthalmos, she suspected Graves disease (or hyperthyroidism).
3. An adrenalectomy was necessary to treat the pheochromocytoma.
4. Hypoparathyroidism is one cause of tetany.
5. Two diagnostic tests were ordered, a thyroid scan and a thyroid function test.
6. Hypersecretion of growth hormone produces gigantism and lack of growth hormone can produce dwarfism.
7. A person with diabetes insipidus often has polydipsia and polyuria.
8. When Mrs. Ruiz developed facial hair and a deeper voice adrenal virilism was suspected.
9. Corticosteroids were prescribed for the patient with rheumatoid arthritis.
10. Mr. McDonald's adrenomegaly was caused by an adenocarcinoma.

C. Build Medical Terms

1. thyroidal; 2. thyroiditis; 3. thyroidectomy; 4. hyperthyroidism; 5. hypothyroidism;
6. hyperglycemia; 7. hypoglycemia; 8. polydipsia; 9. polyuria; 10. adenocarcinoma;
11. adenoid; 12. adenomalacia; 13. pancreatic; 14. pancreatitis; 15. pancreatotomy

D. Labeling Exercises

1. Pineal gland (pineal/o); 2. Parathyroid glands (parathyroid/o); 3. Adrenal glands (adren/o, adrenal/o); 4. Pancreas (pancreat/o); 5. Pituitary gland (pituitar/o); 6. Thyroid gland (thyr/o, thyroid/o); 7. Thymus gland (thym/o); 8. Ovaries (oophor/o, ovari/o); 9. Testes (orch/o, orchi/o, orchid/o, testicul/o)

E. Spelling

1. correctly spelled; 2. ovariocentesis; 3. myxedema; 4. correctly spelled; 5. correctly spelled; 6. tetany; 7. exophthalmos; 8. correctly spelled; 9. correctly spelled; 10. virilism

F. Fill in the Blank

1. homeostasis; 2. hormones, target organs; 3. hypersecretion, hyposecretion; 4. kidney, cortex, medulla, 5. estrogen, menstrual; 6. insulin, glucagon; 7. calcium; 8. melatonin, circadian; 9. pituitary; 10. thymus

G. Abbreviation Matching

1. E; 2. C; 3. H; 4. J; 5. B; 6. I; 7. D; 8. A; 9. G; 10. F

H. Med Term Analysis

1. orchid/o, testes, -pexy, surgical fixation, surgical fixation of the testes;   2. thyr/o, thyroid gland, -megaly, enlarged, enlarged thyroid gland;   3. aden/o, gland, carcin, cancer, -oma, tumor, cancerous gland tumor;   4. hypo-, insufficient, parathyroid, parathyroid gland, -ism, condition, condition of insufficient parathyroid gland;   5. thyr/o, thyroid gland, toxic, poison, -osis, abnormal condition, abnormal condition of thyroid poisoning;   6. pineal, pineal gland, -ectomy, surgical removal, surgical removal of pineal gland;   7. ovari/o, ovary, -rrhexis, rupture, ruptured ovary;   8. thym, thymus gland, -itis, inflammation, inflammation of thymus gland;
9. hyper-, excessive, glyc, sugar, -emia, blood condition; blood condition of excessive sugar;
10. oophor/o, ovary, -plasty, surgical repair, surgical repair of the ovary

I. Photomatch Challenge

1. oste/o, osteoporosis;   2. thyr/o or thyroid/o, thyromegaly;   3. testicul/o, testicular;
4. adren/o or adrenal/o, adrenalitis;   5. ovari/o, ovariorrhexis;   6. mamm/o or mast/o, mastectomy

J. Crossword Puzzle

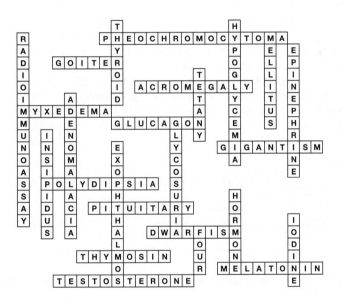

Chapter 16

Word Building

1. a. aqueous   2. a. blepharoptosis; b. blepharoplasty; c. blepharoplegia   3. a. choroidal;
b. choroiditis   4. a. conjunctivitis; b. conjunctival   5. a. coreometer; b. coreometry   6. a. corneal
7. a. cycloplegia; b. cyclotomy   8. a. dacryolith; b. dacryorrhea; c. dacryoadenitis; d. dacryocystitis
9. a. a. iritis   10. a. iridoplegia; b. iridotomy   11. a. keratometer; b. keratometry; c. keratectomy;
d. keratitis; e. keratotomy; g. keratoplasty   12. a. lacrimal; b. nasolacrimal   13. a. intraocular;
b. oculomycosis; c. ocular   14. a. ophthalmic; b. ophthalmology; c. ophthalmologist;
d. ophthalmoscope; e. ophthalmoscopy; f. ophthalmoplegia; g. xerophthalmia   15. a. hemianopia;
b. diplopia   16. a. optic; b. optometer; c. optometry   17. a. phacomalacia; b. phacolysis;
c. phacosclerosis   18. a. pupillary; b. pupillometer   19. a. retinal; b. retinopathy; c. retinitis;
d. cryoretinopexy   20. a. scleral; b. sclerotomy; c. scleromalacia; d. scleritis   21. a. tonometer;
b. tonometry   22. a. vitreous

Case Study

1. pain; excessive tearing; decreased visual acuity–fuzzy or cloudy vision; photophobia–increased sensitivity to light
2. thigh bone
3. The patient had normal 20/20 vision in the left eye, meaning he could see clearly at 20 ft what a normal person would expect to see at 20 ft. However, the right eye had 20/200 vision, meaning he could see at 20 ft what a normal person would expect to see at 200 ft.
4. corneal abrasions appear bright green under a black light
5. abrasion–scrapping away of a layer
   ulcer–an erosion or crater, deeper than an abrasion
6. antibiotic eye drops–to fight infection
   anesthetic eye drops–to reduce eye pain
7. to wear an eye patch; to put a lubricating ointment in his eyes if they are too dry when he wakes up in the morning; to see an ophthalmologist in 24 hours to make sure his eye is healing

Practice Exercises

A. Sound It Out

1. ophthalmic; 2. keratoplasty; 3. retinal; 4. choroidal; 5. oculomycosis; 6. tonometer; 7. conjunctivitis; 8. dacryoadenitis; 9. optometrist; 10. iridotomy; 11. diplopia; 12. fluorescein; 13. achromatopsia; 14. glaucoma; 15. hemianopia; 16. astigmatism; 17. blepharoptosis; 18. hyperopia; 19. intraocular; 20. iritis; 21. scleromalacia; 22. ophthalmoscopy; 23. keratectomy; 24. coreometry; 25. cryoretinopexy; 26. ophthalmic; 27. keratitis; 28. amblyopia; 29. keratotomy; 30. lacrimal; 31. phacolysis; 32. myopia; 33. nasolacrimal; 34. cataract; 35. nyctalopia; 36. pupillary; 37. cycloplegia; 38. corneal; 39. nystagmus; 40. ocular; 41. optician; 42. phacosclerosis; 43. aqueous; 44. photophobia; 45. ophthalmoplegia; 46. scleral; 47. cilia; 48. strabismus; 49. hordeolum; 50. stye

B. Transcription Practice

1. Dr. Cohen decided to use cryoextraction to remove the patient's cataract rather than a phacoemulsification.
2. Mr. Blair's myopia was corrected by radial keratotomy.
3. The head injury caused a retinal detachment that required repair by laser retinal photocoagulation.
4. Because the cornea was abnormally curved, light rays were not evenly refracted, resulting in astigmatism.
5. Examination of the eye with an ophthalmoscope did not reveal any reason for Mr. Mendez's photophobia.
6. Mrs. Capers made an appointment with the optometrist because of scleritis and diplopia.
7. The baby's mother was concerned about her infant when she noticed conjunctivitis and excessive dacryorrhea.
8. Mr. Carpenter decided that it was no longer safe for him to drive because after he developed nyctalopia and macular degeneration.
9. A patient's visual acuity can be evaluated using a Snellen chart.
10. A corneal abrasion occurred when sand became trapped under Karen's contact lens that was identified by using fluorescein.

C. Fill in the Blank

1. Diabetic retinopathy; 2. glaucoma; 3. achromatopsia; 4. hordeolum; 5. nystagmus; 6. Myopia; 7. strabismus; 8. Snellen; 9. Nyctalopia; 10. astigmatism

D. Abbreviation Matching

1. E; 2. I; 3. A; 4. G; 5. C; 6. J. 7. B. 8. F; 9. H; 10. D

E. Labeling Exercise

1. Conjunctiva (conjunctiv/o);   2. Pupil (core/o, pupill/o);   3. Cornea (corne/o, kerat/o);
4. Aqueous humor (aque/o);   5. Iris (ir/o, irid/o);   6. Lens (phac/o);   7. Vitreous body (vitre/o);
8. Suspensory ligament;   9. Ciliary body (cycl/o);   10. Retina (retin/o);   11. Choroid (choroid/o);
12. Sclera (scler/o);   13. Macula lutea;   14. Optic nerve;   15. Central retinal artery and vein

F. Build Medical Terms

1. ophthalmology;   2. ophthalmoscope;   3. ophthalmoplegia;   4. ophthalmic;   5. keratectomy;
6. keratotomy;   7. keratometer;   8. keratoplasty;   9. retinopathy;   10. retinitis;
11. blepharoplasty;   12. blepharoplegia;   13. blepharoptosis;   14. diplopia;   15. amblyopia

G. Medical Term Analysis

1. blephar/o, eyelid, -ptosis, drooping, drooping eyelid;   2. dacry/o, tear, aden, gland, -itis, inflammation, inflammation of a lacrimal gland;   3. nas/o, nose, lacrim, tears, -al, pertaining to, pertaining to the nose and tears;   4. intra-, within, ocul, eye, -ar, pertaining to, pertaining to within the eye;   5. cry/o, cold, retin/o, retina, -pexy, surgical fixation, surgical fixation of the retina using cold;   6. choroid, choroid layer, -itis, inflammation; inflammation of choroid layer;   7. kerat/o, cornea, -plasty, surgical repair, surgical repair of cornea;   8. opt/o, vision, -metry, process of measuring, process of measuring vision;   9. ophthalm/o, eye, -scope, instrument to measure, instrument to measure the eye;   10. phac/o, lens, -sclerosis, hardening, hardening of the lens

H. Spelling

1. stye;   2. correctly spelled;   3. hordeolum;   4. myopia;   5. correctly spelled;   6. correctly spelled;   7. dacryolith;   8. correctly spelled;   9. correctly spelled;   10. strabismus

I. Photomatch Challenge

1. dark spots in visual field, diabetic retinopathy;   2. losing vision around edges, glaucoma;
3. whole image is blurry, cataract;   4. center of image is blurry, macular degeneration

J. Crossword Puzzle

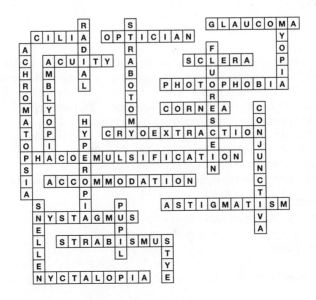

Chapter 17

Word Building

1. a. adenoidectomy; b. adenoiditis 2. a. audiology; b. audiologist; c. audiometry; d. audiometer; e. audiogram 3. a. auditory 4. a. aural 5. a. cochlear 6. a. epiglottic; b. epiglottitis 7. a. laryngeal; b. laryngitis; c. laryngoscopy; d. laryngoscope; e. laryngectomy; f. laryngoplasty; g. laryngoplegia; h. laryngospasm 8. a. myringitis; b. myringectomy; c. myringoplasty; d. myringosclerosis; e. myringotomy 9. a. nasal; b. nasogastric; c. nasopharyngeal 10. a. anosmia 11. a. otic; b. otitis; c. otalgia; d. otology; e. otologist; f. otoscopy; g. otoscope; h. otoplasty; i. otomycosis; j. otopyorrhea 12. a. pharyngeal; b. pharyngitis; c. pharyngoplasty; d. pharyngospasm; e. pharyngotomy 13. a. aphonia; b. dysphonia 14. a. rhinitis; b. rhinoplasty; c. rhinorrhea; d. rhinomycosis 15. a. sinusitis; b. pansinusitis; c. nasosinusitis 16. a. tonsillar; b. tonsillitis; c. tonsillectomy 17. a. tracheal; b. tracheomegaly; c. tracheoplasty; d. tracheotomy; e. tracheostenosis; f. endotracheal 18. a. tympanic; b. tympanometry; c. tympanometer; d. tympanogram; e. tympanoplasty; f. tympanorrhexis; g. tympanotomy

Case Study

1. She has been feeling run-down and having headaches for about 10 years. Pain is over her eyes, but sometimes it moves down and makes her upper teeth hurt. Recently she became unable to detect the strong odor of cooking fish.
2. anosmia
3. b
4. enlargement or disease of the lymph nodes in the neck region
5. *Pan-* is a prefix meaning all; infection has spread to all of the paranasal sinuses
6. temperature, blood pressure, and breathing rate are normal; pulse is high
7. Culture grows sample of infected tissue to determine whether bacteria are present. If bacteria are present, then the culture can be used to identify the specific type. This culture found bacteria but did not find fungus.
8. antibiotic to fight the infection, corticosteroid nose spray to reduce inflammation, repeat culture to check whether treatment is working and infection is gone, stop smoking because smoke irritates the sinuses, go to an allergist to see whether she has allergies that could make her prone to infections

Practice Exercises

A Sound It Out

1. otalgia; 2. anosmia; 3. malleus; 4. audiometer; 5. cochlear; 6. diphtheria; 7. pharyngospasm; 8. myringosclerosis; 9. dysphonia; 10. adenoidectomy; 11. endotracheal; 12. otoplasty; 13. epiglottis; 14. auditory; 15. incus; 16. laryngeal; 17. laryngitis; 18. equilibrium; 19. laryngoplegia; 20. laryngoscope; 21. myringoplasty; 22. pharyngotomy; 23. nares; 24. vertigo; 25. tympanogram; 26. nasogastric; 27. tympanometry; 28. ossicles; 29. croup; 30. otitis; 31. otopyorrhea; 32. otoscopy; 33. pansinusitis; 34. epistaxis; 35. pertussis; 36. aural; 37. pharynx; 38. otologist; 39. pinna; 40. rhinitis; 41. rhinorrhea; 42. stapes; 43. tinnitus; 44. tonsillectomy; 45. tonsillitis; 46. tracheomegaly; 47. audiogram; 48. tracheostenosis; 49. rhinomycosis; 50. tympanorrhexis

B. Transcription Practice

1. The new parents were quite concerned when their baby developed croup.
2. Meilin's deafness was due to an acoustic neuroma.
3. The DPT vaccination protects children against diphtheria and pertussis.
4. The physician ordered supplemental oxygen to be delivered by a nasal cannula.
5. His physician became concerned when Mr. Janssen developed vertigo and tinnitus.

6. Carmen's physician recommended to her parents that she have pressure equalizing tubes because of her repeated otitis media.
7. The paramedics had to quickly determine whether the patient's condition required a tracheotomy or endotracheal intubation.
8. Ursula went to see an otorhinolaryngologist because of her repeated epistaxis.
9. For his deafness, Tariq needed a cochlear implant rather than a hearing aid.
10. After examining the external auditory canal with an otoscope, it was obvious Jackson had otitis externa.

C. Fill in the Blank

1. hearing, equilibrium (balance);   2. epiglottis;   3. larynx;   4. adenoids;   5. tympanic membrane (eardrum);   6. auditory;   7. nares;   8. nosebleed;   9. amplification device;
10. malleus, incus, stapes

D. Abbreviation Matching

1. E;   2. I;   3. A;   4. G;   5. B;   6. J;   7. F;   8. C;   9. H;   10. D

E. Labeling Exercises

1. Pinna;   2. External auditory canal;   3. Mastoid process;   4. Malleus (hammer);   5. Incus (anvil);   6. Semicircular canals (equilibrium);   7. Auditory nerve;   8. Cochlea (hearing) (cochle/o);   9. Oval window;   10. Stapes (stirrup);   11. Eustachian tube;   12. Tympanic membrane (eardrum) (myring/o, tympan/o)

F. Build Medical Terms

1. otology;   2. otomycosis;   3. otoplasty;   4. otitis;   5. otoscopy;   6. pharyngospasm;
7. pharyngeal;   8. aphonia;   9. dysphonia;   10. tracheostenosis;   11. tracheotomy;
12. tracheomegaly;   13. tympanoplasty;   14. tympanometer;   15. tympanorrhexis

G. Med Term Analysis

1. tympan, tympanic membrane, -otomy, cutting into, cutting into tympanic membrane;
2. cochle, coclea, -ar, pertaining to, pertaining to the cochlea;   3. nas/o, nose, gastr, stomach, -ic, pertaining to, pertaining to the nose and stomach;   4. endo-, within, trache, trachea, -al, pertaining to, pertaining to within the trachea;   5. rhin/o, nose, myc, fungus, -osis, abnormal condition, abnormal condition of nose fungus;   6. tonsill, tonsil, -ectomy, surgical removal, surgical removal of tonsils;   7. an-, without, -osmia, smell, without smell;   8. laryng/o, larynx, -plegia, paralysis, paralysis of the larynx;   9. pan-, all, sinus, sinuses, -itis, inflammation, inflammation of all the sinuses;   10. myring/o, tympanic membrane, -sclerosis, hardening, hardening of the tympanic membrane

H. Spelling

1. spelled correctly;   2. epistaxis;   3. diphtheria;   4. otopyorrhea;   5. spelled correctly;
6. spelled correctly;   7. spelled correctly;   8. cannula;   9. spelled correctly;   10. pertussis

I. Photomatch Challenge

1. rhinitis;   2. pharyngitis;   3. tonsillitis;   4. sinusitis;   5. epistaxis;   6. laryngitis

J. Crossword Puzzle

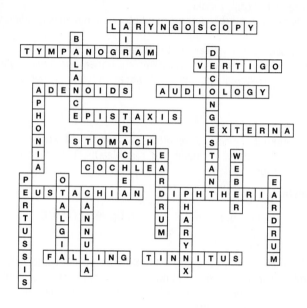

Index

Lacrimal (tear) glands, 340, 341
Lactate dehydrogenase (LDH), 121
Lactiferous glands, 276, 278
Laparoscope, in tubal ligation, 280
Larynx, 193, 361, 363, 365, 368
Laser-assisted in-situ keratomileusis (LASIK), 347
Laser surgery, 66
Last menstrual period (LMP), 280
Lateral, 42
Lateral view, of body, 42, 47
Latin-based medical terms, 1, 2
    plurals, 7
Lazy eye. *See* Amblyopia
Left ear (AS), 371
Left eye (OS), 349
Left hypochondriac region, 49
Left inguinal region, 49
Left lower quadrant (LLQ), 48
Left lumbar region, 49
Left upper quadrant (LUQ), 48
Lens, 337, 339, 343
    cataract, 345
    cylindrical, 349
    intraocular, 347
Lesion, 66
Leukemia, 149
Leukocytes, 141, 143, 149, 150
    basophils, 141, 143
    eosinophils, 141, 143
    lymphocytes, 141, 143
    monocytes, 141, 143
    neutrophils, 141, 143
Ligaments, suspensory, 341
Lingual tonsils, 363, 367
Liver, 213, 215, 219
    cirrhosis, 222
    jaundice, 224
Lobes, of lung, 190
Longitudinal section, 41
Lordosis, 93, 94
Lou Gehrig disease. *See* Amyotrophic lateral sclerosis (ALS)
Lower extremity (LE), 44, 45
Lower GI series, 222
Lumbar puncture (LP), 301
Lungs, 113, 185, 191, 192, 368
    collapsed, 198
    emphysema in, 196
    left, 187
    lobe, 190
    right, 187
    tumor, 195
Luteinizing hormone, 321

Lymph, 167
Lymphatic system, 163
    Hodgkin disease, 171
    organs of, 165
Lymphatic vessels, 165, 168
Lymphedema, 167
Lymph nodes, 165, 168
Lymphocytes (lymphs), 141, 143, 163, 168
Lymphoma, non-Hodgkin, 172

M

Macula lutea, 339, 344
Macular degeneration, 347
Macule, 66
Male reproductive system, 237, 241
    organs, 243, 244, 247
Malignant melanoma (MM), 66
Malleus (hammer), 363, 364
Mandible, 83, 363
Mastoid process, 363
Maxilla, 83
Meatus, 246
Medial, 42
Mediastinum, 47, 187, 190
Medical personnel. *See* Personnel, medical
Medical specialties, suffixes indicating, 18–19
Medical terms
    analysis of, 6–7
    building, 6–7
    defining, 6
    pluralizing, 7
    pronunciation of, 8
    types of, 1
Medications
    antibiotics, 253
    anticonvulsant, 299
    decongestant, 369
Medulla oblongata, 295, 296
Melanin, 62
Melanocytes, 62, 67
Melanocyte-stimulating hormone (MSH), 321
Melatonin, 320
Melena, 224
Ménière disease, 370
Meninges, 47, 297
Meningocele, 302
Menstrual cycle, 272, 319
Menstruation, 273
Metacarpus, 83
Metatarsus, 83
Middle ear, 364
Middle ear infection. *See* Otitis media (OM)